second edition
Pediatric Dermatology
Bernard A Cohen

Bernard A Cohen, MD
Director, Division of Pediatric Dermatology
The Johns Hopkins Medical Institutions
Baltimore, Maryland

Forewords by
Frank A Oski, MD
Chairman and Given Professor of Pediatrics
The Johns Hopkins Medical Institutions
Baltimore, Maryland

and
Nancy B Esterly, MD
Professor of Pediatrics
Professor of Dermatology
Medical College of Wisconsin
Milwaukee, Wisconsin

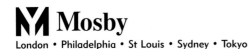
London • Philadelphia • St Louis • Sydney • Tokyo

Publisher	Gina Almond
Development Editor	Maria Stewart
Project Manager	Louise Patchett
Designer	Ian Spick
Layout	Rob Curran
Illustration Manager	Danny Pyne
Illustrator	Mick Ruddy
Cover design	Ian Spick
Copyeditor	John Ormiston
Proofreader	Andrew Baker
Production	Siobhan Egan
Index	Anita Reid

ISBN: 0 7234 3010 1

Printed and bound by Grafos S.A. Arte sobre papel, Barcelona, Spain

Cataloging-in-Publication Data:
Catalogue records for this book are available from the US Library of Congress and the British Library

For full details of Mosby titles please write to:
Mosby International Ltd
Lynton House
7–12 Tavistock Square
London WC1H 9LB
UK

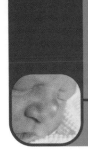

Contents

Acknowledgements

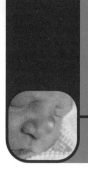

This book would not have been possible without the help of the children and parents who allowed me to photograph their skin rashes, and the practitioners who referred them to me. I am particularly indebted to the faculty at the Johns Hopkins Children's Center and the Dermatology Department at the Johns Hopkins University School of Medicine for their inspiration and support. I would also like to thank my friends at the Children's Hospital of Pittsburgh where this book was first conceived.

I am grateful for the gentle but persistent prodding and sensitive guidance of the Editors at Mosby who are responsible for completion of this book in a timely fashion. I would also like to thank Tracy Shuford for keeping the communication lines open between the Publisher and my office.

Special thanks go to Judy Liggett, the pediatric dermatology and cutaneous laser nurse who continues the gargantuan task of identifying and organizing the clinical slides. She keeps the kids smiling for pictures.

I would like to thank the residents in dermatology and pediatrics, who by their questions and consultations, have helped me to prioritize topics for inclusion in this book.

Finally, I would like to acknowledge Dr Nancy Esterly and Dr Frank Oski, both of whom have contributed forewords to the book. Dr Esterly taught me that pediatric dermatology could be exciting and academically challenging. As a role model and friend, she continues to guide all of us in pediatric dermatology. Dr Oski brought me home to Baltimore where he incorporated pediatric dermatology into the pediatric prgram. Hopefully, we can live up to the high standards which he demanded. To honor him, I have included his foreword from the first edition.

Figure Credits
The following figures have been reprinted from Zitelli BJ, Davis HW, eds. Atlas of Pediatric Physical Diagnosis, 3rd ed. (St. Louis: Mosby–Year Book Inc, 1997)

4.10, 7.8, 7.9, 8.1, 8.14, 8.45, 9.5, 9.7, 9.8, 9.11, 9.13.

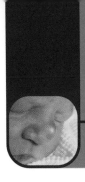

Preface

Since I began taking clinical photographs during my residency training 20 years ago, I have been impressed by the virtually unlimited variation in the expression of skin disease. However, with careful observation, clinical patterns that permit the development of a reasonable differential diagnosis begin to emerge. In the second edition I have been able to use over 600 images, nearly a third of which are new, to demonstrate both the diverse variations and common patterns that are fundamental to an understanding of rashes in children.

Pediatric Dermatology is designed for the pediatrician and primary care practitioner with an interest in dermatology and for the dermatologist who cares for children. The text is organized around practical clinical problems, and most chapters end with an algorithm for developing a differential diagnosis. This book should not be considered an encyclopedic text of pediatric dermatology; it should be used in conjunction with the references suggested at the end of Chapter 1. Classic papers and more recent references are included in the bibliography at the end of each chapter.

During the last 20 years neonatology has blossomed into a respected pediatric discipline. This is reflected in Chapter 2, the longest chapter in the book, which is devoted to the dermatologic disorders of newborns and infants. A number of chapters are organized by morphologic findings: Chapter 3, Papulosquamous Eruptions; Chapter 4, Vesiculopustular Eruptions; and Chapter 5, Nodules and Tumors. Disorders of Pigmentation are covered in Chapter 6, and Disorders of the Hair and Nails in Chapter 8. Reactive Erythema, Chapter 7, includes a series of descriptive diagnoses that are often confusing because of overlapping clinical features. Chapter 9, Factitial Dermatoses, concludes with several disorders that are triggered, exacerbated, or caused primarily by external factors.

Finally, the format of the text should be user friendly. The pages and legends have been numbered in a standard textbook fashion, and the index is completely revised to include all of the disorders listed in the text as well as the legends. The atlas incorporates advances made in diagnosis, evaluation and treatment during the last 5 years since the publication of the first edition. I only hope that students of pediatric dermatology will enjoy reading the book as much as I enjoyed writing and illustrating it.

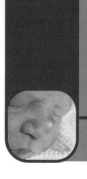

Foreword to 1st Edition

In memory of Dr Oski, this foreword has been taken from the first edition of *Pediatric Dermatology*.

It is estimated that approximately 20 percent of all patients coming to visit a pediatrician, be they sick or well, have a dermatologic problem. The next best thing to having a dermatologist with you when you encounter these patients is to have your own working knowledge of pediatric dermatology. The more you see, the more you know, and just seeing the pictures in Bernard Cohen's *Atlas of Pediatric Dermatology* is one pleasant way to acquire a useful, working knowledge of this field.

Take this book, or at least a mental image of Cohen's clear and colorful pictures, with you every time you see a patient. It can make you a better pediatrician.

Frank A. Oski, MD
Chairman and Given Professor of Pediatrics
The Johns Hopkins Medical Institutions
1985–1995

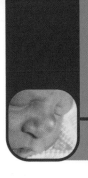

Foreword to 2nd Edition

As those of us who practice pediatric dermatology know full well, nothing surpasses a photograph of vivid color and exquisite detail to instruct the reader in dermatologic diagnosis. What has made *Pediatric Dermatology* so unusual is the combination of beautiful photographs with a concise and informative text. Special features include the extensive chapter on neonatal skin problems, numerous tables and the inclusion of algorithms at the end of each chapter.

This second edition of Bernard Cohen's *Pediatric Dermatology* retains the successful format of the previous volume but adds some two hundred new images, permitting illustration of the less common variants of many skin disorders. There is something here for all of us – the uninitiated and experienced, student and teacher, pediatrician and dermatologist.

Nancy B. Esterly, MD
Professor of Dermatology
Professor of Pediatrics
Medical College of Wisconsin

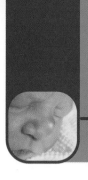

Dedication

To Sherry for her continued patience, love, and understanding during the revision of this book.

To Michael, Jared, and Jenny for keeping me young.

To Dr Frank Oski for bringing me home to Baltimore and supporting my endeavors in pediatric dermatology.

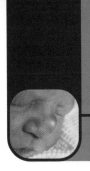

Chapter One

Introduction to Pediatric Dermatology

ANATOMY OF THE SKIN

Most of us think of skin as a simple, durable covering for the skeleton and internal organs. Yet skin is actually a very complex and dynamic organ consisting of many parts and appendages (Fig 1.1). The outermost layer of the epidermis, the stratum corneum, is an effective barrier to the penetration of irritants, toxins, and organisms, as well as a membrane that holds in body fluids. The remainder of the epidermis, the stratum granulosum, stratum spinosum, and stratum basale, manufactures this protective layer. Melanocytes within the epidermis are important for protection against the harmful effects of ultraviolet light, and the Langerhan cells are one of the body's first lines of immunologic defense.

The dermis, consisting largely of fibroblasts and collagen, is a tough, leathery, mechanical barrier against cuts, bites, and bruises. Its collagenous matrix also provides structural support for a number of cutaneous appendages. Hair, which grows from follicles deep within the dermis, is important for cosmesis as well as protection from sunlight and particulate matter. Sebaceous glands arise as an outgrowth of the hair follicles. Oil produced by these glands helps to lubricate the skin and contributes to the protective function of the epidermal barrier. The nails are specialized

organs of manipulation that also protect sensitive digits. Thermoregulation of the skin is accomplished by eccrine sweat glands as well as changes in the cutaneous blood flow regulated by glomus cells. The skin also contains specialized receptors for heat, pain, touch, and pressure. Sensory input from these structures helps to protect the skin surface against environmental trauma. Beneath the dermis, in the subcutaneous tissue, fat is stored as a source of energy and also acts as a soft protective cushion.

EXAMINATION AND ASSESSMENT OF THE SKIN

The skin is the largest, and most accessible and easily examined organ of the body, and it is the organ of most frequent concern to the patient. Therefore, all practitioners should be able to recognize basic skin diseases and dermatologic clues to systemic disease.

Optimal examination of the skin is best achieved in a well lit room. The clinician should inspect the entire skin surface including the hair, nails, scalp, and mucous membranes. This may present particular problems in infants and teenagers, since it may be necessary to examine the skin in small segments to prevent cooling or embarrassment, respectively.

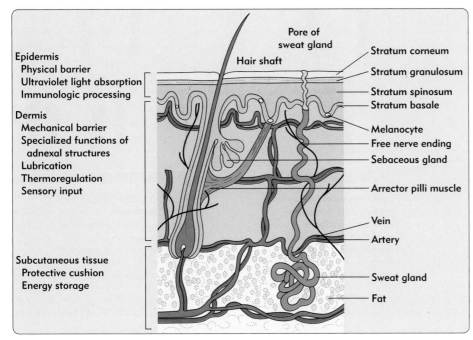

Fig 1.1 Schematic diagram of normal skin anatomy.

Epidermis
 Physical barrier
 Ultraviolet light absorption
 Immunologic processing

Dermis
 Mechanical barrier
 Specialized functions of
  adnexal structures
 Lubrication
 Thermoregulation
 Sensory input

Subcutaneous tissue
 Protective cushion
 Energy storage

Pore of
sweat gland
Hair shaft
Stratum corneum
Stratum granulosum
Stratum spinosum
Stratum basale
Melanocyte
Free nerve ending
Sebaceous gland
Arrector pilli muscle
Vein
Artery
Sweat gland
Fat

Although no special equipment is required, a hand lens and side lighting are useful aids in the assessment of skin texture and small discrete lesions.

Despite the myriad of conditions affecting skin, a systematic approach to the evaluation of a rash facilitates and simplifies the process of developing a manageable differential diagnosis. After assessing the general health of a child, the practitioner should obtain a detailed history of the cutaneous symptoms, including the date of onset, inciting factors, the evolution of lesions, and the presence or absence of pruritus. Recent immunizations, infections, drugs, and allergies may be directly related to new rashes. The family history may suggest a hereditary or contagious process, and the clinician may need to examine other members of the family. A review of nursery records and photographs will help to document the presence of congenital lesions.

Attention should then turn to the distribution and pattern of the rash. The distribution refers to the location of the skin findings, while the pattern defines a specific anatomic or physiologic arrangement. For example, the distribution of a rash may include the extremities, face, or trunk, while the pattern could be flexural or intertriginous areas (Fig 1.2a).

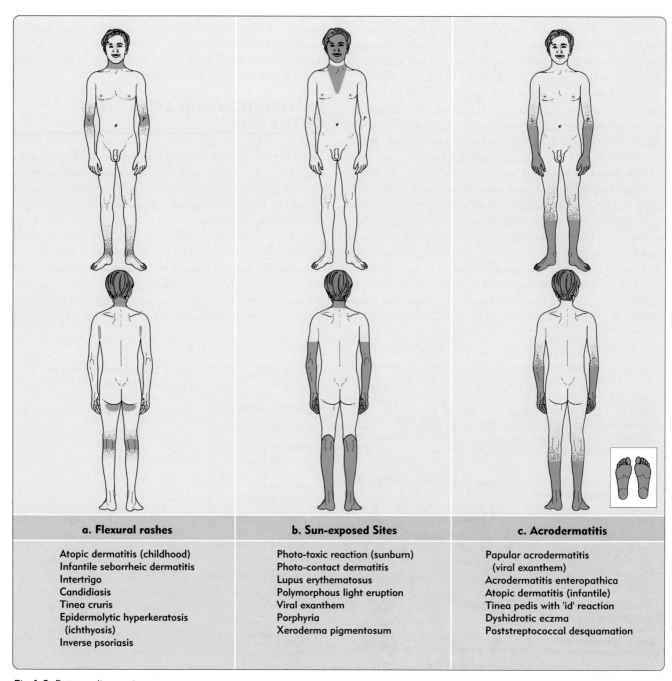

a. Flexural rashes	b. Sun-exposed Sites	c. Acrodermatitis

Atopic dermatitis (childhood)
Infantile seborrheic dermatitis
Intertrigo
Candidiasis
Tinea cruris
Epidermolytic hyperkeratosis
  (ichthyosis)
Inverse psoriasis
	Photo-toxic reaction (sunburn)
	Photo-contact dermatitis
	Lupus erythematosus
	Polymorphous light eruption
	Viral exanthem
	Porphyria
	Xeroderma pigmentosum
		Papular acrodermatitis
		  (viral exanthem)
		Acrodermatitis enteropathica
		Atopic dermatitis (infantile)
		Tinea pedis with 'id' reaction
		Dyshidrotic eczma
		Poststreptococcal desquamation

Fig 1.2 Pattern diagnosis.

Other common patterns include sun-exposed sites, acrodermatitis, pityriasis rosea, clothing protected sites, and acneiform rashes (Figs 1.2b–f).

Next, the clinician should consider the local organization of the lesions, defining the relationship of primary and secondary lesions to one another in a given location (Fig 1.3). Are the lesions diffusely scattered or clustered (herpetiform)? Are they linear, serpiginous, annular, or dermatomal?

The depth of the lesions in the skin, as noted by both observation and palpation, may also give further clues (Fig 1.4). Disruption of the normal skin markings by scale,

papules, vesicles, or pustules points to the involvement of the epidermis. Alterations in skin color alone can occur in epidermal and dermal processes. In disorders of pigmentation, the color of the pigment may suggest the anatomic depth of the lesion. Shades of brown are present in flat junctional nevi, lentigines, and café au lait spots where the increased pigment resides in the epidermis or superficial dermis. In Mongolian spots and nevus of Ota the Tyndal effect results in bluish-green to gray macules from melanin in the mid-dermis. If the epidermal markings are normal but the lesion is elevated, the disorder usually involves the

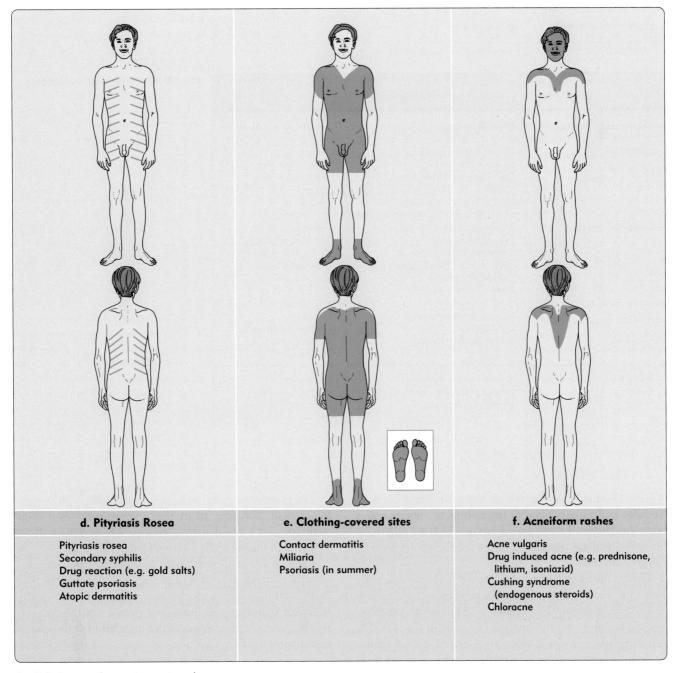

d. Pityriasis Rosea	**e. Clothing-covered sites**	**f. Acneiform rashes**
Pityriasis rosea Secondary syphilis Drug reaction (e.g. gold salts) Guttate psoriasis Atopic dermatitis	Contact dermatitis Miliaria Psoriasis (in summer)	Acne vulgaris Drug induced acne (e.g. prednisone, lithium, isoniazid) Cushing syndrome (endogenous steroids) Chloracne

Fig 1.2 Pattern diagnosis *continued*.

Fig 1.3 Organization of lesions.

Organization of lesions			
Linear	**Dermatomal**	**Serpiginous**	**Annular**
Epidermal nevi	Herpes zoster	Psoriasis	Ringworm
Lichen striatus	Vitiligo	Erythema marginatum	Granuloma annulare
Contact dermatitis	Nevus depigmentosus	Cutaneous larvae migrans	Lupus
Warts	Becker nevus		Atopic dermatitis
Ichthyosis	Café au lait spot	Elastosis perforans serpiginosa	Erythema annulare centrificum
Psoriasis	Port wine stain		Erythema chronicum migrans
Porokeratosis			
Incontinentia pigmenti			

Fig 1.4 Anatomic depth of lesions.

Anatomic depth of lesions		
Cutaneous structure	**Physical findings**	**Specific skin disorders**
Epidermis	Altered surface markings Scale, vesicle, crust Color changes (black, brown, white)	Impetigo Café au lait spot Atopic dermatitis Vitiligo Freckle
Epidermis+dermis	Altered surface markings Scale, vesicle, crust Distinct borders Color changes (black, brown, white, and/or red) Edema	Psoriasis Atopic dermatitis Contact dermatitis Cutaneous lupus erythematosus
Dermis	Normal surface markings Color changes Altered dermal firmness	Urticaria Granuloma annulare Hemangioma Blue nevus
Subcutaneous tissue	Normal surface markings Normal or red skin color Altered skin firmness	Hematoma Cold panniculitis Erythema nodosum

dermis. Dermal lesions have well demarcated firm borders. Nodules and tumors deep in the dermis or subcutaneous tissue can distort the surface markings, which are otherwise intact. Some deep seated lesions can only be appreciated by careful palpation.

Finally, the clinician may develop a differential diagnosis using the morphology of the cutaneous lesions. Primary lesions (macules, papules, plaques, vesicles, bullae, pustules, wheals, nodules, and tumors) arise *de novo* in the skin (Fig 1.5). Secondary lesions (scale, crust, ulcers, scars, excoriations, and fissures) evolve from primary lesions or result from scratching of primary lesions by the patient (Fig 1.6).

The practitioner who becomes comfortable with dermatology will integrate all of these approaches into their evaluation of a child with a skin problem. This will be reflected in the clinically focused format of this text.

Each chapter will finish with an algorithm that summarizes the material in a differential diagnostic flow pattern. The limited bibliography includes comprehensive, historically significant, and/or well organized reviews of the subject. Readers may also find some of the texts listed at the end of this chapter useful.

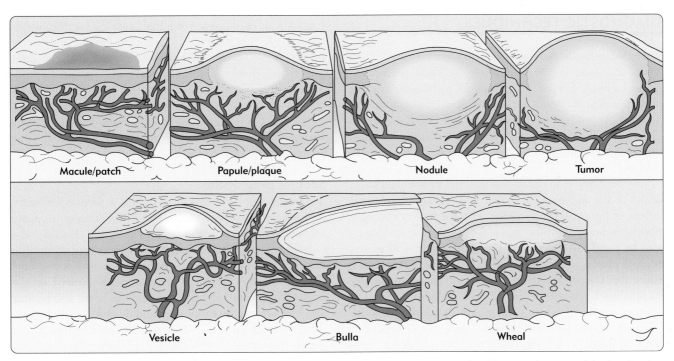

Fig 1.5 Primary skin lesions. Macule: a small (usually ≤ 1 cm), flat lesion showing an alteration in color or tone. Large macules are referred to as patches. Papule: a small (≤ 1 cm), sharply circumscribed, elevated lesion. An elevated lesion over 1 cm is referred to as a plaque. Nodule: a soft or solid mass in the dermis or subcutaneous fat. Tumor: a large module, localized and palpable, of varied size and consistency. Vesicle: a blister containing transparent fluid. Bulla: a large blister. Wheal: an evanescent, edematous, circumscribed elevated lesion that appears and disappears quickly. (Adapted from CIBA.)

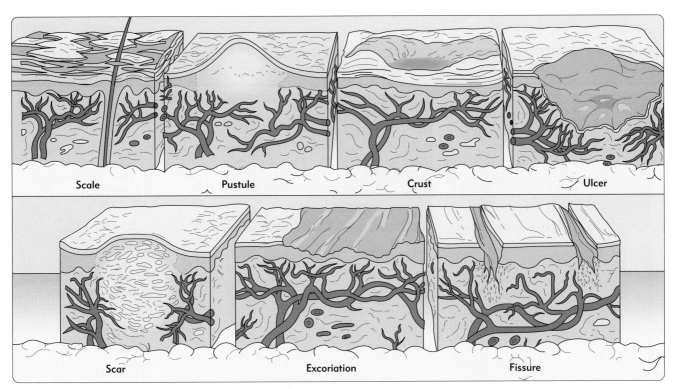

Fig 1.6 Secondary skin lesions. Scale: a dry, greasy fragment of dead skin. Pustule: a sharply circumscribed lesion containing free pus. Crust: a dry mass of exudate from erosions or ruptured vesicles/pustules, consisting of serum, dried blood, scales, and pus. Ulcer: a clearly defined, deep erosion of the epidermis and cutis. Scar: a permanent skin change resulting from new formation of connective tissue after destruction of the epidermis and cutis. Excoriation: any scratch mark on the surface of the skin. Fissure: any linear crack in the skin, usually accompanied by inflammation and pain. (Adapted from CIBA.)

DIAGNOSTIC TECHNIQUES

Potassium hydroxide preparation

There are a number of rapid, bedside diagnostic procedures in dermatology. One of the most useful techniques is a wet mount of skin scrapings for microscopic examination (Fig 1.7). Twenty per cent potassium hydroxide (KOH) is used to change the optic properties of skin samples and make scales more transparent. The technique requires practice and patience.

The first step is to obtain the material by scraping loose scales at the margin of a lesion, nail parings, subungual debris, or the small pearly globules from a molluscum body. Short residual hair stubs (black dots in tinea capitis) may also be painlessly shaved off the scalp with a #15 blade. Scale is placed on the slide and moved to the center with a cover slip. One or two drops of KOH are added and gently warmed with a match or the microscope light. Boiling the specimen will introduce artifact and should be avoided. Excess KOH can be removed with a paper towel applied to the edge of the cover slip. Thick specimens may be more easily viewed after gentle, but firm pressure is applied to the cover slip with a pencil eraser. Thick scale will also dissolve after being set aside for 15–20 minutes.

View the preparation under a microscope, with the condenser and light at low levels to maximize contrast, and with the objective at 10×. Focus up and down as the entire slide is rapidly scanned. True hyphae are long branching green hyaline rods of uniform width that cross the borders of epidermal cells. They often contain septae. False positives may be vegetative fibers, cell borders, or other artifacts. Yeast infections show budding yeast and pseudohyphae. Molluscum bodies are oval discs that have homogeneous cytoplasm and are slightly larger than keratinocytes. In hair fragments, the fungi appear as small round spores packed within or surrounding the hair shaft (see Fig 8.11f). Hyphae are only rarely seen on the hair.

Scabies preparation

A skin scraping showing a mite, its egg, or feces is necessary to diagnose infestation with *Acarus scabei*, because many other skin rashes resemble scabies clinically (Fig 1.8). The most important factor for obtaining a successful scraping is the choice of site. Burrows and papules, which are most likely to harbor the mite, are commonly located on the wrists, fingers, and elbows. In infants, primary lesions may also be found on the trunk, palms, and soles. A fresh burrow can be identified as a 5–10 mm elongated papule with a vesicle or pustule at one end. A small dark spot resembling a fleck of pepper may be seen in the vesicle. This spot is the mite and it can be lifted out of its burrow with a needle or the point of a scalpel. Usually it is best to hold the skin taut between the thumb and index finger while vigorously scraping the burrow. Although this may induce a small amount of bleeding, if performed with multiple, short, rapid strokes, it is usually painless. A drop of mineral oil should be applied

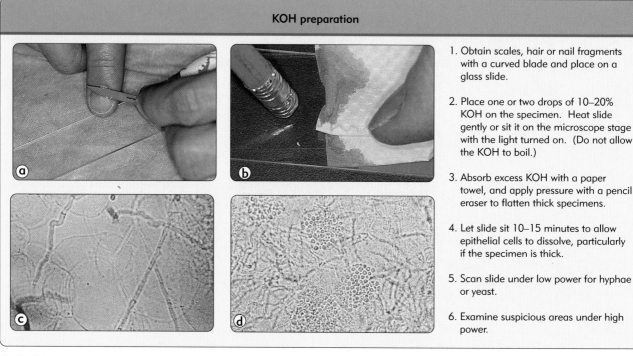

KOH preparation

1. Obtain scales, hair or nail fragments with a curved blade and place on a glass slide.

2. Place one or two drops of 10–20% KOH on the specimen. Heat slide gently or sit it on the microscope stage with the light turned on. (Do not allow the KOH to boil.)

3. Absorb excess KOH with a paper towel, and apply pressure with a pencil eraser to flatten thick specimens.

4. Let slide sit 10–15 minutes to allow epithelial cells to dissolve, particularly if the specimen is thick.

5. Scan slide under low power for hyphae or yeast.

6. Examine suspicious areas under high power.

Fig 1.7 Potassium hydroxide (KOH) preparation. **(a)** Small scales are scraped from the edge of the lesion onto a microscopic slide. **(b)** The scales are crushed to form a thin layer of cells in order to visualize the fungus easily. **(c)** In this positive KOH preparation of skin scrapings, fungal hyphae are seen as long septate, branching rods at the margins and center of the scales. **(d)** Pseudohyphae and spores typical of tinea versicolor give the appearance of spaghetti and meatballs.

to the skin before scraping to ensure adherence of the scrapings to the blade. The scrapings are then placed on the slide, another drop of mineral oil is added, and a cover slip is applied. Gentle pressure with a pencil eraser may be used to flatten thick specimens.

Mites are eight-legged arachnids easily identified with the scanning power of the microscope. Care must be taken to focus through thick areas of skin scrapings so as not to miss any camouflaged mites. The presence of eggs (smooth ovals, approximately one half the size of an adult mite) or feces (brown pellets, often seen in clusters) are also diagnostic. If eggs or feces are found first, perusal of the entire slide usually reveals the adult mite.

Lice preparation

Lice are six-legged insects visible to the unaided eye that are commonly found on the scalp (Fig 1.9), eyelashes, and pubic areas. Pubic lice are short and broad, with claws spaced far apart for grasping the sparse hairs on the trunk, pubic area, and eyelashes, whereas scalp lice are long and thin, with claws closer together to grasp the denser hairs found on the head. The lice are best identified close to the skin, where their eggs are more numerous and more obvious. Diagnosis can be made by identifying the louse, or by plucking hairs and confirming the presence of its eggs or 'nits' by microscopic examination.

Tzanck smear

The Tzanck smear is an important diagnostic tool in the evaluation of blistering diseases. It is most commonly used to distinguish viral diseases, such as herpes simplex, varicella, and herpes zoster, from non-viral disorders (Fig 1.10).

The smear is obtained by removing the 'roof' of the blister with a curved scalpel blade or scissors, and scraping the base to obtain the moist, cloudy debris. The material is then spread on a glass slide, air dried, and stained with Giemsa or Wright stain. The diagnostic finding of viral blisters is the multinucleated giant cell. The giant cell is a syncytium of epidermal cells, with multiple overlapping nuclei; it is much larger than other inflammatory cells. A giant cell may be mistaken for multiple epidermal cells piled on top of each other.

Wood light

Wood light is an ultraviolet source that emits at a wavelength of 365 nm. Formerly, its most common use was in screening patients with alopecia for tinea capitis, as the most common causative organism, *Microsporum* (M.) *audouinii*, was easily identified by its blue-green fluorescence under Wood light. However, today *Trichophyton tonsurans* is the most common fungus associated with tinea capitis, but it does not fluoresce. In the USA fewer than 10% of cases are caused by *M. canis* and other *Microsporum* species. In Europe, Africa, and Asia organisms that cause ectothrix scalp infection and which fluoresce include *M. ferrugineum*, *M. audouinii*, and *M. canis*.

Wood light is still of value in diagnosing a number of other diseases. Erythrasma is a superficial bacterial infection of moist skin in the groin, axilla, and toe webs. It appears as a brown or red flat plaque, and is caused by a corynebacterium that excretes a pigment which contains a porphyrin. This pigment fluoresces coral red or pink under Wood light. Tinea versicolor, a superficial fungal infection with hypopigmented macules and plaques on the trunk, also fluoresces under

---

Scabies preparation

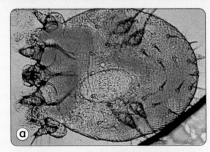
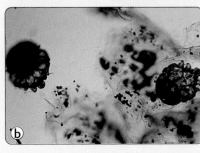

1. Using a cotton-tip applicator, apply a drop of mineral oil on a suspicious lesion that has not been scraped.

2. Vigorously scrape the lesion with a curved blade while the skin is held taut between the opposite index finger and thumb.

3. Place material on a glass slide and apply a cover slip. Examine the slide under low power for the mite, eggs, and feces.

Fig 1.8 (a) Microscopic appearance of the adult scabies mite. Note the small oval egg within the body. **(b)** Scraping from an adolescent with crusted scabies shows two mites and multiple fecal pellets.

Lice preparation

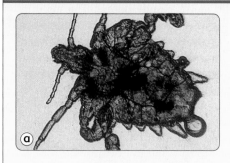

1. Search the involved area with the unaided eye or a hand lens.

2. Grasp any moving objects with a forceps or snip hairs with nits and place on a glass slide under a piece of clear tape.

3. Examine under low power for viable organisms or unhatched nits.

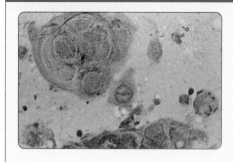
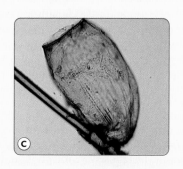

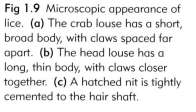

Fig 1.9 Microscopic appearance of lice. **(a)** The crab louse has a short, broad body, with claws spaced far apart. **(b)** The head louse has a long, thin body, with claws closer together. **(c)** A hatched nit is tightly cemented to the hair shaft.

Tzanck smear

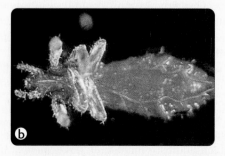

1. Gently unroof blisters with a curved blade or scissors.

2. Blot fluid from vesicle.

3. Gently scrape base of blister or erosion with a curved blade.

4. Spread material thinly on glass slide.

5. Air dry and if possible fix for 2 minutes in 95% alcohol.

6. Cover slide with Wright's or Giemsa stain.

7. Scan slide under low power to find an area with epithelial cells; then examine under high power.

Fig 1.10 Tzanck smear. Note the multinucleated giant cells characteristic of viral infection with herpes simplex and varicella/zoster.

Wood light with a green-yellow color. *Pseudomonas* infection of the toe web space and colonization of the skin in burn patients will fluoresce yellow-green. Patients with porphyria cutanea tarda excrete uroporphyrins in their urine, and examination of a urine specimen will show an orange-yellow fluorescence. Adequate blood levels of tetracycline produce yellow fluorescence in the opening of hair follicles, while lack of fluorescence indicates poor intestinal absorption or poor patient compliance.

Wood light also emits purple light in the visible spectrum. This wavelength can be used to accentuate subtle changes in pigmentation. The purple light is absorbed by melanin in the skin, and variably reflected by patches of hypopigmentation and depigmentation. This may be particularly useful in evaluating light pigmented individuals with vitiligo or ash leaf macules.

DERMATOLOGIC THERAPEUTICS

General Principles

Single component generic preparations are often effective and inexpensive. Fixed multiple component preparations are occasionally useful, but the practitioner must be aware of all the constituent agents and the increased risk of adverse drug reactions. Specially formulated medications are often prohibitively expensive and seldom indicated in general practice.

The practitioner must calculate the quantity of medication required for the patient to comply with instructions. In a child, 15–30 g of an ointment is needed to cover the entire skin surface once. This quantity will vary with the vehicle used and the experience of the individual applying the preparation.

Topical vehicles

Two variables are particularly important in the selection of effective topical therapy: the active medication and the vehicle.

Ointments

In general, ointments are occlusive and allow for high transcutaneous penetration of the active drug. Ointments are stable for long periods and require few preservatives and bacteriostatic additives. As a consequence, they are least likely to cause contact allergy or irritation.

Open wet dressings

Open wet dressings, using tap water or normal saline, provide symptomatic relief by cooling and drying acute inflammatory lesions. They cleanse the skin by loosening exudates and crusts that can be painlessly removed before the dressing dries. Various astringents and antiseptics, such as vinegar or 5% aluminum acetate solution (e.g. Burrow solution), may be added to compression solutions in a 1:20–40 dilution.

Powders and lotions

Powders promote drying and are especially useful in the intertriginous areas. Lotions are powders suspended in water (e.g. calamine lotion). When these preparations dry, they cool the skin and provide a uniform covering of the suspended agent.

Gels

Gels are aqueous preparations that liquefy on contact with the skin and leave a uniform film on drying. Gels are well tolerated in hair-bearing areas.

Aerosols

Aerosols and sprays act in a manner similar to lotions and gels. Active ingredients are incorporated into an aqueous phase. A convenient delivery system usually allows for easy dispersion over the skin surface. Aerosols are also particularly useful on the scalp.

Creams

Traditional creams are suspensions of oil in water. As the proportion of oil increases, the preparation approaches the consistency of an ointment, which is the most lubricating vehicle. Creams are water washable and hygroscopic. They may be drying and occasionally sensitizing.

Pastes

Pastes, which are mixtures of powder in ointment, are messy and may be difficult to remove from the skin. They are used to protect areas prone to irritation, such as the diaper area. Pastes can be removed with mineral oil.

Topical corticosteroids

Topical steroids are available in every type of vehicle. A good approach is to become familiar with one or two products in each of the potency ranges (Fig 1.11). A check of local pharmacies is useful in determining the availability and cost of medications.

Most childhood skin eruptions requiring topical steroids can be readily managed with twice daily applications of low- or medium-potency preparations. Only low-potency medications should be used on the face and intertriginous areas, because more potent preparations may produce atrophy, telangiectasias, and hypopigmentation. Regardless of the potency of a medication, patients should be followed carefully for steroid-induced changes, even though they are only rarely produced by therapy restricted to 2–4 weeks. Patients receiving chronic therapy should take frequent 'time outs' from their topical steroids (e.g. 1 week per month) and should taper them when possible. Tapering may be achieved by decreasing the frequency of application as well as by mixing the active preparation with a bland emollient such as petrolatum.

Steroids may mask infections and suppress local and systemic immune responses. Consequently, they are contraindicated in most patients with viral, fungal, bacterial, or mycobacterial infection.

Emollients (lubricants)

Any preparation that reduces friction and leaves a smooth, occlusive film that prevents drying is classified as a lubricant (Fig 1.12). In patients with chronic dermatitis, ointments (or water in oil-based products) provide the best lubrication, especially during the dry winter months. Less oily preparations (oil in water creams) are often preferred by patients during the spring and summer. Cultural preferences should also be taken into account when selecting a lubricant. Preparations containing topical sensitizers such as fragrance, neomycin, and benzocaine should be avoided, particularly in patients with inflamed skin.

A number of other topical and oral agents are used in the treatment of skin disorders. They will be discussed in detail in later chapters. The most commonly recommended agents are listed in *Pocket Guide to Medications Used in Dermatology*, by Scheman. This frequently updated guide includes detailed lists of oral and topical prescriptions and over-the-counter products used in the management of skin disorders.

Fig 1.11 Topical corticosteroids.

Topical corticosteroids			
Group	**Generic name**	**Trade name**	

1	Betamethasone dipropionate, augmented 0.05%
	Clobetasol propionate 0.05%
	
	Diflorasone diacetate 0.05%
	Halobetasol propriate
		Diprolene 0.05%
		  Diproline AF 0.05%
		Temovate 0.05%
		  Dermovate 0.05%
		Psorcon 0.05%
		Ultravate 0.05%
			High potency

2	Amcinonide
	Betamethasone dipropionate
	Diflorasone diacetate
	
	Halcinonide
	
	Fluocinonide
	
	Desoximetasone
	Mometasone furoate
		Cyclocort ointment 0.1%
		Diprosone ointment 0.05%
		Florone ointment 0.05%
		  Maxiflor ointment 0.05%
		Halog cream 0.1%
		  Halciderm 0.1%
		Lidex cream 0.05%
		  Metosyn 0.05%
		Lidex ointment 0.05%
		Topicort cream 0.25 %
		Elocon ointment 0.1%	

3	Betametasone dipropionate Betametasone benzoate Betametasone valerate Fluticosone propionate	Diprosone cream 0.05% Benisone gel 0.025% Valisone ointment 0.1% Betacap 0.1% Cutivate ointment 0.05%	
4	Triamcinolone acetonide Fluradrenolide Triamcinolone acetonide Fluocinolone acetonide	Aristocort ointment 0.1% Cordran ointment 0.05% Kenalog ointment 0.1% Adocortyl 0.1% Synalar cream 0.025%	

5	Desonide
	Triamcinolone acetonide
	Fluradrenolide
	Fluocinolone acetonide
	
	Triamcinolone acetonide
	Betamethasone valerate
	Hydrocortisone valerate
	Hydrocortisone butyrate
		Tridesilon ointment 0.05%
		Aristocort cream 0.1%
		Cordran SP cream 0.05%
		Fluonid cream 0.01%
		  Synalar 0.025%
		  Synalar cream 0.01%
		Kenalog cream 0.1%
		Valisone cream 0.1%
		Westcort cream 0.2%
		Locoid cream 0.1%
			Low potency

6	Hydrocortisone 1%, urea 10% Flumetasone pivalate Desonide Alclometasone dipropionate	Alphaderm cream 1% Locorten cream 0.03% Tridesilon cream 0.05% Aclorate cream 0.05% Modrasone 0.05%	
7	Hydrocortisone 1% Dexamethasone Methylprednisolone acetate Prednisolone	Hytone cream 1% Cobadex 1% Dioderm 1% Mildison 1% Hydrocortisyl 1% Hytone ointment 1% Hexadrol cream 0.04% Medrol ointment 0.25% Meti-derm cream 0.5%	
8	Hydrocortisone 0.5%	Cortaid cream	

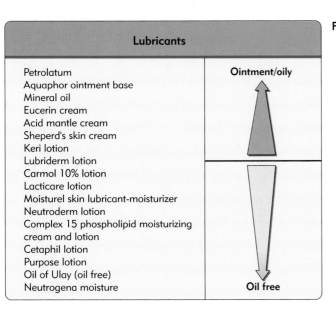

Fig 1.12 Lubricants.

BIBLIOGRAPHY

Arndt KA, LeBoit PE, Robinson JK, Wintroub BU. *Cutaneous medicine and surgery: an integrated program in dermatology.* W. B. Saunders, Philadelphia, 1996.

Champion RH, Burton JL, Ebling FJG: Rook/Wilkinson/ Ebling. *Textbook of dermatology,* 5th edn. Blackwell Scientific, Oxford, 1992.

Fitzpatrick TB, Eisen AZ, Wolff K, Freedberg IM, Austen KF. *Dermatology in general medicine,* 4th edn. McGraw Hill, New York, 1993.

Hurwitz S. *Clinical pediatric dermatology,* 2nd edn. W. B. Saunders, Philadelphia, 1994.

Lever WF, Schaumburg-Lever. *Histopathology of the skin,* 8th edn. Lippincott, Philadelphia, 1997.

Meneghini CL, Bonifazi E. *An atlas of pediatric dermatology.* Yearbook Medical Publishers, Chicago, 1986.

Moschella SL, Hurley HJ. *Dermatology.* W. B. Saunders, Philadelphia, 1992

Ruiz-Maldonado R, Parish LC, Beare JM. *Textbook of pediatric dermatology.* Grune and Stratton, Philadelphia, 1989.

Schachner LA, Hansen RC. *Pediatric dermatology,* 2nd edn. Churchill Livingstone, New York, 1995.

Scheman AJ. *Pocket Guide to Medication Used in Dermatology.* Baltimore: Williams & Wilkins, 1997.

Verbov J, Morley N. *Color atlas of pediatric dermatology.* Lippincott, London, 1983.

Weinberg S, Leider M, Shapiro L. *Color atlas of pediatric dermatology.* McGraw-Hill, London, 1975.

Weston WL. *Practical pediatric dermatology.* Little, Brown, Boston, 1985.

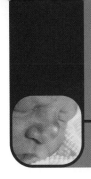

Chapter Two

Neonatal Dermatology

INTRODUCTION

The skin of the newborn differs from that of the adult in several ways (Fig 2.1). It is less hairy, has less sweat and sebaceous gland secretions, is thinner, has fewer intercellular attachments, and fewer melanosomes. These differences are magnified in the preterm neonate. As a consequence, newborns are not as well equipped to handle thermal stress and sunlight, have increased transepidermal water loss and penetration of toxic substances and medications, and are more likely to develop blisters or erosions in response to heat, chemical irritants, mechanical trauma, and inflammatory skin conditions.

BARRIER PROPERTIES AND USE OF TOPICAL AGENTS

The barrier properties of the skin reside primarily in the stratum corneum, the compact layer of flattened keratinocytes that cover the surface. Although keratinization begins at 24 weeks, it is not complete until close to term. Transepidermal water loss and drug absorption through the epidermis at term are similar to those in older children and adults. Skin barrier properties in babies of gestational age 36 weeks approximate those of term infants within several days, but may be delayed by 14–21 days in children of gestational age less than 32–34 weeks. Barrier maturation may be further delayed when epidermal injury, inflammation, or hyperemia are present. Sepsis, ischemia, and acidosis in the severely ill newborn may also compromise barrier function. Moreover, even in healthy term infants the increased surface-to-volume ratio compared with older children and adults may result in relatively high transcutaneous penetration of topical agents.

Percutaneous absorption of toxic substances in newborns, particularly preterm infants and term infants with disruption of barrier function, has been well documented. Aniline dyes used to mark diapers have caused methemoglobinemia and death. Topical corticosteroids may produce adrenal suppression and systemic effects. Vacuolar encephalopathy has been demonstrated in infants bathed with hexachlorophene, particularly premature infants exposed repeatedly.

Pentachlorophenol poisoning occurred in 20 infants who were accidentally exposed to this chemical in nursery linens. Topical application of povidone–iodine to the perineum before delivery and the umbilical cord after delivery

	Adult	Term	Preterm (30 weeks)	Significance
Structural and functional differences of adult, term, and preterm infant skin				
Epidermal thickness	50 μm	50 μm	27.4 μm	Permeability to topical agents ⇑ Transepidermal water loss
Cell attachments (desmosome, hemidesmosome)	Normal	Normal	Fewer	⇑ Tendency to blister
Dermis	Normal	⇓ Collagen and elastic fibers	⇓⇓ Collagen and elastic fibers	⇓ Elasticity ⇑ Blistering
Melanosomes	Normal	Fewer	One-third term infant	⇑ Photosensitivity
Eccrine glands	Normal	Delayed activity for 1–7 days ⇓ Neurologic control for 2–3 years	Total anhidrosis	⇓ Response to thermal stress
Sebaceous glands	Normal	Normal	Normal	Barrier properties? Lubricant? Antibacterial?
Hair	Normal	⇓ Terminal hair	Persistent lanugo	Helpful in assessing gestational age

Fig 2.1 Structural and functional differences of adult, term and preterm infant skin.

has resulted in elevated plasma iodine levels and thyroid dysfunction in the neonate. Other substances, which include isopropyl alcohol, ethyl and methyl alcohol, and chlorhexidine, are readily absorbed and may produce toxic reactions.

In general, topical agents should be used in newborns and infants only if systemic administration of the agent is not associated with toxicity. Antiseptic agents must be used only with great caution and to limited areas of the skin, particularly in premature infants under 30 weeks gestational age during the first several weeks of life. Injuries to the skin induced by tape, monitors, adhesives, and cleansing agents must be kept to a minimum as these tend to compromise barrier function. When lubrication is necessary, small amounts of petrolatum or other fragrance-free, bland emollients are adequate. Some investigators advocate the routine use of barrier products in tiny, premature infants to reduce heat and insensible water loss. Bubble blankets and humidified air also help to minimize energy requirements.

At birth the skin is covered with a greasy white material of pH 6.7–7.4. Although the function of this vernix caseosa is unknown, it may have lubricating and antibacterial properties. Beneath the vernix the skin has a pH of 5.5–6.0. Over washing of the baby, particularly with harsh soaps, may result in irritation, alkaline pH, and a decrease in normal barrier function of the stratum corneum. As a consequence, bathing is done gently several times a week with tap water, and mild soaps are restricted to areas in which cutaneous bacteria are most numerous, such as the umbilicus, diaper area, neck, and axillae. In ill newborns, bathing may be limited to saline compresses of areas of irritated, macerated skin, which occur commonly in intertriginous areas.

Thermoregulation

Cold stress is the major risk to naked preterm infants nursed in a dry incubator. Decreased epidermal and dermal thicknesses result in increased heat loss from radiation and conduction. Minimal subcutaneous fat and an immature nervous system also decrease the premature infant's ability to respond to cooling. Although heat loss may be minimized by increasing ambient humidity and temperature and by covering the child with a plastic bubble, increasing postnatal age and weight approaching 2000g are associated with maintenance of normal body temperature.

In growing premature and full-term infants hyperthermia may be a problem in warm climates, particularly when additional thermal stresses such as insulated clothing and phototherapy are present. Although sweat glands are anatomically complete at 28 weeks' gestation, they may not be fully functional until several weeks after delivery, even in the full-term neonate. At birth, sweating has been demonstrated in response to thermal stress in term babies. However, it may not be detectable in infants under 35 weeks' gestational age for several weeks. Consequently, sweating may not be an effective mechanism for thermoregulation in term or premature infants for at least several weeks, so thermal stress must be minimized.

Pigmentation and photoprotection

Although melanocytes are actively synthesizing and transferring pigment to epidermal keratinocytes by 20–24 weeks of intrauterine life, the skin surface tends to be less pigmented during the first few postnatal months than in later childhood. As a consequence, infants have less natural protection from sunlight and are more likely to develop sunburn.

Several investigators have expressed concern about using sunscreens in children under 6 months of age. However, as these infants are not ambulatory sun avoidance and protective clothing are effective barriers to excessive sun exposure.

Certain children are particularly sensitive to sunlight, and for these prolonged sun avoidance beyond infancy and aggressive use of sunscreens may be mandatory (see Chapter 7). Hereditary porphyrias, xeroderma pigmentosum, Bloom syndrome, Cockayne syndrome, and a number of other photosensitivity disorders may present with exaggerated sunburn reactions in infancy. In some infants tingling and burning of the skin may occur after sun exposure with no obvious physical findings. In neonatal lupus erythematosus the skin rash is often triggered by sun exposure. Although some of these children benefit from broad-spectrum sunscreens or sunscreens with sun protective factors above 15, photoreactions may be caused by wavelengths of light that are not absorbed by currently available sunscreens. In some patients, oral β-carotene may provide additional protection.

CUTANEOUS COMPLICATIONS OF THE INTENSIVE CARE NURSERY

Scars and burns are inevitable complications of nursery care and monitoring. Careful management of the skin in the nursery and after discharge minimizes the risk of serious functional impairment and cosmetic disfigurement.

Surgical scars

Wounds from subclavian and jugular venous lines generally heal with barely noticeable scars. Occasionally, scars are more obvious, but usually they fade over the first 2 years of life, particularly if the wounds conform to the normal skin lines. However, dimpling may result from sutures used to keep the lines in place (Fig 2.2). Scarring and dimpling may also be minimized by gentle massage of the area.

Frequently, chest tubes are placed in such an emergent setting that little time is taken to consider optimal site selection. Lateral placement beyond the breast tissue may eliminate the need for later surgical repair. Gentle massage after removal may prevent the formation of adhesions and dimpling. As with other surgical scars, these lesions tend to improve spontaneously over the first several years of life.

Arterial catheters

In addition to local scarring, arterial catheters may be associated with serious systemic and cutaneous complications in the areas distal to their placement. Extensive ischemia and necrosis of the genital and buttock skin is an unusual complication of umbilical artery spasm and thromboembolism. Ensuing ulcerations may take months to heal and require surgical repair (Fig 2.3). Radial artery catheters have rarely been associated with the necrosis of digits. However, more subtle findings, such as discrepancies in hand size, may not be evident for a year.

Chemical and thermal burns

Infiltration of the soft tissues by intravenous fluids often produces cutaneous inflammation and necrosis. Hypertonic fluids, such as glucose and calcium, may result in full-thickness sloughing of the skin and in contractures (Fig 2.4). These lesions usually heal over weeks to months and may require splinting, physical therapy, and surgical repair, particularly if they are located over joints.

Removal of adhesives used with dressings, of endotracheal and nasotracheal tubes, and of monitor leads results in extensive trauma to the skin (Fig 2.5). Although full-thickness sloughs may rarely develop, postinflammatory hyperpigmentation and hypopigmentation are common. Pigmentary changes may persist for years, particularly in dark-pigmented individuals, but usually fade markedly within the first year of life. Other topical agents, such as iodophors, soaps,

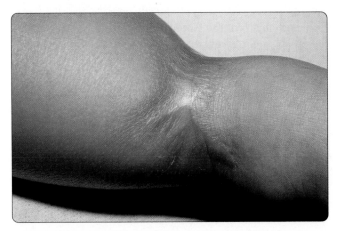

Fig 2.2 Effect of surgical scars. (a) Scar from an arterial cut down site. Recurrent drainage ended after a small fistulous tract in the scar was excised from the wrist of this 2-year-old girl. (b) This 6-year-old girl has a hypertrophic scar in the right antecubital space. She developed prurigo nodules in the center of the scar from chronic scratching.

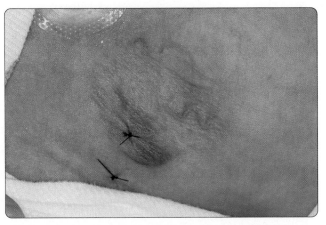

Fig 2.3 Several hours after an umbilical artery catheter was removed from this infant a purple area developed unilaterally on the scrotum, perineum, and perirectal skin. After 1 day, the area became ulcerated. Note the formation of granulation tissue and early scarring 1 week later.

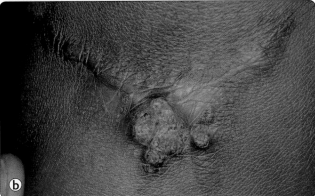

Fig 2.4 Infiltration of the antecubital skin with 20% glucose resulted in an ulcer that healed with severe scarring. The scar was surgically revised at 4 years of age.

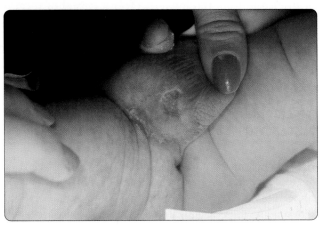

Fig 2.5 Repeated trauma from removal of monitor leads produced a round, atrophic patch on the lower abdominal wall of this 29-week premature infant. Note the wrinkling of the skin, prominent vessels, and purpura (which was present before a biopsy was taken).

detergents, and solvents, may produce severe irritant reactions, particularly in premature infants or children with an antecedent cutaneous injury (Fig 2.6).

Accidental thermal burns have been reported following exposure to heated water beds, radiant warmers, transcutaneous oxygen monitors, and heated, humidified air. Although cold stress must be minimized in the small premature infant, extensive burns that have cutaneous and airway involvement may be prevented by close monitoring of these devices.

Heel-stick nodules

Repeated blood sampling from the heel leads to the formation of papules and nodules in many graduates of the neonatal intensive care unit (Fig 2.7). Although the most prominent lesions occur in children who have had frequent heel sticks, these scars are also detected in infants who have had only a few. Lesions may be palpable at the time of discharge from the nursery. Over a period of several months, they generally become more superficial and resemble milia. Papules typically calcify over the ensuing months and resolve spontaneously in 18–30 months. During this time infants are asymptomatic, and walking is not delayed.

TRANSIENT ERUPTIONS OF THE NEWBORN

A number of innocent rashes occur in infants. Although they are usually transient, they may be very dramatic and a major source of parental anxiety. Early recognition is important to differentiate these lesions from more serious disorders and to provide appropriate counseling to parents.

Transient vascular phenomena

During the first 2–4 weeks of life, cold stress may be associated with acrocyanosis and cutis marmorata (Fig 2.8). In acrocyanosis, the hands and feet become variably and symmetrically blue in color without edema or other cutaneous changes. Cutis marmorata is identified by the characteristic reticulated cyanosis or marbling of the skin, which symmetrically involves the trunk and extremities. Both patterns usually resolve with warming of the skin, and recurrence is unusual after 1 month of age. Acrocyanosis is readily differentiated from persistent central cyanosis (cyanosis of the lips, face, and/or trunk), which occurs in association with pulmonary or cardiac disease. Cutis marmorata that persists beyond the neonatal period may be a marker for trisomy 18, Down syndrome, Cornelia de Lange syndrome, and hypothyroidism. Cutis marmorata telangiectatica congenita (or congenital phlebectasia; Fig 2.9) may mimic cutis marmorata. However, the lesions are persistent in a localized patch on the trunk or extremities. The eruption may extend in a dermatomal pattern, and occasionally widespread lesions and reticulated cutaneous atrophy are present. Although congenital phlebectasia may be an isolated cutaneous finding, it may also occur in association with other mesodermal and neuroectodermal anomalies.

The harlequin color change is noted when the infant lays horizontally and the dependent half of the body turns bright red in contrast to the pale upper half (Fig 2.10). The color shifts when the infant is rolled from side to side. This phenomenon lasts from seconds to 20 minutes, and recurrences are common until 3–4 weeks of life. The cause is unknown, and it is not associated with serious underlying disease.

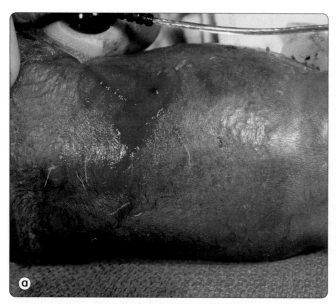

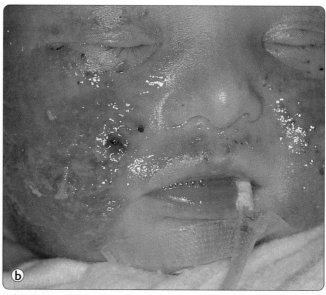

Fig 2.6 Severe irritant reactions. **(a)** Application of a solution containing topical iodophor produced an erosive irritant dermatitis on the flank of a premature infant in the intensive care nursery. Fortunately, this area healed with only minimal scarring. **(b)** A chemical burn resulted from a solvent that was applied to this child's face to remove adhesive tape.

Benign pustular dermatoses

Several innocent pustular eruptions must be differentiated from potentially serious infectious dermatoses.

Erythema toxicum neonatorum

Erythema toxicum neonatorum (ETN) is the most common pustular rash; it occurs in up to 70% of full-term infants (Fig 2.11). Although lesions usually appear on the second or third day of life, onset has been reported up to 2–3 weeks of age. Typically, ETN begins with 2–3 mm diameter erythematous, blotchy macules and papules, which may evolve over several hours into pustules on a broad erythematous base to give affected infants a 'flea-bitten' appearance. Lesions may be isolated or clustered on the face, trunk, and proximal extremities, and usually fade over 5–7

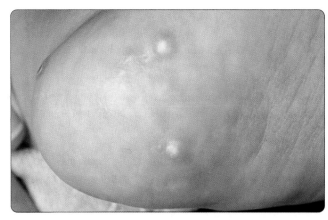

Fig 2.7 Heel-stick papules on the feet of this graduate of the intensive care nursery resolved without treatment.

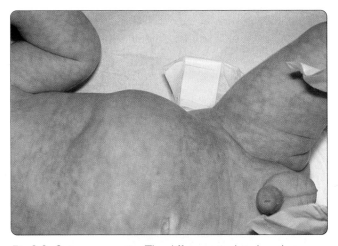

Fig 2.8 Cutis marmorata. The diffuse, reticulated erythema disappeared with warming of this newborn.

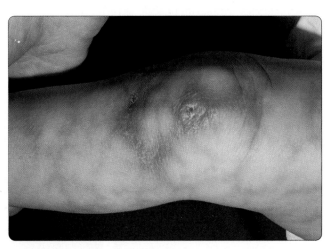

Fig 2.9 Cutis marmorata telangiectatica congenita was associated with some cutaneous atrophy on the left leg of a newborn. A careful medical evaluation failed to reveal any associated anomalies.

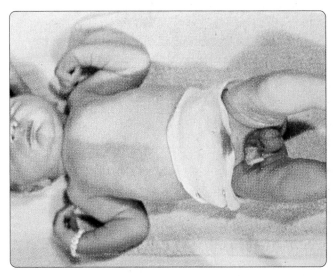

Fig 2.10 The dependent side is bright red in this infant with the harlequin color change.

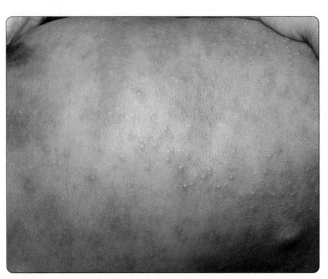

Fig 2.11 Erythema toxicum neonatorum. Numerous yellow papules and pustules are surrounded by large, intensely erythematous rings on the trunk of this infant.

days. Recurrences, however, may occur for several weeks. A Wright stain of the pustule contents reveals sheets of eosinophils and occasional neutrophils, and 15–20% of patients have a circulating eosinophilia.

Transient neonatal pustular melanosis

Transient neonatal pustular melanosis (TNPM) occurs in 4% of newborns, particularly in black male infants (Fig 2.12). Unlike ETN, lesions are usually present at birth and probably evolve in many children prenatally. Characteristically, TNPM appears as 2–5 mm diameter pustules on a non-erythematous base on the chin, neck, upper chest, sacrum, abdomen, and thighs. Over several days, lesions develop a central crust, which desquamates to leave a hyperpigmented macule with a collarette of fine scale. Lesions at different stages of development may be present simultaneously. Often the only manifestation of the eruption is the presence of brown macules with a rim of scale at birth. A Wright stain of the pustular smear shows numerous neutrophils and rare eosinophils.

Acropustulosis of infancy

Acropustulosis of infancy is a chronic, recurrent pustular eruption that appears on the palms and soles, but may also involve the scalp, trunk, buttocks, and extremities (Fig 2.13). Onset may occur during the newborn period or in early infancy, and episodes typically last 1–3 weeks with intervening remissions of 1–3 weeks. Disease-free periods tend to lengthen until the rash resolves by 2–3 years of age. During flares infants are usually fussy and pruritus is severe. Histopathology of the lesions reveals sterile, intraepidermal pustules. A Wright stain shows numerous neutrophils and occasional eosinophils. Although oral dapsone (1–3 mg/kg/day) suppresses lesions and symptoms in 24–48 hours, brief courses of moderate- or high-potency topical corticosteroids to the palms and soles may provide safe temporary relief.

Eosinophilic pustular folliculitis

Eosinophilic pustular folliculitis (EPF), or Ofuji disease, is a rare, self-limiting vesiculopustular eruption of infancy

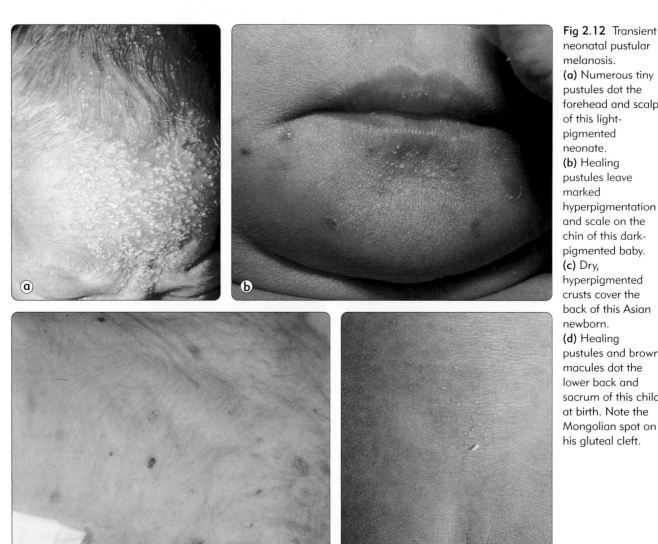

Fig 2.12 Transient neonatal pustular melanosis.
(a) Numerous tiny pustules dot the forehead and scalp of this light-pigmented neonate.
(b) Healing pustules leave marked hyperpigmentation and scale on the chin of this dark-pigmented baby.
(c) Dry, hyperpigmented crusts cover the back of this Asian newborn.
(d) Healing pustules and brown macules dot the lower back and sacrum of this child at birth. Note the Mongolian spot on his gluteal cleft.

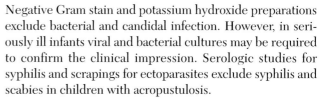

characterized by recurrent episodes of 2–3 mm diameter white vesicles and pustules on a red base on the scalp and forehead. Occasionally, lesions spread to the trunk. It occurs almost exclusively in boys of age 5–10 months and can recur for months to years. Several neonatal cases have also been described. Although affected infants experience intense pruritus and irritability, EPF is not associated with systemic disease, and treatment is symptomatic. Wright stain preparations of material from pustules show large numbers of eosinophils, but no evidence of bacterial, fungal, or viral organisms. The strong association of EPF with human immunodeficiency virus infection seen in adults has not been noted in infants. The clinical findings and course may overlap with some cases of ETN and acropustulosis of infancy.

Other papulopustular rashes

Benign pustular dermatoses can be differentiated from Herpes simplex infection by the absence of multinucleated giant cells on Wright stained smears of pustular contents.

Negative Gram stain and potassium hydroxide preparations exclude bacterial and candidal infection. However, in seriously ill infants viral and bacterial cultures may be required to confirm the clinical impression. Serologic studies for syphilis and scrapings for ectoparasites exclude syphilis and scabies in children with acropustulosis.

The benign pustular dermatoses may also be confused with several other innocent papulopustular rashes, which include sebaceous gland hyperplasia, miliaria, milia, and acne.

Sebaceous gland hyperplasia

Sebaceous gland hyperplasia is a common finding over the nose and cheeks of term infants (Fig 2.14). Lesions consist of multiple 1–2 mm diameter yellow papules that result from maternal or endogenous androgenic stimulation of sebaceous gland growth. Parents are counseled that the eruption resolves within 4–6 months.

Miliaria

Miliaria results from obstruction to the flow of sweat and rupture of the eccrine sweat duct. In miliaria crystallina, superficial, 1–2 mm diameter vesicles appear on noninflamed skin when the duct is blocked by keratinous debris just beneath the stratum corneum (Fig 2.15). Small papules and pustules are typical of miliaria rubra (prickly heat), in which the obstruction occurs in the mid epidermis (Fig 2.16). Deep-seated papulopustular lesions of miliaria profunda occur only rarely in infancy, when the duct ruptures at the dermal–epidermal junction.

Miliaria occurs frequently in term and preterm infants after the first week of life in response to thermal stress. Lesions erupt in crops in the intertriginous areas, scalp, face, and trunk. In older infants, lesions appear most commonly in areas of skin occluded by tight-fitting clothing. Cooling the skin and loosening clothing results in prompt resolution of the rash.

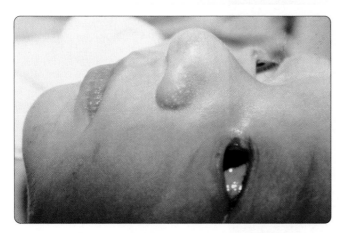

Fig 2.13 Acropustulosis of infancy. Multiple 2–3 mm pustules covered the hands and feet of this otherwise healthy infant. Lesions recurred episodically until this child was 3 years old.

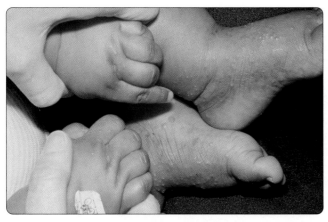

Fig 2.14 Sebaceous gland hyperplasia. Note the yellow papules on the nose of this newborn.

Fig 2.15 Miliaria crystallina. Tiny, thin-walled vesicles quickly desquamated when this child was placed in a cooler environment.

Milia

Milia appear as pearly, yellow, 1–3 mm diameter papules on the face, chin, and forehead of 50% of newborns (Fig 2.17). Occasionally, they erupt on the trunk and extremities. Although milia usually resolve during the first month of life

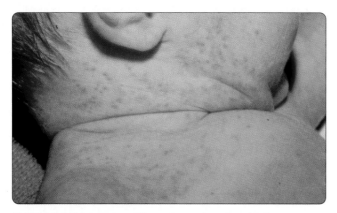

Fig 2.16 Miliaria rubra. The red papules of prickly heat are readily visible on this infant.

without treatment, they may persist for several months. Histology demonstrates miniature epidermal inclusion cysts that arise from the pilosebaceous apparatus of vellus hairs. Large numbers of lesions distributed over a wide area or persistence beyond several months of age suggest the possibility of the oral–facial–digital syndrome or hereditary trichodysplasia (Marie Unna hypotrichosis). Increasing numbers of lesions, particularly in areas of normal trauma such as the hands, knees, and feet, may occur in patients with mild variants of scarring epidermolysis bullosa where blistering is subtle.

Acne

Mild acne develops in up to 20% of newborns. Lesions may be present at birth or appear in early infancy. Although closed comedones (white heads) predominate, open comdones (black heads), red papules, pustules, and (rarely) cysts may also occur (Fig 2.18). As in sebaceous hyperplasia, maternal and endogenous androgens probably play

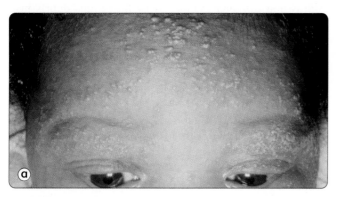
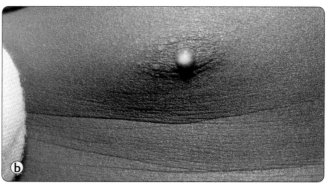

Fig 2.17 Milia. **(a)** Widespread milia were noted on the forehead and eyelids of this vigorous newborn. The white papules resolved spontaneously before the 2-month pediatric

check-up. **(b)** The milium on this infant's nipple also cleared without treatment.

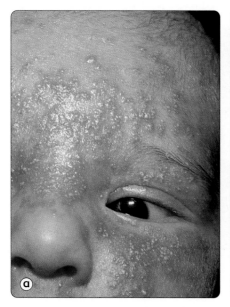
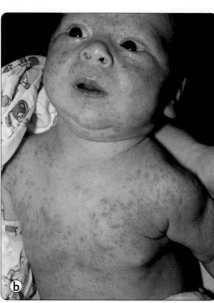

Fig 2.18 Neonatal acne. **(a)** Red papules and pustules covered the face of this 4-week-old boy. **(b)** Acne spread to the trunk of this healthy infant. In both children the eruption cleared by 4 months of age.

a role in the pathogenesis of neonatal acne. Treatment is usually unnecessary as lesions involute spontaneously within 1–3 months. Risk of acne in adolescence does not seem to be increased.

Occasionally, the onset of acne is delayed until 3–6 months of age. Lesions tend to be more pleiomorphic and inflammatory papules and pustules are common. Although infantile acne usually resolves by 3 years of age, lesions may persist until the child is 11 years old. As with neonatal acne, infantile acne is probably triggered by endogenous androgens. Children with early onset, persistent disease, and a positive family history of severe acne tend to have a more severe course with resurgence at puberty. Severe infantile acne prompts a search for other signs of hyperandrogenism and an abnormal endogenous or exogenous source of androgens.

Subcutaneous fat necrosis of the newborn

Fat necrosis is a benign, self-limited process that usually occurs in otherwise healthy infants (Fig 2.19). Discrete red or hemorrhagic nodules and plaques up to 3 cm in diameter appear most commonly over areas exposed to trauma, such as the cheeks, back, buttocks, arms, and thighs, during the first few weeks of life. Lesions are usually painless, but marked tenderness may be present. Although the cause is unknown, difficult deliveries, hypothermia, perinatal asphyxia, and maternal diabetes predispose to the development of fat necrosis.

Nodules usually resolve without scarring in 1–2 months. However, lesions occasionally become fluctuant, drain, and heal with atrophy. When calcification occurs, infants are evaluated for primary hyperparathyroidism, and calcium levels must be monitored.

Histopathology demonstrates necrosis of fat with a foreign body giant cell reaction. Remaining fat cells contain needle-shaped clefts, and calcium deposits are scattered throughout the subcutis. Occasionally, early lesions of scleredema neonatorum are confused with subcutaneous fat necrosis. However, in a severely ill newborn, scleredema is usually differentiated from fat necrosis by the presence of diffuse, wax-like hardening of the skin. Unlike subcutaneous fat necrosis, skin biopsy shows only minimal inflammation in the fat. Thickening of the skin occurs from the increased size of fat cells and interlacing bundles of collagen in the dermis and subcutis.

MINOR ANOMALIES

Minor anomalies occur in up to half of all newborns and are of no physiologic consequence. Their presence, particularly in association with other minor anomalies, prompts an evaluation for more serious multisystem disease.

Dimpling

Dimpling is a common finding over bony prominences, particularly the sacral area (Fig 2.20). Although skin dimples may be the first sign of several dysmorphic syndromes,

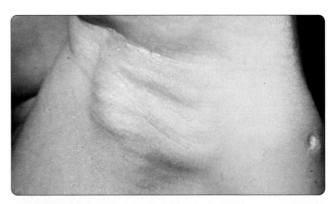

Fig 2.19 Subcutaneous fat necrosis. Red nodules are evident on the arm of this neonate. Lesions resolved without atrophy by 2 months of age.

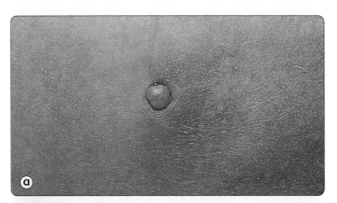

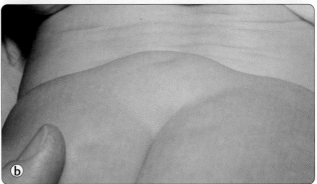

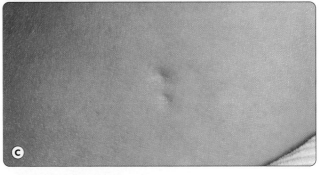

Fig 2.20 Dimples. **(a)** A sacral dimple was noted in this healthy infant. Computed tomography scan of the lumbosacral spine was normal. **(b)** At birth a spongy mass was palpable in the sacral area of this baby. A magnetic resonance image of this tumor revealed a lipoma and normal spine. **(c)** These dimples on the thigh of an otherwise healthy infant may have resulted from amniocentesis-induced trauma.

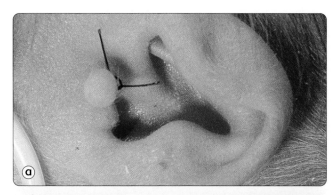

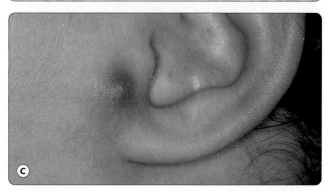

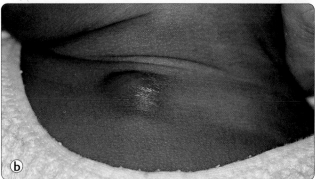

Fig 2.21 Skin tags and cysts. **(a)** This preauricular skin tag was tied off in the nursery. **(b)** Congenital cyst on the supraclavicular area. **(c)** Congenital cyst on the preauricular area. The cysts on these children became apparent when they became infected. Both required surgical excision.

these lesions are usually of only cosmetic consequence. Spinal anomalies should be excluded when deep dimples, sinus tracts, or other cutaneous lesions (such as lipomas, hemangiomas, nevi, and tufts of hair) involve the lumbo-sacral spine.

Periauricular sinuses, pits, tags, and cysts

Periauricular sinuses, pits, tags, and cysts occur when brachial arches or clefts fail to fuse or close normally (Fig 2.21). Defects may be unilateral or bilateral and are occasionally associated with other facial anomalies. Although occult lesions may be discovered when they present with secondary infection, many of these anomalies are noted at birth and readily excised during childhood.

Supernumerary digits

Supernumerary digits appear most commonly as rudimentary structures at the base of the ulnar side of the fifth finger (Fig 2.22). They are usually familial and asymptomatic. Histology demonstrates bundles of peripheral nerves extending in various directions and sharply demarcated from dermal connective tissue. A good cosmetic result is best achieved by local surgical excision.

Supernumerary nipples

Supernumerary nipples may appear unilaterally or bilaterally anywhere along a line from the mid axilla to the inguinal area (Fig 2.23). Accessory nipples may develop without areolae, which results in their misdiagnosis as congenital nevi. Malignant degeneration rarely occurs, and many are excised for cosmetic purposes.

Umbilical granulomas

Umbilical granulomas occur commonly during the first few weeks of life. Normally, the cord dries and separates in 7 days. The open surface epithelializes and scars down in an additional 1–2 weeks. Excessive moisture and low-grade infection may result in the growth of exuberant granulation tissue to form an umbilical granuloma (Fig 2.24).

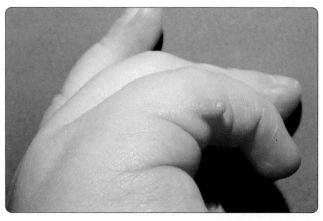

Fig 2.22 This rudimentary, supernumerary digit was present at birth. It was surgically excised at 6 months of age.

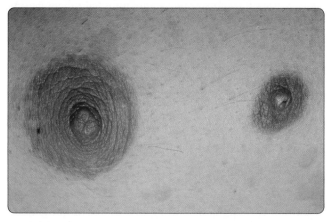

Fig 2.23 This accessory nipple was an incidental finding on a healthy teenager with tinea versicolor.

Cauterization with silver nitrate or desiccation with repeated applications of isopropyl alcohol usually produces rapid healing of the granuloma.

In some infants, secondary infection results in omphalitis (Fig 2.25). Aggressive antibiotic therapy is necessary to prevent peritonitis and sepsis.

Umbilical granulomas must be differentiated from umbilical polyps, which result from persistence of the omphalomesenteric duct or urachus. A mucoid discharge may occur at the tip of the firm, red polyp, which histologically demonstrates gastrointestinal or urinary tract mucosa. Surgical excision is necessary.

THE SCALY NEWBORN

At delivery the skin is smooth, moist, and velvety. Desquamation begins at 24–36 hours of age and may not be complete for 3 weeks (Fig 2.26). As peeling progresses, the underlying skin appears normal and cracking and fissuring is absent. Desquamation at birth or during the first day of life is abnormal and suggests postmaturity, intrauterine stress, or congenital ichthyosis.

Collodion baby

Collodion infants are born encased in a thick, cellophane-like membrane (Fig 2.27). Although the collodion membrane may desquamate to leave normal skin, 60–70% of these infants go on to develop congenital ichthyosiform erythroderma. Less commonly, this membrane is a prelude to lamellar ichthyosis, Netherton disease, or Conradi disease. The association with other variants of ichthyosis is less clear.

Although the horny layer is markedly thickened in collodion babies, barrier function is compromised by cracking

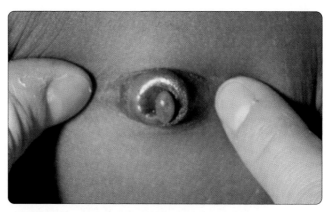

Fig 2.24 An umbilical granuloma responded to cautery with silver nitrate. Note the bright red, friable nodule at the umbilical stump.

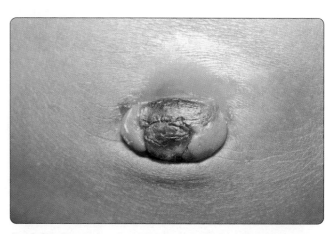

Fig 2.25 Omphalitis developed in this 10-day-old infant shortly after the cord separated from the umbilicus. The infection cleared after a 10-day course of parenteral antibiotics.

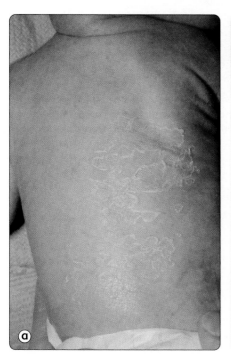

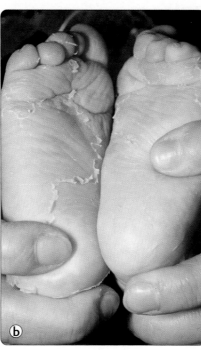

Fig 2.26 Scaling in a 1-week-old healthy infant. (a) Scaling was present on the trunk. (b) Similar scaling was present on the hands and feet. A week later the scaling had resolved completely.

and fissuring. Increased insensible water loss, heat loss, and risk of cutaneous infection and sepsis are minimized by placing affected newborns in a high humidity, neutrally thermal environment. Débridement of the membrane is contraindicated, and topical applications should be restricted to bland emollients such as petrolatum. Desquamation is usually complete by 2–3 weeks of life.

A severe variant of ichthyosis, the harlequin baby, occurs rarely (Fig 2.28). Although these infants appear normal at birth, within minutes they develop a thick, generalized membrane, deep cracks and fissures, and marked ectropion and eclabium. Most infants succumb to respiratory distress or infection, but children who survive the neonatal period may develop scale reminiscent of lamellar ichthyosis.

Ichthyosis

The ichthyoses are a heterogeneous group of scaling disorders that may be differentiated by mode of inheritance, clinical features, histology, and biochemical markers (Fig 2.29). Rarely, ichthyosis is a marker of multisystem disease in the newborn (Fig 2.30).

Congenital ichthyosiform erythroderma and lamellar ichthyosis

Congenital ichthyosiform erythroderma (Fig 2.31) and lamellar ichthyosis (Fig 2.32) present with a collodion membrane at birth. Both are autosomal recessive and occur in fewer than 1/100,000 deliveries. The erythroderma of congenital ichthyosiform erythroderma and the generalized, thick, brown scales of lamellar ichthyosis develop after the membrane desquamates at 2–4 weeks of age. Infants with epidermolytic hyperkeratosis (also referred to as bullous congenital ichthyosiform erythroderma; Fig 2.33) demonstrate widespread blistering at birth and may be misdiagnosed as having a primary blistering dermatosis such as staphylococcal scalded skin syndrome or

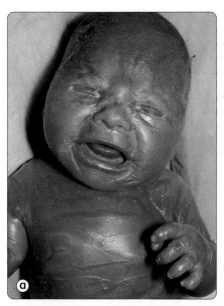
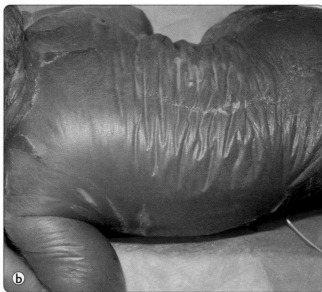

Fig 2.27 Collodion baby. A shiny transparent membrane covered this baby at birth; she later developed lamellar ichthyosis.

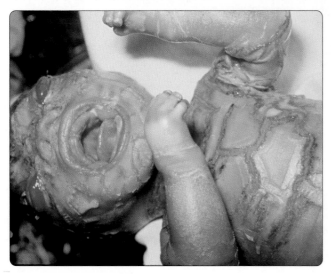

Fig 2.28 Harlequin baby. This baby developed thick, plate-like scales immediately after drying in the delivery room. Respiratory failure resulted in death during the first week. Note the ectropion and eclabium.

			Ichthyoses			
Variant	Inheritance	Incidence	Clinical feature	Onset	Histology	Molecular/biochemical marker
Congenital ichthysiform erythroderma	Autosomal recessive	1/100 000 to 1/50 000	Collodion baby Fine white scale on trunk, face and scalp Large scale on legs Variable erythroderma Variable scarring, alopecia, nail dystrophy	Birth	⇑ Stratum corneum ⇑ Granular layer	Accelerated epidermal turnover
Lamellar ichthyosis	Autosomal recessive	1/100 000	Collodion baby Generalized, large, dark, plate-like scale Ectropion, eclabium Mild palmar–plantar hyperkeratosis	Birth	⇑⇑⇑ Stratum corneum	Normal epidermal turnover
Epidermolytic hyperkeratosis	Autosomal dominant (sporadic)	Rare	Widespread blisters at birth ⇑ Erythema, ⇑ scale with ⇑ age Marked scale in intertriginous areas, palms, soles Foul odor, bacterial overgrowth	Birth	Epidermocytic hyperkeratosis	Accelerated epidermal turnover Mutations in K1 or K10 keratin genes
Ichthyosis vulgaris	Autosomal dominant (variable expression)	1/250 (may be much higher)	Generalized mild scales Spares flexures Improves with age	After 3 months	⇑ Stratum corneum ⇓ Granular layer	Normal epidermal turnover Defect in profilaggrin expression)
X-linked ichthyosis	X-linked recessive	1/6000 to 1/2000 males	Large 'dirty' scales on trunk, extremities Spares flexures Variable in female carriers Corneal opacities on Descemet's membrane Cryptorchidism Placental sulfatase deficiency syndrome Contiguous gene syndromes	Within first 3 months	⇑ Stratum corneum	⇓ Corticosteroid sulfatase in amniocytes, fibroblasts, leukocytes, keratinocytes Corticosteroid sulfatase gene defect

Fig 2.29 Ichthyoses.

Ichthyosis syndromes		
Syndrome/disease	Biochemical marker	Associated defects
Netherton syndrome		Hair shaft anomaly, ichthyosis linearis circumflexa
Refsum disease	⇓ Phytanic oxidase ⇑ Phytanic acid	Retinitis pigmentosa, chronic polyneuritis with deafness, flaccid paralysis, ataxia
Rud syndrome		Mental retardation, seizures, dwarfism, sexual infantilism
Sjögren–Larsson syndrome	⇓ Fatty alcohol oxidoreductase	Spastic paralysis, mental retardation, seizures, glistening dots on retina, dental–bone dysplasia
Conradi disease	Peroxisome deficiency, X-linked	Chondrodysplasia punctata, alopecia, skeletal anomalies, cataracts, dysmorphic facies, ichthyosiform erythroderma
KID (keratitis, ichthyosis, deafness)		Fixed keratotic plaques, keratoderma, atypical ichthyosis with prominent keratoses on extremities and head, neurosensory deafness, keratoconjunctivitis

Fig 2.30 Ichthyosis syndromes.

epidermolysis bullosa. During the first few weeks and months of life, blisters give way to increasing hyperkeratoses, especially in intertriginous and flexural areas. In these ichthyotic disorders, increased insensible water loss, temperature instability, and increased risk of infection may persist for weeks. Involvement of the face may result in ectropion formation, particularly in lamellar ichthyosis, and aggressive eye care is necessary to preserve visual acuity. Decreased sweating as a result of the obstruction of eccrine ducts in the epidermal scale often interferes with effective cooling of the skin. Aggressive management of fever, air conditioning, and cooling suits reduce the risk of hyperthermia associated with self-limited childhood illnesses and increased physical activity, especially during the summer.

Ichthyosis vulgaris and X-linked ichthyosis

Children with ichthyosis vulgaris (Fig 2.34) and X-linked ichthyosis (Fig 2.35) may not develop scaling until 3 months of age or later. The generally mild scales of ichthyosis vulgaris

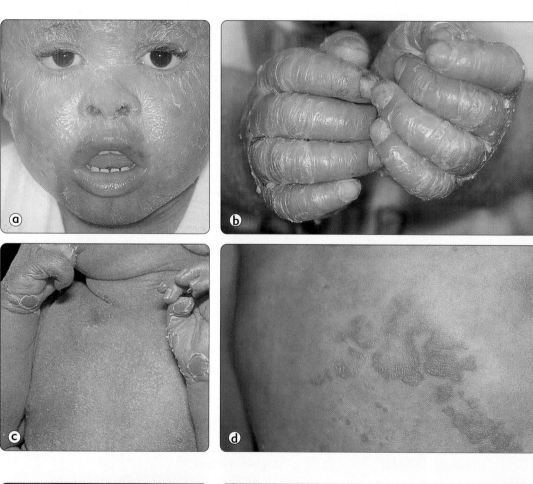

Fig 2.31 Congenital ichthyosiform erythroderma. (a) Congenital erythroderma persisted in this child. (b) Note the marked scaling on her hands. (c) Generalized erythema with fine scaling was noted on the first day of life. (d) Shortly after his first birthday he developed a new pattern of migrating, scaly, erythematous plaques typical of Netherton's syndrome. Microscopic examination of his hair revealed trichorrhexis invaginata (bamboo hair).

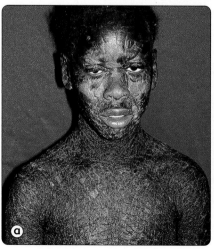
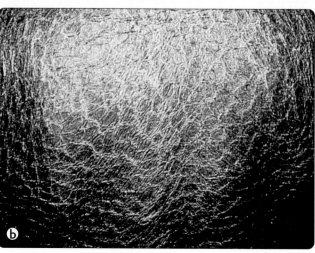

Fig 2.32 Lamellar ichthyosis. (a) Typical appearance. (b) Note the thick, brown scales that cover the entire skin. This child was born with a collodion membrane.

tend to spare the flexures and improve with age. The 'dirty' brown scales of X-linked ichthyosis also spare the flexures, but typically involve much of the body surface. The skin lesions do not usually impair epidermal barrier function.

Mild scaling responds well to lubricants, urea-containing preparations (Carmol®, Ureacin®), and α-hydroxy acids in emollients (lactic acid [LactiCare®, LacHydrin®], glycolic acid [Acqua Glycolic®, Glycolix®]). Although topical salicylic acid and phenol are also potent keratolytics, their use is restricted to small areas because of the risk of transcutaneous absorption and systemic toxicity.

Recent trials with oral retinoids (isotretinoin, etretinate) have demonstrated marked improvement of cutaneous lesions in severe ichthyosis. However, clinical benefits must be weighed against the risk of systemic effects, particularly hepatic and skeletal toxicity.

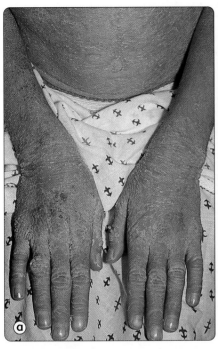
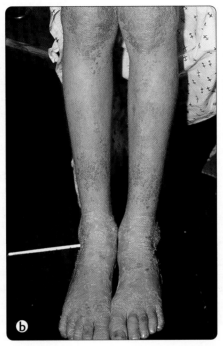
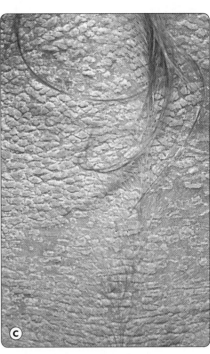

Fig 2.33 Epidermolytic hyperkeratosis in a 6-year-old girl. **(a, b)** Generalized, thick, greasy scales accentuate the normal skin markings on the extremities. **(c)** Similar scales on the trunk and neck. Flexures were most severely involved.

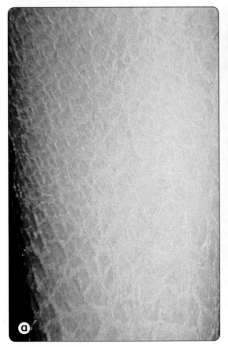
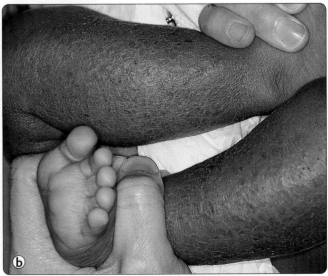

Fig 2.34 Ichthyosis vulgaris. **(a)** Typical fish-scale appearance on the lower extremities of a light-pigmented child. **(b)** The appearance on a dark-pigmented child. Both children had at least one parent with similar findings.

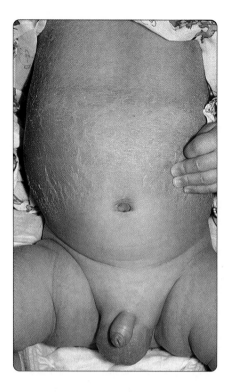

Fig 2.35 X-linked ichthyosis: 'dirty' tan scales are evident on the trunk of this infant.

DIAPER DERMATITIS AND RELATED DISORDERS

The dermatitides are characterized by acute changes (erythema, edema, and vesiculation) and/or chronic changes (scale, lichenification, and increased or decreased pigmentation) in the skin. Microscopically, these disorders show infiltration of the dermis with inflammatory cells, variable thickening of the epidermis, and scale.

Irritant contact dermatitis

Diaper dermatitis is one of the most common skin disorders of infancy. In its most usual form it is an irritant contact dermatitis (Fig 2.36). The diaper area is a prime target for an irritant dermatitis, because it is bathed in urine and feces and occluded by plastic diaper covers. Although ammonia from urine was first thought to play a leading role in the pathogenesis of diaper dermatitis, recent evidence points to feces as the principal culprit. Once the epidermal barrier is disrupted, the skin may become sensitive to other irritants such as soap, powder, and detergents. Watery stools, particularly after antibiotic exposure or viral infections, often trigger severe dermatitis that is recalcitrant to conservative measures.

Red, scaly, and occasionally erosive irritant reactions are usually confined to convex surfaces of the perineum, lower abdomen, buttocks, and proximal thighs. The intertriginous areas are invariably spared. Gentle, thorough cleansing of the area and the application of lubricants (e.g. petrolatum) and barrier pastes (e.g. zinc oxide) usually result in clearing of the dermatitis. A tapering course of low-potency topical corticosteroid ointment (e.g. hydrocortisone) in severe dermatitis may speed resolution of symptoms and clinical findings.

Allergic contact dermatitis

Although less common than irritant dermatitis, allergic contact dermatitis may account for occasional diaper rashes. Fragrance, preservatives, and emulsifiers in topical baby products may be associated with allergic reactions in the diaper area, as well as on the face, trunk, and extremities. Avoidance of the offending agent, aggressive use of emollients, and judicious use of topical corticosteroids clear these reactions within several days.

Infected contact dermatitis

Contact diaper dermatitis is occasionally complicated by secondary staphylococcal infection, or pustules may appear as primary lesions, especially in the first few weeks of life (Fig 2.37). The presence of thin-walled pustules on an erythematous base should alert the clinician to the diagnosis of staphylococcal pustulosis. Typically, the lesions rupture rapidly and dry, to produce a collarette of scale around a denuded red base. Gram stain of pustule contents demonstrates Gram-positive cocci in clusters and neutrophils. Bacterial cultures are confirmatory.

Seborrheic dermatitis

Persistent diaper dermatitis may result from other disorders such as seborrheic dermatitis, infantile psoriasis and candidiasis. In particular, these should be considered when the intertriginous areas are involved.

Seborrheic dermatitis is characterized by salmon-colored patches with greasy, yellow scale beginning in the intertriginous areas, especially the diaper area, axillae, and scalp (Fig 2.38). Fissuring, maceration, and weeping develop occasionally. Thick, adherent scales on the occiput are referred to as 'cradle cap'. Although oval, red patches may spread to the

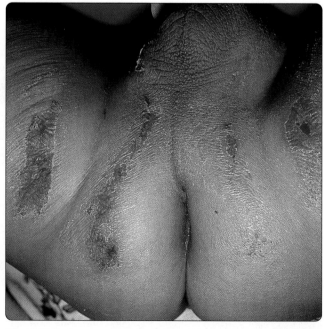

Fig 2.36 Irritant contact dermatitis involves the convex surfaces and spares the creases in the diaper area.

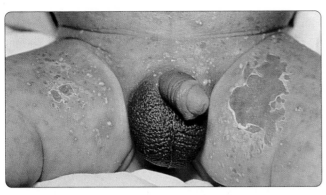

Fig 2.37 Staphylococcal diaper dermatitis. Numerous, intact, thin-walled pustules surrounded by red halos are present, as well as multiple areas in which pustules have ruptured to leave a collarette of scaling around a denuded red base.

trunk, proximal extremities, and postauricular areas, affected infants remain healthy and asymptomatic. In dark-pigmented children, postinflammatory hypopigmentation is marked, but transient.

In the diaper area, red, greasy, scaly patches extend from the skin creases to involve the genitals, perineum, suprapubic area, and thighs. Secondary candidiasis or impetigo may mask the underlying process.

The cause of seborrheic dermatitis is unknown. However, the yeast *Pityrosporum* has been implicated in adult seborrhea and identified in the scalp of infants with 'cradle cap'. This organism tends to proliferate in areas where sebaceous glands are most numerous and active, which probably explains the timing and distribution of the eruption. Seborrheic dermatitis may clear without treatment by 2–3

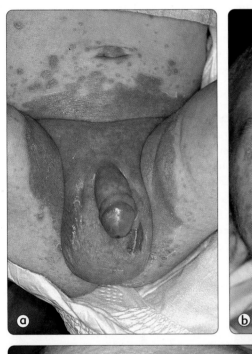

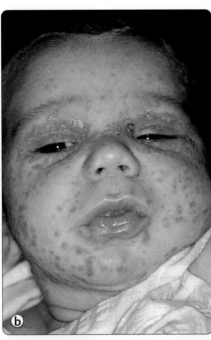

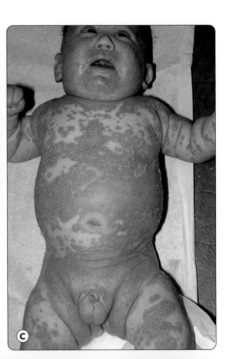

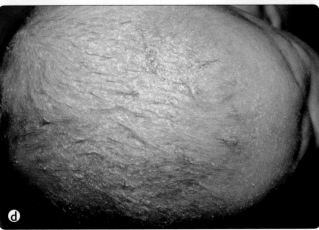

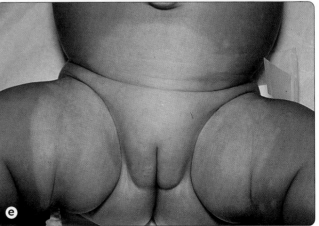

Fig 2.38 Seborrheic dermatitis. **(a)** The slightly greasy, red, scaling eruption typically begins in the groin creases and spreads throughout the diaper area. **(b, c)** In florid cases, the dermatitis involves the trunk, face, and creases of the neck and extremities. **(d)** 'Cradle cap' consists of thick, tenacious scaling of the scalp. **(e)** Postinflammatory hypopigmentation may be marked, particularly in darkly pigmented individuals.

months of age, but often persists until 8–12 months. Mild keratolytics found in antiseborrheic shampoos (zinc pyrithione, sulfur, and salicylic acid) are helpful in the management of 'cradle cap'. Emollients and low-potency topical corticosteroids hasten the resolution of cutaneous lesions. Topical ketoconazole has been approved for treating adult seborrheic dermatitis and may be useful in infants, particularly in patients with associated candidiasis.

Psoriasis

Psoriasis occasionally begins as a persistent diaper dermatitis (Fig 2.39), and there may be considerable clinical overlap with seborrheic dermatitis. Although lesions may disseminate to the trunk and extremities, the rash may continue in the diaper area alone for months. The eruption is typically bright red, scaly, and well demarcated at the diaper line. Although topical corticosteroids result in temporary improvement, lesions tend to persist or recur for months. Infants remain well, and the eruption may be asymptomatic. Skin biopsy is the only way to confirm the diagnosis.

Candidiasis

Candidiasis appears as a brilliant red eruption with sharp borders, satellite red papules, and pustules (Fig 2.40). Lesions typically involve the skin creases. *Candida* is a common complication of systemic antibiotic therapy, seborrheic dermatitis, psoriasis, and chronic irritant dermatitis. Examination of material from a pustule by Gram stain or potassium hydroxide preparation reveals pseudohyphae. Diaper candidiasis may be accompanied by oral thrush, candidal paronychia of the fingers or toes, and candidiasis of other intertriginous areas such as the neck and axillae. Diaper

candidiasis responds rapidly to topical antifungals such as nystatin, ciclopirox olamine, and the imidazoles (miconazole, clotrimazole, econazole, sulconazole, ketoconazole). Although a brief course of topical corticosteroids (1–2 times a day for 3–4 days) may speed clinical improvement, high-potency agents can produce atrophy in a short period of time. Several products that incorporate a combination of topical corticosteroid and antifungal agents are available. Unfortunately, several of these agents include high-potency corticosteroids and should be avoided.

Histiocytosis X

Severe multisystem disease may begin with a progressive diaper dermatitis. A seborrheic dermatitis-like eruption is characteristic of histiocytosis X (Fig 2.41). However, the rash tends to become hemorrhagic and erosive, particularly in the diaper area. Scaly, crusted, purpuric plaques also develop on the scalp, trunk, and extremities. Diagnostic skin biopsies demonstrate infiltrates of atypical S-100 protein OKT6-positive histiocytes containing Langerhan cell granules. Similar infiltrates may involve the bone marrow, liver, lungs, kidneys, and nervous system, resulting in severe organ dysfunction and death.

'Benign' histiocytosis

Several benign variants of histiocytosis have been described in newborns and infants (Fig 2.42). Reddish-yellow patches and papules erupt most commonly on the head and neck, but lesions may involve the trunk and extremities. No evidence of systemic disease is present. The histologic findings are indistinguishable from those of histiocytosis X, although Langerhan cell markers have been absent in some patients. Cutaneous lesions generally involute without therapy within

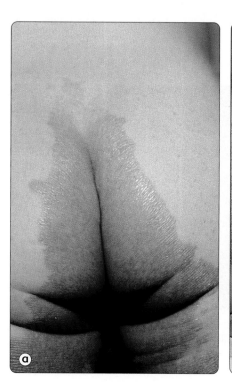

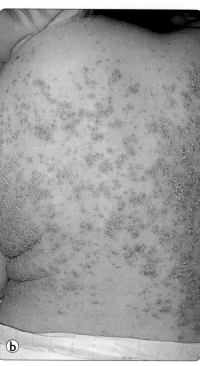

Fig 2.39 Psoriasis. This diaper dermatitis failed to respond to routine topical therapy. **(a)** A skin biopsy demonstrated histologic changes of psoriasis. **(b)** In some infants with psoriasis, thick, disseminated plaques appear.

several years. However, infants should receive long-term pediatric follow-up, because histiocytosis X may rarely present with self-limited skin disease in infancy and systemic complications in later childhood or adolescence.

Acrodermatitis enteropathica

Acrodermatitis enteropathica (AEP) classically presents with an erosive diaper dermatitis, diarrhea, and hair loss during the first few months of life (Fig 2.43). Weeping, crusted, erythematous patches also appear in a periorificial, acral, and intertriginous distribution. Affected infants are irritable, grow poorly, and are prone to infection and septicemia.

Since AEP is an autosomal recessive disorder of zinc metabolism, affected infants have either defective or low levels of a zinc-binding protein in the gastrointestinal tract and resultant zinc malabsorption. Breast milk contains a compensatory zinc-binding ligand that facilitates absorption. Consequently, breast-fed infants do not develop symptoms until nursing is discontinued. Zinc is stored in the fetal liver, particularly during the last month of gestation. As a result, affected premature infants who are not breast fed become zinc deficient quickly. Normal infants who require hyperalimentation, as well as those with zinc losses from other malabsorption states (e.g. cystic fibrosis, chronic infectious diarrhea, short bowel syndrome), also develop an AEP-like rash if they do not receive zinc supplementation. Similar rashes have also been reported with biotin deficiency, essential fatty acid deficiency, and urea enzyme cycle defects, which result in essential amino acid deficiency.

AEP responds to high doses of oral or intravenous zinc within several days. Although dietary zinc without supplementation may be adequate in older children with AEP, these patients require close monitoring of growth and development. Some patients require lifelong zinc supplements.

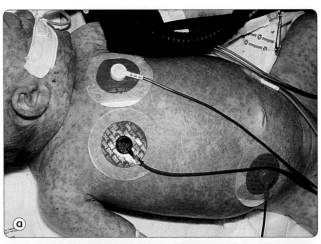

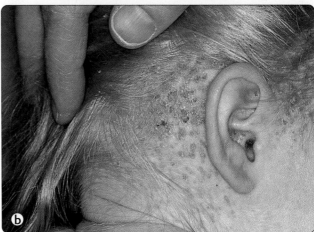

Fig 2.41 Histiocytosis X. **(a)** A hemorrhagic diaper dermatitis rapidly generalized to the entire skin surface in this 3-week-old infant with diarrhea, poor weight gain, lymphadenopathy, and hepatosplenomegaly. This child died of disseminated histiocytosis at 6 weeks of age. **(b)** This toddler with chronic histiocytosis X had an episodic, erosive diaper dermatitis associated with papules and plaques in the scalp.

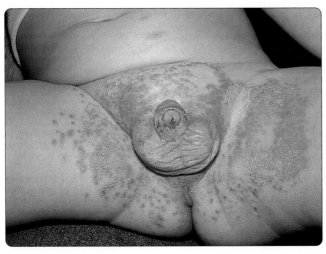

Fig 2.40 Diaper candidiasis. The eruption is bright red, with numerous pinpoint satellite papules and pustules. The urethra and intertriginous areas are prominently involved.

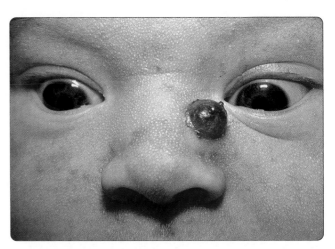

Fig 2.42 Benign cephalic histiocytosis. Although this nodule demonstrated typical microscopic changes of histiocytosis X, this infant developed no evidence of systemic disease, and several other skin nodules resolved without treatment.

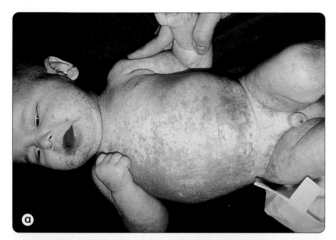

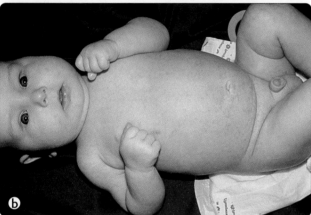

Fig 2.43 Acrodermatitis enteropathica. **(a)** A bright red, scaling dermatitis spread to the intertriginous areas, face, and extremities of this 4-week-old infant. **(b)** After 4 days of zinc supplementation, many lesions were healing with desquamation.

CONGENITAL SYPHILIS

Although the incidence of neonatal syphilis decreased in the 1970s and 1980s, a resurgence has occurred, particularly in urban centers. Infants born to mothers who have syphilis late in their pregnancy are at high risk for contracting the disease.

Although clinical manifestations of syphilis may be delayed until several years of age, common findings in the newborn include mucocutaneous lesions, prematurity, poor growth, and hepatosplenomegaly. Occasionally, severe systemic disease presents with generalized lymphadenopathy, pneumonitis, nephritis, enteritis, pancreatitis, osteochondritis, hematologic abnormalities, and meningitis.

Mucocutaneous lesions usually appear between 2 and 6 weeks of age. The most common finding in the skin is a papulosquamous eruption beginning on the palms and soles and spreading over the extremities, face and trunk (Fig 2.44). These lesions are comparable to the secondary syphilitic eruption of adults and may be associated with vesiculation, ulceration, and desquamation. Moist, warty excrescences may develop in the intertriginous and periorificial areas.

Smooth, round, moist mucous patches are characteristic of early neonatal syphilis and commonly involve the mouth and perianal area. Such lesions are highly infectious and readily demonstrate treponemes on dark-field examination. 'Snuffles' or rhinitis with profuse and occasionally bloody rhinorrhea is invariably present in symptomatic babies.

Diagnosis may be confirmed by darkfield examination of mucocutaneous lesions and serologic studies of the serum and cerebrospinal fluid. Screening of babies at risk for syphilis should include both specific treponoma (fluorescent treponemal antibody absorption tests) and nontreponemal (rapid plasma reagin or Venereal Disease Research Laboratory) studies. Early diagnosis and treatment with high-dose penicillin prevents late complications of syphilis, including skeletal and dental anomalies, neurologic deterioration, eighth nerve deafness, and ophthalmologic disease.

VESICULOPUSTULAR DERMATOSES

Vesiculobullous and pustular eruptions may present a confusing clinical picture. Their diagnosis is critical, and early therapeutic intervention may be lifesaving.

Infections and infestations
Viral infections, including herpes simplex and varicella-zoster, produce characteristic vesiculopustular eruptions. Herpes simplex is a common cause of self-limited oral and cutaneous lesions in toddlers and older children. However, in neonates there is a high risk of dissemination. Varicella is less common, but if lesions appear during the first week of life the risk of mortality approaches 30%.

Herpes simplex infection
Herpes simplex infection occurs in 1 out of 3500 deliveries. Inoculation occurs from lesions on the cervix or vaginal area in most cases. However, the disease may be acquired postnatally from nursery personnel and family members. The incubation period varies from 2 to 21 days and peaks at 6 days. Consequently, infants may appear normal in the nursery and develop lesions after discharge home. Manifestations vary from subclinical disease to widely disseminated infection and death. Of infected babies, 70% develop the skin rash and 90% of these children go on to develop systemic disease with involvement of the lungs, liver, gastrointestinal tract, and brain.

Cutaneous lesions typically begin as 1–2 mm diameter, clustered, red papules and vesicles, which may become pustular, denuded, crusted, and hemorrhagic over the following 2–3 days (Fig 2.45). The first lesions commonly develop on the face and scalp in head deliveries and on the feet or buttocks after breech presentation.

Blisters reveal multinucleated giant cells when their contents are prepared on a glass slide with Giemsa or Wright stain. Viral cultures from blister fluid or denuded areas of skin often demonstrate a cytopathic effect within 12–24 hours. Diagnosis can be rapidly confirmed by polymerase chain reaction or electron microscopy studies in some medical

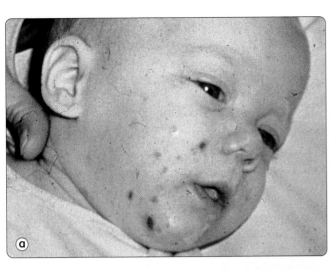

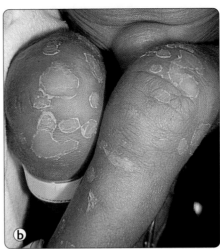

Fig 2.44 Neonatal syphilis. (a,b) A scaly eruption reminiscent of the lesions of secondary syphilis appeared on the face, trunk, and extremities of these infants.

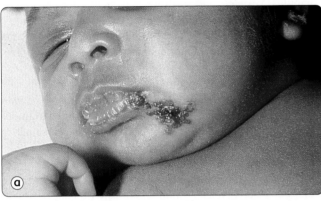

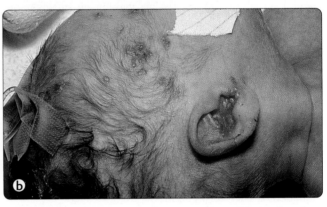

Fig 2.45 Herpes simplex. (a) The eroded vesicles at the corner of the mouth were the first signs of herpes infection in this neonate.

(b) An infant with respiratory distress and hepatitis developed herpetic vesicles on the face, scalp, and ear.

centers. Early intervention with parenteral acyclovir may decrease the risk of disseminated disease, and of morbidity and mortality when dissemination has already occurred. Skin lesions are gently cleansed and excess blister fluid absorbed with a gauze pad to reduce cutaneous spread. Skin lesions may recur for up to 5 years; recurrence prompts a trial of oral acyclovir, particularly when recurrences are frequent.

Varicella

When a mother has varicella within 3 weeks of delivery, her baby has a 25% risk of acquiring disease during the neonatal period. Early exposure during the first trimester rarely leads to the development of the neonatal varicella syndrome, with linear scars, limb anomalies, ocular defects, and central nervous system involvement (Fig 2.46).

As in herpes simplex, infants are usually well at birth and develop vesicles at 3–10 days of life. Dissemination may result in pneumonitis, encephalitis, and purpura fulminans, with widespread bleeding, hypotension, and death. When neonates develop the rash before 5 days of life or mothers develop lesions at least 5 days before delivery, the disease in neonates tends to be mild because of the presence of protective transplacental antibody.

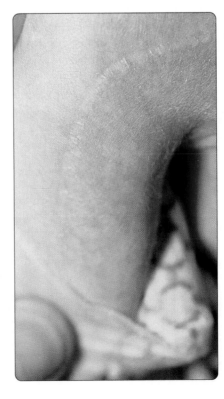

Fig 2.46 Varicella. A linear scar was evident on the arm of this newborn whose mother developed chickenpox during the first trimester.

Varicella-zoster immune globulin and parenteral acyclovir may improve the outcome and should be considered early in the course. As with herpes simplex, the Tzanck smear shows multinucleated giant cells. These two viral infections can only be definitively differentiated by culture of the blister contents or by molecular studies.

Impetigo and staphylococcal scalded skin syndrome

Several common bacterial infections present with vesiculo-pustular eruptions in infancy. The rash tends to be localized in impetigo (see Fig 4.11) and generalized in staphylococcal scalded-skin syndrome (SSSS) (Fig 2.47, also see Fig 4.12).

In classic streptococcal impetigo, honey-colored crusts overlie infected insect bites, abrasions, and other skin rashes, such as diaper dermatitis. Bullous impetigo, however, is characterized by slowly enlarging, blistering rings that surround central, umbilicated crusts. Lesions may appear anywhere on the skin surface. However, in young infants areas prone to trauma, such as the diaper area, circumcision wound, and umbilical stump, are frequent sites of primary infection. Bullous lesions are caused by certain epidermal toxin-producing types of *Staphylococcus*. Although lesions may remain localized, they are highly infectious and may be inoculated to multiple sites on the patient as well as on other family members. In newborns and young infants, dissemination of the toxin may result in widespread erythema and blistering typical of SSSS (see Fig 2.47). Gentle pressure on the skin causes the upper epidermis to slide off leaving a denuded base (Nikolsky sign).

In localized impetigo, bacteria are identified in Gram-stained material obtained directly from the rash. In SSSS, the practitioner may be unable to identify a primary cutaneous site of infection. In these children, noncutaneous sources, which include lungs, bone, meninges, and ears, must be sought.

Small patches of impetigo respond well to topical antibiotic therapy (e.g. mupirocin, bacitracin, bacitracin– polymixin B) and normal saline compresses. Healthy infants with recalcitrant or widespread impetigo require oral antibiotics with broad-spectrum Gram-positive coverage (erythromycin, dicloxacillin, cephalexin, cotrimoxazole, amoxicillin–clavulanate [co-amixoclav]). Neonates and young infants may not localize infection to the epidermis and superficial dermis. Any signs of progressive cellulitis or visceral dissemination require immediate hospitalization, parenteral antibiotics, and supportive care. When infants develop infection in the first 2–3 weeks of life, even after discharge from the hospital, a nursery source should be suspected. Breeches in nursery hygiene and skin colonization of personnel must be investigated.

Disseminated candidiasis

Disseminated candidiasis in the newborn may be confused with bacterial infection. In congenital candidiasis, which develops during the first day of life, generalized erythematous papules, vesicles, and pustules may slough to leave large, denuded areas reminiscent of SSSS. The organism is acquired by ascending vaginal or cervical infection. The presence of oral thrush in some infants at birth and the identification of pseudohyphae and spores from pustules and scale are diagnostic. When infants acquire infection at delivery, the onset of lesions may be delayed by 7–10 days and erosive patches with satellite pustules are usually limited to intertriginous areas. Full-term infants often go on to heal with desquamation without treatment, although topical antifungals may help. Preterm infants are at high risk for dissemination, and early diagnosis and initiation of parenteral amphotericin may be lifesaving. As increasing numbers of tiny premature infants survive the first few weeks of life and undergo long term systemic antibiotic therapy, infection with other opportunistic fungal organisms should be considered (Fig 2.48).

Scabies

Scabies is a common, well-characterized infectious dermatosis produced by the *Sarcoptes scabiei* mite. The impregnated female burrows through the outer epidermis,

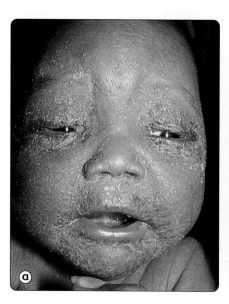
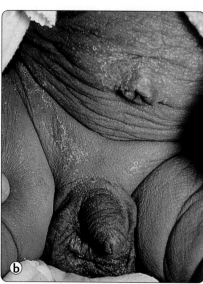

Fig 2.47 Staphylococcal scalded-skin syndrome developed in this neonate who was being treated for mastitis. **(a)** Erosive patches were most marked on the face and **(b)** diaper areas.

where she deposits her eggs. The resultant diagnostic rash consists of pruritic, linear burrows on the finger webs, wrists, elbows, belt line, areola, scrotum, and penis. In infants, burrows are widespread with involvement of the trunk, scalp, and extremities, including the palms and soles (Fig 2.49). Although infants may be otherwise healthy and well grown, chronic infestation may result in poor feeding, fussiness, and failure to thrive. Chronic and recurrent infection, with pustules, crusting, and cellulitis, is a frequent complication.

The diagnosis is considered for any infant with a widespread dermatosis that involves the palms and soles, particularly if other family members are involved. The presence of burrows is pathognomonic, and an ectoparasite preparation is confirmatory. A drop of mineral oil is applied to a burrow, and the skin surface is stretched between the examiner's

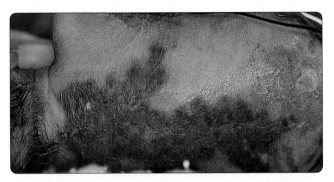

Fig 2.48 Primary cutaneous *Aspergillus* infection developed in this tiny premature infant who had extensive skin breakdown and was receiving parenteral antibiotics for pneumonia. The black eschars were loaded with hyphae.

thumb and index finger. A #15 blade is used to scrape vigorously until the burrow is no longer palpable. This may leave a small bleeding point at the center of the burrow. The material is subsequently spread with the blade on a glass slide and pressed under a coverslip. The female mite, eggs, and fecal material are readily visualized under a scanning 10× lens (see Fig 1.8).

Until approximately 10 years ago, topical 1% lindane (γ-benzene hydrochloride) was the mainstay of treatment. Although the risk of toxicity with lindane is low when it is used appropriately in the medical setting, severe central nervous reactions have been reported in young infants, particularly wasted, chronically ill children. Alternative agents are either ineffective (crotamiton, benzyl benzoate), potentially toxic (sulfur ointment, benzyl benzoate), or cosmetically unacceptable (sulfur ointment). In 1989, permethrin 5% cream was introduced. Studies have shown that permethrin has a higher cure rate than lindane and that it may be used safely in children as young as 2 months.

At the start of therapy parents are given careful instructions and limited quantities of the scabicide. The entire family and any others who have contact with the infant (such as baby-sitters) are treated simultaneously. Topical lubricants are necessary for several weeks after treatment to counteract drying and irritation produced by the scabicide and to resolve cutaneous lesions. Persistent pruritic nodules may arise from some burrows, particularly in intertriginous areas. Nodular scabies requires symptomatic treatment only. The appearance of new inflammatory lesions suggests reinfestation or inadequate therapy. Secondary infection responds to tap water compresses and antibiotics.

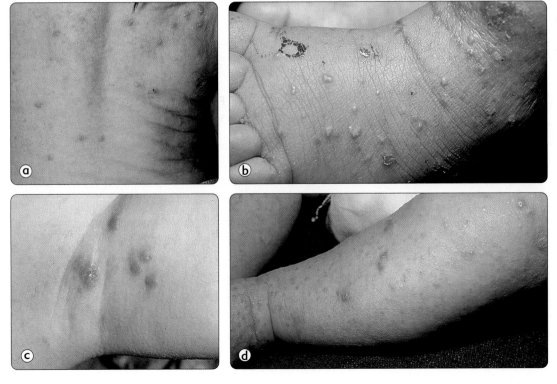

Fig 2.49 Infants with widespread scabies. Burrows were present on (a) the trunk, and (b) feet. Nodules persisted on the axillae (c) and legs (d) of these infants for 4 months.

Mechanobullous diseases (epidermolysis bullosa)

Mechanobullous diseases (epidermolysis bullosa [EB]) are a heterogeneous group of blistering dermatoses characterized by the development of lesions after trauma to the skin. Variants of EB are differentiated by their inheritance pattern, clinical presentation, histopathology, and biochemical markers (Fig 2.50). Although blisters may appear at birth or in the neonatal period, in mild, localized forms the onset of lesions is often delayed until later childhood or adult life.

Categorization of EB is into three major types based upon the cleavage plane of the blister. In EB simplex, or epidermolytic EB, blisters are intraepidermal, and the clinical course is usually mild (Fig 2.51). In junctional EB, blisters form at the dermal–epidermal junction, usually through the

Selected hereditary mechanobullous disorders						
Type	Pattern	Variant	Site of blister	Inheritance	Onset	Clinical features
Epidermolysis bullosa simplex (epidermolytic)	Localized	Weber–Cockayne syndrome	Intraepidermal (suprabasal)	Autosomal dominant	Infancy to childhood	Nonscarring blisters on hands and feet; hyperhidrosis
	Generalized	Koebner	Intraepidermal (basal cell cytolysis)	Autosomal dominant	Birth to early infancy	Nonscarring generalized blisters, worse on hands and feet
		Herpetiformis, Dowling–Meara	Intraepidermal	Autosomal dominant	Birth	Grouped blisters, generalized denudation; nail dystrophy, milia, scarring may occur; keratoderma; improvement in adulthood
Junctional epidermolysis bullosa	Localized	Inversa	Lamina lucida	Autosomal recessive	Nail changes at birth; Skin changes at school age	Localized blistering of hands, feet; nail dystrophy; bullosa enamel dysplasia
	Generalized	Gravis (letalis, Herlitz disease)	Lamina lucida (reduced in number, abnormal hemidesmosomes)	Autosomal recessive	Birth	Often lethal by 2 years; nonscarring widespread blisters; ⇑ granulation tissue; nail dystrophy, loss; severe oral–dental involvement
		Mitis (atrophic/benign)	Lamina lucida	Autosomal recessive	Birth	Blisters heal with atrophy; nail dystrophy; enamel dysplasia
Dystrophic epidermolysis bullosa (Dermolytic)	Localized	Dominant, pretibial	Dermis	Autosomal dominant	Infancy, childhood	Lichen planus-like papules, plaques on shins; intense pruritus; nail dystrophy
		Recessive, inversa	Dermis (⇓ or absent anchoring fibrils)	Autosomal recessive	Infancy, childhood	Lateral neck, intertriginous areas; pseudosyndactyly; severe oral esophageal involvement
	Generalized	Dominant (Pasini, Cockayne–Touraine syndrome)	Dermis (50% ⇓ in anchoring fibrils)	Autosomal dominant	Birth to early childhood	Pasini-variant–albopapuloid skin lesions; mild esophageal, oral involvement; normal life span
		Recessive (Hallopeau–Siemens)	Dermis (absent anchoring fibrils)	Autosomal recessive	Birth	Marked skin fragility; widespread blisters, atrophy, scarring; nail dystrophy, loss; risk of squamous cell carcinoma; severe oral, dental, esophageal, intestinal, genitourinary involvement
		Mitis	Dermis (⇓ anchoring fibrils)	Autosomal recessive	Birth	Mild widespread lesions; mild oral involvement; normal life span

Fig 2.50 Selected hereditary mechanobullous disorders.

lamina lucida in the basement membrane zone. Although patients may have mild disease comparable to EB simplex, in some children progressive blistering with involvement of the mucous membranes and gastrointestinal tract leads to inanition, sepsis, and death in the first 2 years of life (Fig 2.52). Dystrophic EB, or dermolytic EB, is characterized by scarring blisters that form in the dermis beneath the basement membrane zone. Blisters may be localized to the hands and feet or widespread with involvement of the dentition, nails, airway, and esophagus (Fig 2.53).

When infection has been excluded, EB should be considered in infants with recurrent blistering. Family history and examination of other family members aids in clinical diagnosis. A skin biopsy for electron microscopy and immunomapping provides precise identification of the

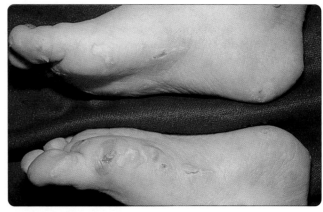

Fig 2.51 Epidermolysis bullosa simplex. Numerous blisters form primarily in pressure areas on the hands and feet.

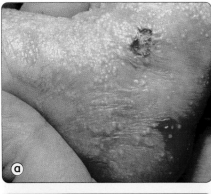

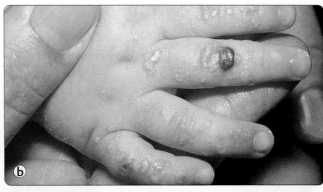

Fig 2.52 Junctional epidermolysis bullosa. Widespread involvement was seen in this infant at birth. **(a)** Note the erosions and the large, intact blister over the thumb and dorsum of the hand. **(b)** Large, denuded areas occur over the back and buttocks.

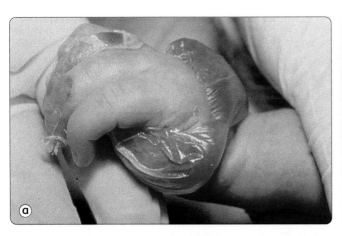

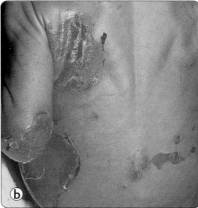

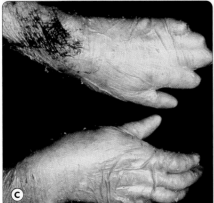

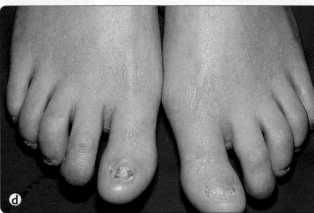

Fig 2.53 Dystrophic epidermolysis bullosa. **(a)** Blisters, erosions, and hundreds of milia are seen on the foot and ankle and **(b)** hand of this newborn. **(c)** In this child, severe scarring encased the fingers, resulting in syndactyly. **(d)** Recurrent blistering resulted in scarring and permanent nail loss in this adolescent.

cleavage plane in the skin (Fig 2.54). Genetic counseling and prenatal diagnosis, particularly in severe variants, should be discussed with the family. Prenatal diagnosis is possible in some variants, using gene markers on amniocytes or electron microscopy on fetal skin biopsies.

In children with no family history of EB, it may be difficult to determine a prognosis in the newborn period. Infants with dystrophic EB may do very well, and children with junctional disease may develop a downhill course after a period of stabilization. In this setting, the practitioner should be reassuring and postpone discussion of prognosis until after a period of observation.

Treatment is dependent on the severity of EB. In mild variants, patients learn to avoid trauma that triggers bullae formation. Pain and progression of large blisters may be controlled by gently unroofing lesions or cutting a square skin window and covering with a topical antibiotic ointment and sterile gauze. Adhesives are applied from dressing to dressing and kept out of direct contact with the skin.

In severely affected children, the practitioner must orchestrate a multidisciplinary approach to management. The dermatologist, ophthalmologist, gastroenterologist, otolaryngologist, plastic surgeon, thoracic surgeon, dentist, and physical therapist may be involved in care. Preventive care includes avoidance of trauma to the skin and mucous membranes, and early treatment of infection with topical and oral antibiotics. Iron may be required to replace chronic blood losses through the skin. Adaptic®, Vaseline® gauze, and Telfa® dressings help to retain moisture, reduce pain, and facilitate healing of erosions and ulcers. Topical dressings are gently held in place by clean wraps, such as gauze or Kling®, and soaked off without tearing at fresh granulation tissue. Semipermeable dressings (N-ter-face®, Ensure®, Vigilon®) and occlusive dressings (Duoderm®, Comfeel®) may be useful in the treatment of recalcitrant wounds. Good nutrition is mandatory for cutaneous healing and normal growth and development.

Aplasia cutis congenita

Aplasia cutis congenita is a heterogeneous group of disorders, the common feature of which is congenital absence of the skin. Although the cause is unknown this entity has been recognized for over 150 years. In the classic form one or several erosions or ulcerations covered with a crust or thin membrane involve the vertex of the scalp (Fig 2.55). Healing with atrophic, hairless scars occurs over 2–6 months, depending on the size and depth of the ulceration (which may extend through the soft tissue into bone). This benign variant is usually inherited as an autosomal dominant trait. Less commonly, the trunk and extremities are involved and lesions may be associated with limb defects, EB, and chromosomal aberrations (Fig 2.56).

In uncomplicated aplasia cutis congenita, the defect is amenable to simple excision during later childhood or adult life. Large lesions may require staged excision and the use of tissue expanders (Fig 2.57). In the newborn, care must be taken to evaluate the depth of the defect, prevent further tissue damage and infection, and search for associated anomalies. Gentle normal saline compresses, topical antibiotics, and sterile dressings are adequate for most patients. Large defects may respond to occlusive dressings (Duoderm®, Comfeel®). Occasionally, early surgical intervention is necessary.

Perinatal trauma to the scalp may result in similar defects noted at birth or within the first month of life. Scalp blood sampling, monitor electrodes, and forceps may produce small ulcers that heal with scarring (Fig 2.58). Halo scalp ring is another form of localized scalp injury rarely associated with caput succedaneum and cephalohematoma, which occasionally resolves with a scarring alopecia (Fig 2.59). Other nevoid malformations, which commonly present as hairless patches on the scalp, resemble aplasia cutis congenita. However, these birthmarks do not appear crusted or atrophic and usually develop distinctive clinical features

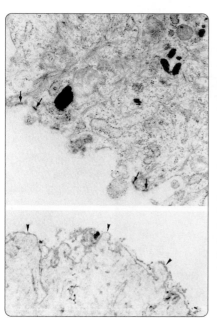

Fig 2.54 Electron microscopic examination of a skin biopsy from a newborn with junctional epidermolysis bullosa revealed hypoplastic hemidesmosomes (top, arrows) in the basal keratinocyte and lamina densa (bottom, arrowheads) on the dermal side due to separation within the lamina lucida.

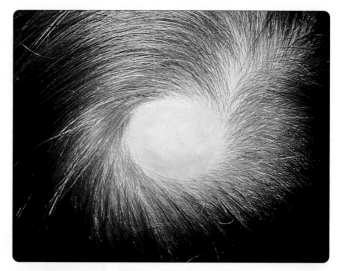

Fig 2.55 Aplasia cutis congenita. This child, his mother, and his grandfather had similar hairless, atrophic plaques on the occiput. A thin, hemorrhagic membrane was noted at birth.

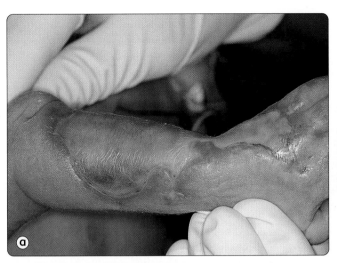

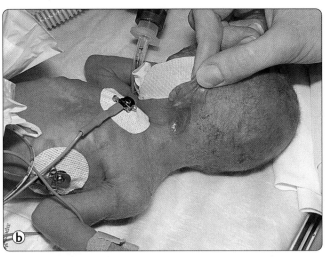

Fig 2.56 Aplasia cutis congenita. **(a)** An isolated cutaneous defect was evident on the arm of this newborn. **(b)** This premature infant with a small defect on the back of the neck had hemiatrophy of the right side of the body (Adams–Oliver syndrome).

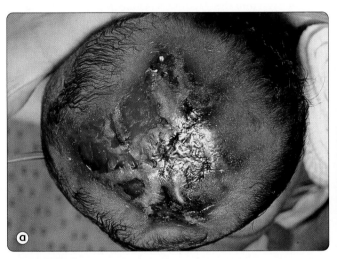

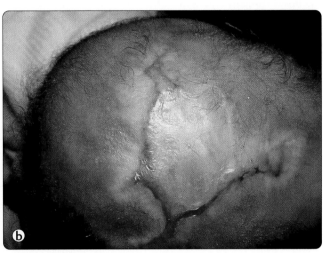

Fig 2.57 Aplasia cutis congenita. **(a)** An extensive area of aplasia cutis was noted on the scalp of this newborn. **(b)** After 5 months the scalp was almost completely healed. When the child was 5 years old, the residual scar was repaired following tissue expansion.

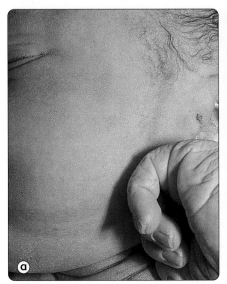

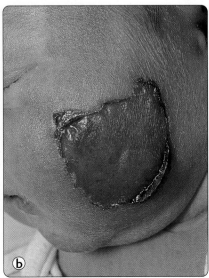

Fig 2.58 Similar defects to aplasia cutis congenita. **(a)** Forceps injuries are most commonly associated with bruising. **(b)** However, pressure necrosis occurs rarely.

(see Fig 2.77c; epidermal nevus and Fig 2.78a; sebaceous nevus). The hair collar sign is diagnostic for a neural nevus which is comprised of meningeal structures (Fig 2.60). Some congenital pigmented nevi on the scalp that are lightly pigmented can also mimic aplasia cutis congenita.

Congenital erosive and vesicular dermatosis healing with supple reticulated scarring

Congenital erosive and vesicular dermatosis healing with supple reticulated scarring must be distinguished from EB and aplasia cutis congenita. Affected infants demonstrate widespread erythema, blistering, and erosions at birth, which heal within a few weeks to a few months with widespread reticulated scars (Fig 2.61). Nails, scalp, and the tongue and oral mucosa may be involved. Although most children grow and develop normally, the risk of prematurity and associated problems is increased.

Cases occur sporadically, and no inheritance pattern has been established. Extensive evaluations have excluded bacterial, fungal, and viral infections. Some infants have shown evidence of vascular insults in visceral sites and/or the placenta. However, the relationship between these findings and cutaneous lesions is unclear.

Unlike EB, new blisters do not occur. The pattern of blisters and erosions and subsequent scarring differs markedly from aplasia cutis congenita and incontinentia pigmenti.

Mastocytosis

Mastocytosis may first come to clinical attention when cutaneous lesions blister. The disorder typically presents at birth or in the first few months of life as a solitary mastocytoma or multiple lesions of urticaria pigmentosa (Fig 2.62a,b). Although the trunk is most commonly involved, these benign macules, papules, and plaques that contain mast cells may involve any cutaneous site, as well as the gastrointestinal tract, bone marrow, lungs, kidneys, and nervous system. Skin lesions range from under 1 cm in

diameter to large, infiltrated plaques that cover the entire chest or back (Fig 2.62c). Although the overlying epidermis may appear normal at birth, increasing age is associated with progressive localized hyperpigmentation.

Nonspecific triggers of mast-cell degranulation, such as rubbing, hot water, vigorous physical activity, and certain medications (e.g. aspirin, anesthetic agents, radiography contrast material), may produce urtication of cutaneous lesions. Darier sign is a reliable physical finding in mastocytosis and refers to the hive that forms after stroking affected skin. Infants are particularly prone to blister formation, and widespread blistering can be associated with fluid and electrolyte losses and increased risk of infection. Rarely, the release of histamine and other vasoactive mediators from mast cells triggers acute or chronic symptoms, including chronic diarrhea, gastric ulceration, uncontrolled pruritus, bleeding, and hypotension.

Pruritus and systemic symptoms are usually controlled with antihistamines. In infants with bullous mastocytosis and/or systemic disease, oral cromolyn sodium 20–40mg/kg/day may be lifesaving. In severe cases, topical corticosteroids under occlusion, systemic corticosteroids, or photochemotherapy (psoralen–ultraviolet A) may be useful. In many children the number of papules and plaques increases for 1–2 years. During childhood, mastocytomas often become less reactive and tan or brown overlying pigmentation fades slowly. Hyperpigmentation, urtication, and systemic symptoms may persist, however, in some individuals.

Incontinentia pigmenti

Incontinentia pigmenti is a neurocutaneous syndrome named for the peculiar marble-cake swirls of brown pigment that appear on the trunk and occasionally the extremities in later infancy and early childhood. In the newborn, patches of erythema and blisters are scattered on the trunk, scalp, and extremities. Blisters are typically oriented in reticulated lines and swirls that follow the lines of Blaschko, special embryonic

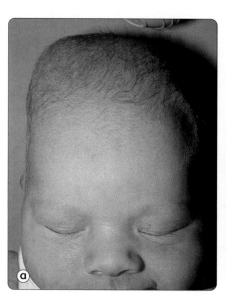

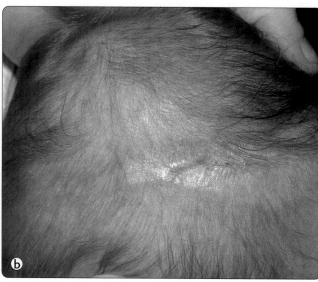

Fig 2.59 Perinatal trauma. **(a)** Cephalo-hematoma, a subperiosteal bleed which usually resolves uneventfully. **(b)** Rarely, perinatal trauma to the scalp results in a 'halo scalp ring' with scarring and permanent hair loss.

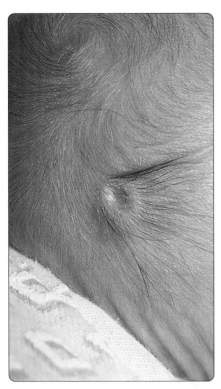

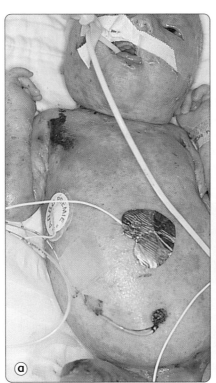

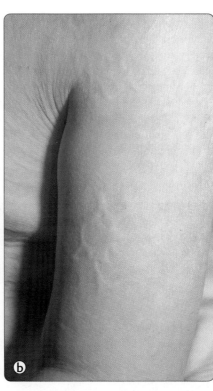

Fig 2.60 Hair collar sign on the scalp of a newborn.

Fig 2.61 Congenital erosive and vesicular dermatosis. **(a)** Extensive vesicles and erosions were noted on the skin of this child in the delivery room. **(b)** Erosions and crusts healed with widespread reticulated, supple scarring.

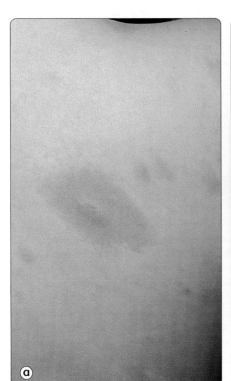

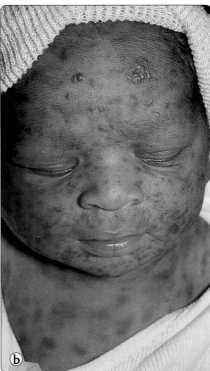

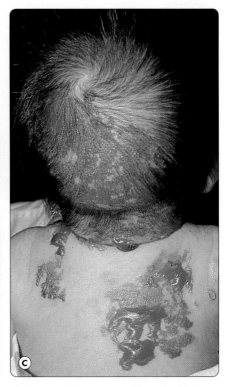

Fig 2.62 Mastocytosis. **(a)** Brown macules and plaques typical of urticaria pigmentosa were scattered on the trunk of this infant. A Darier sign became evident in a single lesion on the back after rubbing. **(b)** Hyperpigmentation is prominent in this healthy black infant with urticaria pigmentosa. Note the blisters on her forehead. **(c)** This infant with diffuse infiltrative lesions had widespread blistering and bleeding into lesions.

cleavage planes (Fig 2.63a,b). Although inflammatory lesions may recur for months, they usually give way to hyperkeratotic, warty plaques by several weeks to several months of age (Fig 2.63c). The hyperkeratotic stage is typically followed by increasing pigmentation at 2–6 months of age (Fig 2.63d). During later childhood, brown streaks often fade to leave atrophic hypopigmented patches. These subtle scars may be the only manifestation of cutaneous disease in older children and adults (Fig 2.63e).

Histopathology of blisters in the newborn demonstrates characteristic intraepidermal edema and vesicles loaded with eosinophils. When incontinentia pigmenti is suspected, the child must be evaluated for associated defects, which may involve the central nervous system, heart, eye, skeletal system, and dentition. Incontinentia pigmenti is inherited as an X-linked dominant disorder that is lethal in males; 97% of affected infants are female. A careful examination of mothers often reveals subtle cutaneous findings.

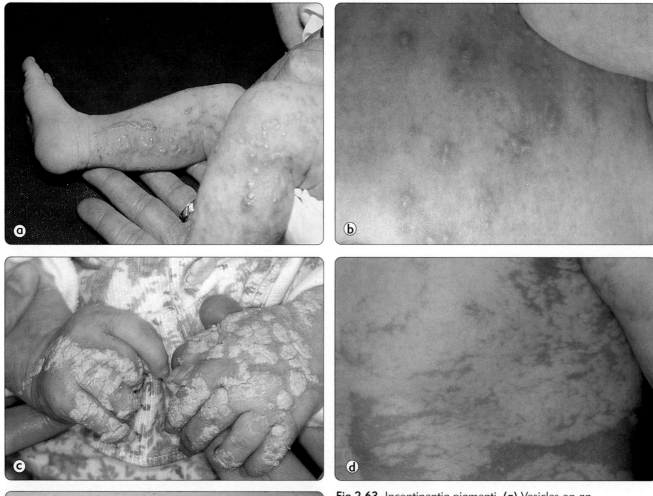

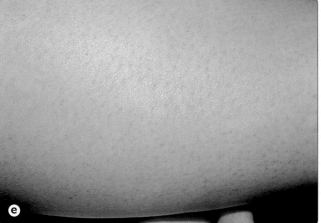

Fig 2.63 Incontinentia pigmenti. **(a)** Vesicles on an erythematous base extended in a linear pattern down the legs and **(b)** trunk of an 8-day-old girl. **(c)** Warty papules developed on the fingers of this 4-month-old girl in the site of earlier vesicles. **(d)** Progressive 'marble cake' hyperpigmentation was first noted on the trunk of this infant at 4 months of age. **(e)** Subtle scarring on the legs was the only sign of incontinenta pigmenti in the mother of the child. Note the absence of hair follicles in the linear scars.

NEVI

Nevus is a term used to describe a group of skin lesions that appear at birth or in the first month of life. Nevi are composed of mature or nearly mature cutaneous elements organized in an abnormal fashion. These hamartomas may comprise virtually any epidermal or dermal structure.

Vascular nevi

For therapeutic and prognostic reasons, clinicians must distinguish between vascular malformations and true hemangiomas in infancy. Vascular malformations, including salmon patches and port-wine stains (PWSs), are stable vascular nevi that comprise mature vascular structures, which are present at birth. Endothelial cell proliferation is not present and vascular lumina become increasingly dilated with increasing age. Lymphatic malformations are also nonproliferative lesions present at birth which slowly enlarge because of increasing ectasia of the lymphatic spaces.

Hemangiomas represent true neoplasms which typically appear within the first 2–4 weeks of life, grow for 6–12 months, and resolve spontaneously over the following years. Early in infancy hemangiomas contain rapidly proliferating endothelial cells with few capillary lumina. As growth slows endothelial cells flatten and capillary lumina increase in size and number. This is followed by involution of capillaries and eventual fibrosis.

Vascular malformations

Salmon patches occur in 60–70% of newborns (Fig 2.64). Lesions are usually located on the nape of the neck, glabella, forehead, or upper eye lids. Although salmon patches usually fade during the first year of life and tend to be camouflaged by normal pigmentation, they may persist indefinitely, particularly on the neck. The pink patches also darken with crying, breath holding, and physical exertion.

At birth, 0.2–0.3% of newborns have PWSs. Unlike salmon patches, PWSs tend to persist unchanged during childhood and to darken in adolescence and adulthood (Figs 2.65–2.67). Small angiomatous papules and underlying soft tissue hypertrophy develop gradually over years.

Although unilateral lesions on the head and neck are most common, any part of the body surface and mucous membranes may be involved. Occasionally, PWSs present in association with extracutaneous defects. Children with involvement of the first division of the trigeminal nerve may have a vascular malformation of the ipsilateral meninges, cerebral cortex, and eye (Sturge–Weber syndrome; Fig 2.65). Seizures, mental retardation, hemiplegia, and glaucoma may develop during the first several years of life. Superficial vascular lesions associated with limb or segmental trunk hypertrophy are typical of Klippel–Trénaunay–Weber syndrome (Fig 2.66). These patients may have underlying malformations of the deep venous system as well. More than 30 other named syndromes have also been described in association with cutaneous vascular malformations.

Infants with PWSs deserve a thorough physical examination for signs of systemic disease. Children with forehead and periorbital involvement require careful neurodevelopmental follow-up, an eye examination to exclude glaucoma, and further neurologic studies as indicated.

Rehabilitative cosmetics (e.g. Dermablend®, Covermark®) provide reasonable, safe, but temporary camouflage of PWSs (Fig 2.67). Definitive treatment eluded practitioners until approval of the flashlamp, pumped, pulsed, yellow-dye laser (see Fig 2.65b). Unlike previous modalities, including the argon and carbon dioxide lasers, the pulsed-dye laser has an extremely low risk of scarring. By selective photothermolysis the yellow beam damages vascular structures while leaving the surrounding skin virtually unscathed. This device is safe, relatively painless, and effective in infants and children, as well as in adults. Maximal improvement of PWSs requires an average of five to ten treatments separated by a 2–3 month healing period. Unfortunately, the laser penetrates only 1.5–2 mm deep into the skin, which results in

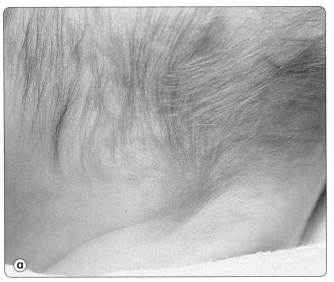
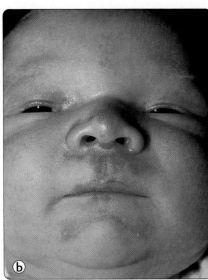

Fig 2.64 Salmon patches.
(a) Typical, light-red, splotchy patch at the nape of the neck in a healthy newborn.
(b) Similar patches were present on this child's eyelids, nose, upper lip, and chin.

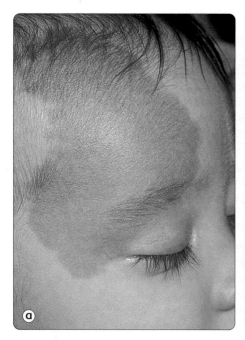

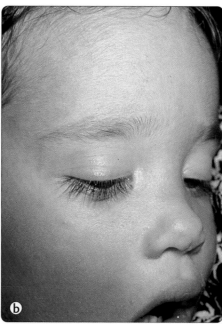

Fig 2.65 Port-wine stains. (a) A port-wine stain involved the ophthalmic distribution of the trigeminal nerve on the face of this infant with Sturge–Weber syndrome. (b) After four treatments with the yellow-pulsed dye laser the lesion had almost completely resolved.

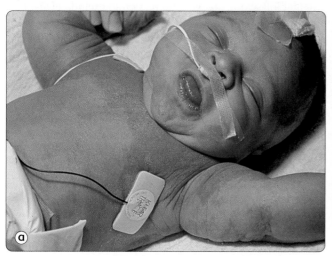

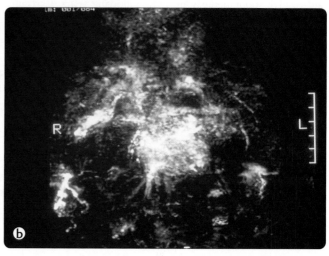

Fig 2.66 Port-wine stains. (a) At birth this newborn had a port-wine stain that involved his upper chest, neck, and portions of both arms and was associated with soft-tissue hypertrophy (Klippel–Trénaunay–Weber syndrome) and high-output cardiac failure. (b) This composite magnetic resonance image of his body demonstrates increased blood flow to the right side of his neck and both upper extremities, with the greatest flow to the right shoulder and arm.

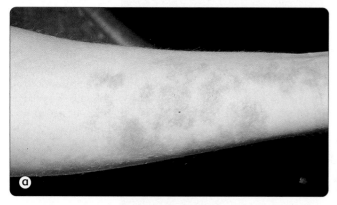

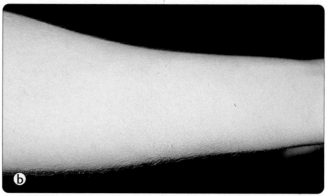

Fig 2.67 Port-wine stains. (a) An extensive port-wine stain on the arm of this teenager. (b) It was readily camouflaged with a corrective cosmetic.

little improvement in those nevi with a deep component. Consequently, early treatment in childhood produces the best outcome with the fewest number of treatments and the least cost.

Hemangiomas

Although rarely present at birth, hemangiomas occur in up to 10% of infants by 4 weeks of age (Fig 2.68). Nearly 75% occur in girls, and premature infants are more commonly affected. Lesions typically begin as barely visible telangiectasias or red macules that rapidly grow into 0.5–4.0 cm diameter bright red compressible tumors or 'strawberry' hemangiomas. Many hemangiomas have a deep dermal or subcutaneous component (Fig 2.69). Occasionally, lesions lack a superficial component altogether and can only be differentiated from vascular malformations by the growth pattern (Fig 2.70).

Growth of hemangiomas usually stops at 6–12 months of age, and signs of involution, such as graying of the surface and flattening of the deeper component, subsequently develop. Regression occurs in 25% by age 2 years, 40–50% by age 4 years, 60–75% by age 6 years, and 95% by adolescence. Involution is independent of sex, location, size, number, and depth of the hemangiomas. Unfortunately, scarring, loose skin, or telangiectasias remain in 30–50% of children.

Although hemangiomas are benign tumors and regression is the rule, these lesions may rarely compromise vital functions when they are located near the anus, urethra, airway,

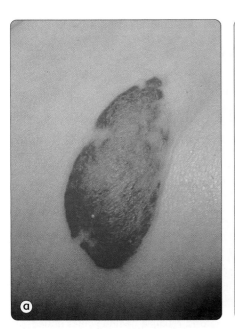
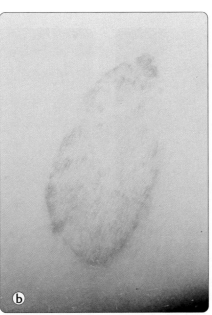

Fig 2.68 Resolving capillary hemangioma. **(a)** Appearance at age 5 months. **(b)** Appearance 2 years later. **(c)** Almost complete resolution at age 5 years.

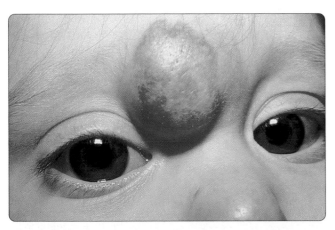

Fig 2.69 The hemangioma on this child's nasal bridge has both a superficial and a deep dermal component. The hemangioma involuted over 3 years without leaving a scar.

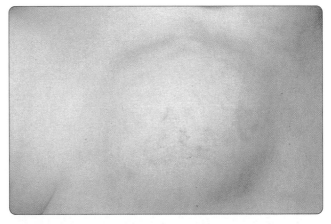

Fig 2.70 Subcutaneous hemangioma. The vessels that make up this large, partially compressible lesion are deep beneath the skin surface, but still impart a bluish hue to the overlying skin. Note the indistinctness of the margins.

and orbit. Hemangiomas around the eye or extending into the orbit may be associated with obstruction amblyopia or direct damage to orbital contents (Fig 2.71). Multiple hemangiomas or single, large, rapidly growing lesions in young infants may be associated with high-output cardiac failure or disseminated intravascular coagulation (Kasabach–Merritt syndrome). In children with widespread multiple nevi or hemangiomatosis, lesions may involve internal organs, including the lungs, liver, gastrointestinal tract, kidneys, and central nervous system (Fig 2.72). In these children, treatment with high-dose corticosteroids (prednisone 3–5mg/kg/day) and/or interferon may be life-saving. Hemangiomas in the diaper area and other skin creases are prone to ulceration and infection (Fig 2.73). Careful hygiene, topical and systemic antibiotics, occlusive

dressings, and barrier pastes may be required to prevent cellulitis and scarring.

In general, hemangiomas are not associated with extra-cutaneous syndromes, but there are some notable exceptions. Midline hemangiomas, particularly in the lumbosacral area, may be associated with underlying vertebral and spinal cord anomalies (Fig 2.74). Large hemangiomas on the upper face and scalp have been associated with midline thoracic and posterior intracranial anomalies, respectively. Magnetic resonance imaging (MRI) has proved particularly useful for delineating the extent of these defects.

Although the yellow pulsed-dye laser was originally approved for treating PWSs, it appears to be particularly useful in treating early, thin hemangiomas and residual telangiectasias later in childhood. The superficial component

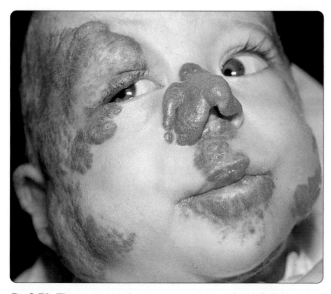

Fig 2.71 This regressing hemangioma extended into the orbit and produced a large refractive difference between the two sides. The tumor also produced destruction of the nasal septum and obstructed the airway, which resulted in the need for tracheostomy.

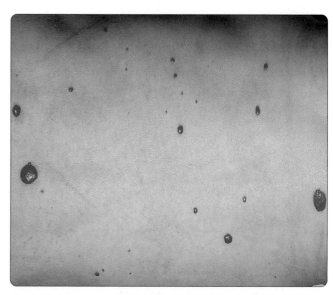

Fig 2.72 Hemangiomatosis. Multiple hemangiomas dotted the back and extremities of this 3-month-old girl.

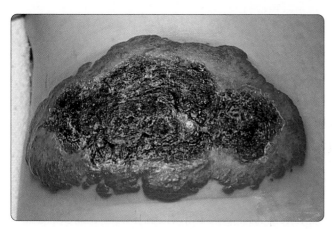

Fig 2.73 A large hemangioma on the back of a 10-month-old girl developed an area of central necrosis that was associated with secondary bacterial infection and sepsis.

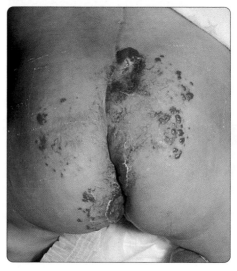

Fig 2.74 This extensive sacral hemangioma was associated with a tethered cord. Note the scar from correction of the spinal defect. Ulceration of the hemangioma from irritation in the diaper area was a recurrent problem.

of rapidly growing hemangiomas can be shut off with the pulsed-dye laser, and overlying ulcerations, which have failed to respond to topical measures, heal quickly after laser therapy.

Lymphangiomas

Congenital defects of the lymphatic system may present as localized lymphangiomas or widespread lesions with involvement of the soft tissues, bones, and viscera.

Lymphangioma circumscriptum consists of one or several patches of thick-walled vesicles that resemble fish eggs or frog spawn (Fig 2.75). Lesions appear at birth or during infancy and may be associated with an underlying soft-tissue fullness or extensive swelling of the involved area. Lesions may occur at any cutaneous site. Cavernous lymphangiomas develop as localized, subcutaneous, cystic swellings, most commonly in the head and neck. These lesions may surround and compress vital structures in the anterior neck. Their presence may be marked by overlying lymphangioma circumscriptum or PWSs.

Lymphangiomas may be associated with complex congenital vascular malformations (Fig 2.76). In the proteus syndrome, extensive dermal and subcutaneous lymphatic and venous malformations are associated with cutaneous PWSs, soft-tissue tumors, and epidermal nevi. Vascular malformations may extend into the mediastinum, peritoneum, retroperitoneal space, and viscera. Organ dysfunction, recurrent soft-tissue infection, and musculoskeletal involvement may be debilitating and life threatening.

Unlike progressive hemangiomas, which respond to corticosteroids, lymphangiomas have eluded medical therapy. Surgical management of lymphangiomas is difficult, because they often extend around vital structures, and recurrence rates are high. Superficial lesions may be ablated with the carbon dioxide laser.

Hamartomatous nevi

Hamartomatous nevi include a number of birthmarks that contain various epidermal, dermal, and subcutaneous structures.

Epidermal nevi

Epidermal nevi occur in 0.1–1% of children and consist of proliferating epidermal keratinocytes. Most epidermal nevi appear at birth or during early infancy as localized, linear, warty, subtly to markedly hyperpigmented plaques (Fig 2.77). Lesions may involve any cutaneous site and extend onto mucous membranes. Epidermal nevi range in size from a few millimeters to extensive lesions that involve a large portion of the trunk and extremities. Infants with large lesions must be evaluated for associated defects, which include seizures, mental retardation, and skeletal and ocular defects (epidermal nevus syndrome). Occasionally, children with small epidermal nevi also demonstrate extracutaneous anomalies. Skin lesions may respond to the application of topical keratolytics such as lactic acid, salicylic acid, and urea. Small lesions can be excised or ablated by carbon dioxide laser.

Sebaceous nevi

Sebaceous nevus of Jadassohn is characterized by a 1–4 cm diameter linear or round, hairless, yellow, cobblestone-like plaque on the scalp (Fig 2.78). Although lesions usually involve the head and neck, nevi occasionally appear on the trunk and extremities. Rarely, lesions extend over a large portion of the body surface and are associated with multiple neuroectodermal and mesodermal defects (nevus sebaceous syndrome). Histology demonstrates multiple sebaceous glands, ectopic apocrine glands, and incompletely differentiated hair structures.

Although 10–15% of patients develop benign neoplasms in adult life (Fig 2.78b), a recent study shows that the risk of

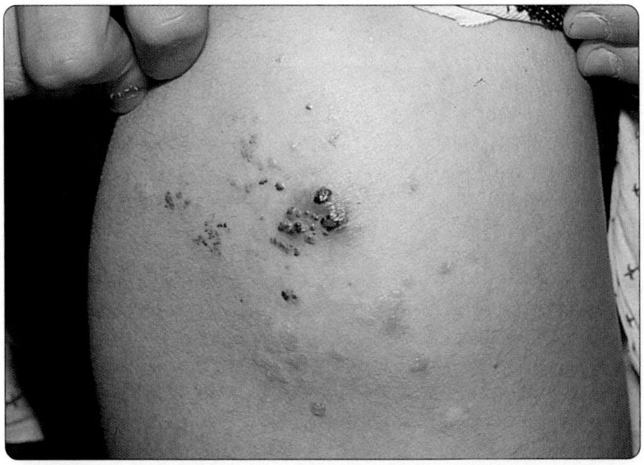

Fig 2.75 Lymphangioma circumscriptum. A small cluster of grayish-purple vesicles on the knee of an adolescent demonstrates the typical 'frog spawn' appearance.

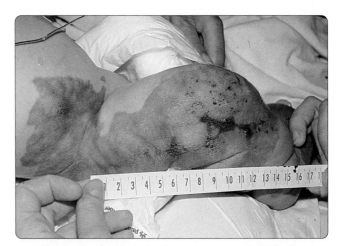

Fig 2.76 Proteus syndrome. Massive hypertrophy of the leg was associated with an extensive cutaneous port-wine stain, soft-tissue tumors, and a deep lymphangiohemangioma that involved the thigh, peritoneal cavity, and retroperitoneal space in this 1-month-old boy.

malignant neoplasms arising in sebaceous nevi, such as basal cell carcinoma and sebaceous carcinoma, is extremely low. Benign hypertrophy of the sebaceous and apocrine components associated with the development of warty nodules and plaques can occur transiently at birth, but is often progressive at puberty.

Smooth muscle and pilar hamartomas

Smooth muscle and pilar hamartomas contain smooth muscle bundles and may be associated with prominent hair follicles (Fig 2.79). Clinically, these innocent nevi are characterized by minimally hyperpigmented, supple 1.0–5.0 cm diameter plaques on the trunk. A pseudo-Darier sign or rippling of the skin occurs with rubbing. Hyperpigmentation and hair may become prominent.

Connective tissue nevus

Connective tissue nevus defines a group of hamartomas with increased quantities of dermal collagen and variable changes in elastic tissue (Fig 2.80). Lesions appear in the newborn as 1.0–10 cm diameter plaques composed of fibrotic papules and nodules, which often give a peau d'orange texture to the skin. Although typically located on the trunk, lesions may be widely disseminated and any cutaneous site may be involved.

Connective tissue nevi may occur as isolated skin findings or in association with asymptomatic osteopoikilosis or radiographic densities in the long bones and the bones of the hands and feet (Bushke–Ollendorff syndrome). The shagreen patch of tuberous sclerosis cannot be differentiated clinically and histologically from an innocent connective

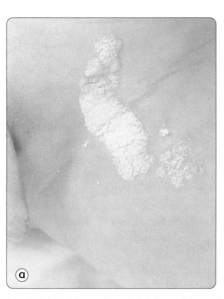
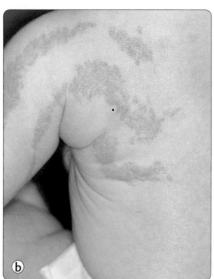
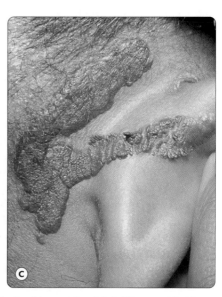

Fig 2.77 Epidermal nevi. **(a)** An epidermal nevus on the upper thigh of a newborn still covered with vernix caseosa.
(b) Three linear, warty plaques extend across the upper chest and down the arm of a healthy toddler. **(c)** A 10-year-old girl complained of itching from a congenital, V-shaped, warty plaque behind her ear.

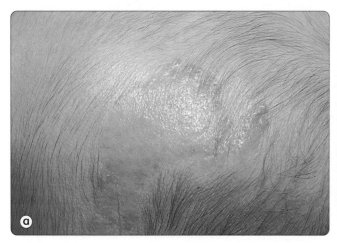
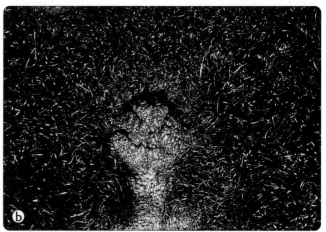

Fig 2.78 Sebaceous nevi. **(a)** Sebaceous nevus of Jadassohn. A yellow, cobblestone-like, hairless patch present since birth.
(b) Syringocystadenoma papilliferum arose in this sebaceous nevus on the scalp of a teenage boy. Local excision gave an excellent cosmetic result.

tissue nevus. Consequently, a careful search for other stigmata of tuberous sclerosis must be performed in all children with these hamartomas.

Congenital pigmented nevi

Congenital pigmented nevi are pigmented macules or plaques, often with dense hair growth noted at birth or during the first few months of life (Fig 2.81). Pigmented nevi contain nevomelanocytic nevus cells, cells derived from neural crest and that share with normal skin melanocytes the ability to produce melanin. At birth, the lesions may be light tan with lightly pigmented vellus hairs. During infancy the nevus darkens and hair may become prominent. Occasionally, darkly pigmented lesions lighten during the first 1–2 years of life. Small dark macules or nodules may also appear within the borders of the nevus (Fig 2.81b).

Giant, congenital pigmented nevi may reach over 20 cm in diameter and are associated with a 2–10% lifetime risk of melanoma (Fig 2.81b,c). The highest risk of malignant change occurs in the first 3–15 years of life. Other tumors of neural-crest origin rarely arise within large lesions (Fig 2.81c). Multistage procedures with tissue expansion may be feasible in selected patients. Unfortunately, large areas of the

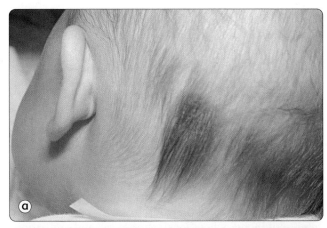

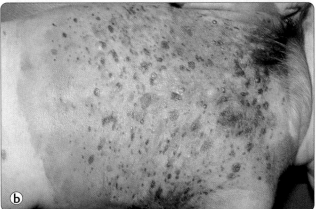

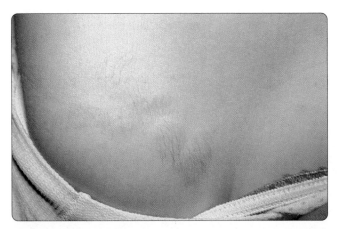

Fig 2.79 Congenital smooth muscle hamartoma. This slightly hairy plaque on the left buttock of a 3-year-old girl demonstrates a pseudo-Darier's sign.

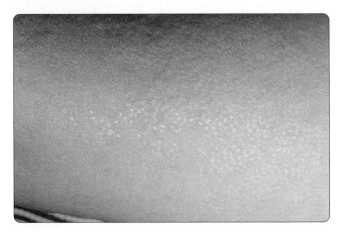

Fig 2.80 Connective tissue nevus. This reticulated fibrotic plaque on the arm of a 10-year-old boy remained unchanged since birth. A medical evaluation for associated disorders was unrevealing.

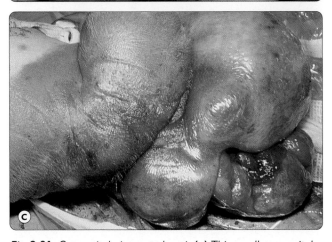

Fig 2.81 Congenital pigmented nevi. (a) This small congenital pigmented nevus was associated with a tuft of dark hair on the scalp of an infant. (b) This giant pigmented nevus contained numerous darkly pigmented nodules. (c) A large tumor developed within a giant pigmented nevus which involved the diaper area of this newborn. The tumor contained structures that arose from various neuroectodermal elements. The tumor was excised in several stages.

nevus may not be amenable to surgical management, and close observation with photographs is required. Trials with dermabrasion and laser surgery in infancy have been disappointing. Regular examinations include careful palpation of the entire lesion, because melanomas may arise deep within the nevus. Some practitioners recommend periodic magnetic resonance imaging (MRI) or computed tomography (CT) scans to follow large nevi. Radioimaging studies can also be used to document leptomeningeal involvement, which is commonly associated with giant pigmented nevi that cover the scalp, neck, and/or back. The presence of inaccessible central nervous system lesions is important when assessing the risk of malignancy and planning surgical intervention.

Medium size (2–10 cm diameter) and small (under 2 cm diameter) congenital pigmented nevi may also be associated with a higher risk of malignant change than acquired moles. However, the incidence is unknown, and there are no uniformly accepted guidelines for their management. Small size and high parental anxiety may dictate early surgical excision, but removal of these nevi is usually safely left until later childhood when local anesthetic and outpatient surgery is possible.

TUMORS

In addition to nevi, a number of other disorders present as lumps and bumps in the newborn. Many of these lesions are self-limited (fat necrosis, juvenile xanthogranuloma, hematoma) or innocent (dermoid cyst, lipoma), but some tumors herald the onset of serious systemic disease (leukemia, neuroblastoma, rhabdomyosarcoma).

Juvenile xanthogranulomas

Juvenile xanthogranulomas (JXGs) commonly present at birth or within the first year of life (Fig 2.82). Enlarging, 0.5–4.0 cm diameter, yellow papules, plaques, and nodules with overlying telangiectasias involve the head, neck, trunk, and occasionally the extremities. Nearly half of the lesions are solitary, but multiple nodules may be scattered over the skin surface.

A confirmatory skin biopsy demonstrates characteristic lipid-laden histiocytes. Generally, JXGs are asymptomatic, and laboratory studies, which include a serum lipid profile, are normal. However, the presence of cutaneous lesions prompts a search for extracutaneous lesions, particularly in the eye. JXGs are the most common cause of spontaneous anterior chamber hemorrhage in children.

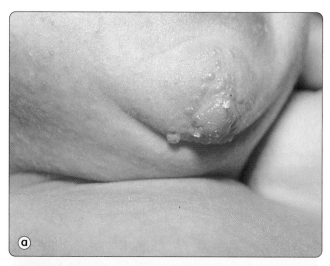

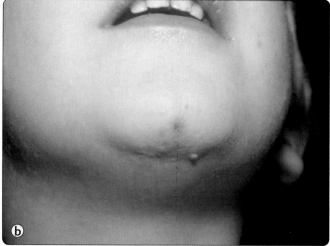

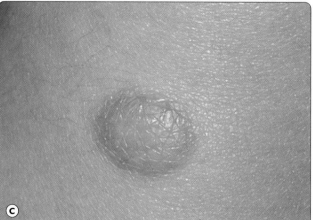

Fig 2.82 Juvenile xanthogranuloma. **(a)** This tumor developed abruptly on the chin of a 3-month-old boy. Numerous tiny papules developed around the primary lesion. **(b)** After 1 year the tumor and satellites had almost completely resolved without treatment. **(c)** A solitary xanthogranuloma on the leg of an infant shows the typical yellow plaque with surrounding telangiectasias.

In most children no therapy is required. Surgical excision can lead to unnecessary scarring, and in early infancy to recurrent lesions at the operative site; also, new lesions may continue to erupt for several months. After a period of growth in infancy, JXGs slowly flatten, and involution is often complete by mid childhood (Fig 2.82b).

Dermoid cysts

Dermoid cysts appear as 1.0–4.0 cm diameter compressible or rubbery subcutaneous nodules at the site of closure of embryonic clefts. Although the lesions are usually noted in the newborn, subtle cysts may escape detection until they become inflamed in later infancy or early childhood. The forehead and periorbital area (Fig 2.83a) are the most common sites of involvement, but dermoids occasionally present on the mid chest, sacrum, perineum, and scrotum (Fig 2.83b).

Dermoid cysts are lined by an epidermis that contains mature adnexal structures, which include sebaceous glands, eccrine glands, and apocrine glands. Although there is no risk of malignancy, lesions on the head may extend to the periosteum and cause erosion of the underlying bone. Cysts may be surgically excised during infancy or childhood.

Lesions on the head must be differentiated from hematomas, encephaloceles, and malignant tumors. A CT scan and MRI of the head demonstrate the cystic nature of the dermoid cyst and exclude the possibility of communication with the central nervous system or infiltrative tumor.

Dermoids that overlie the sacrum may be associated with occult defects of the vertebral column and spinal cord. The tumor and associated anomalies can be visualized with MRI.

Recurrent infantile digital fibroma

In recurrent infantile digital fibroma, single or multiple fibrous nodules appear on the fingers and toes (Fig 2.84). Although these tumors may occur in older children, 85% are diagnosed before 1 year of age and many are noted at birth or in the first month of life. Lesions rarely exceed 2.0 cm in diameter. Skin biopsy demonstrates numerous fibroblasts and interlacing collagen bundles. The presence of perinuclear intracytoplasmic inclusion bodies was considered to suggest a viral etiology, but this has been refuted by electron-microscopy studies. Although excision is followed by recurrence in 75% of cases, most digital fibromas involute spontaneously within several years.

Infantile myofibromatosis

Infantile myofibromatosis, also referred to as congenital fibromatosis, usually presents as a solitary, firm, red or blue, mobile, subcutaneous tumor (Fig 2.85). However, multiple tumors may involve muscle and bone, and visceral lesions may produce organ dysfunction, particularly in the lungs. Histologically, these well-circumscribed tumors contain fibroblasts and smooth muscle cells with no

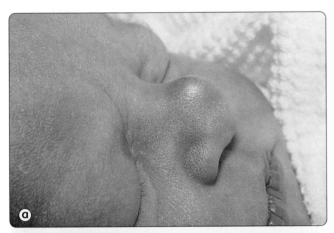

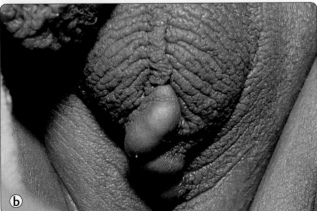

Fig 2.83 Dermoid cyst. (a) This partially compressible mass was present on the nose at birth. A computed tomography scan of the head (to exclude a communication with the underlying central nervous system) was normal. (b) This cyst on the median raphe of the scrotum of a 4-month-old remained unchanged from birth.

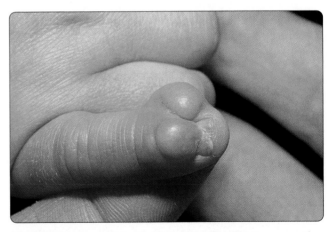

Fig 2.84 Recurrent infantile digital fibroma. This tumor on the finger of a 7-month-old boy recurred after local excision. However, after an initial growth phase, it began to involute without further therapy.

cytologic atypia. Solitary lesions are usually excised without recurrence, but new tumors may erupt for the first several months of life. In the majority of infants who do not have severe visceral disease, spontaneous involution occurs in the first year of life.

Malignant tumors

Malignant tumors rarely present at birth or in the newborn period. Of patients with neuroblastoma, 50% are diagnosed in the first 2 years of life, and many develop clinical disease before 6 months of age. Although cutaneous metastases are seen in only about 3% of all patients with neuroblastoma, nearly a third of affected newborns present with skin lesions as their initial manifestation. Metastases usually appear as 0.5–2.0 cm diameter, firm bluish-red papules and nodules on the trunk and extremities. Stroking results in blanching and a red halo, probably because of the release of catecholamines from tumor cells. These 'blueberry muffin' lesions must be differentiated from areas of extramedullary hematopoiesis seen in infants with congenital infections, such as rubella, cytomegalovirus, and toxoplasmosis (Fig 2.86).

Cutaneous plaques and tumors may also be the earliest finding in newborns with leukemia (Fig 2.87), rhabdomyosarcoma (Fig 2.88), lymphoma, and a number of other carcinomas and sarcomas. Skin biopsy of rapidly growing or infiltrative lesions may lead to early diagnosis and therapy.

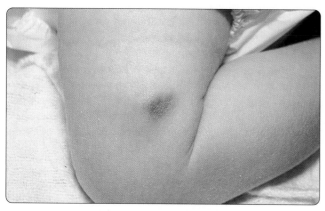

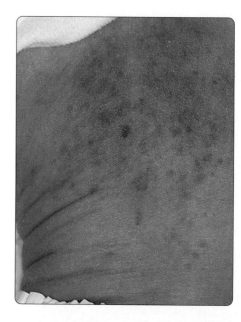

Fig 2.86 Blueberry muffin rash. This infant with congenital rubella demonstrated the typical cutaneous lesions of extramedullary hematopoiesis.

Fig 2.85 Myofibromatosis. An infiltrating subcutaneous tumor on the thigh of a 1-month-old infant demonstrated histologic features of myofibromatosis. Other benign and malignant tumors, which include neuroblastoma, leukemia, and lymphoma, should be considered in the differential diagnosis.

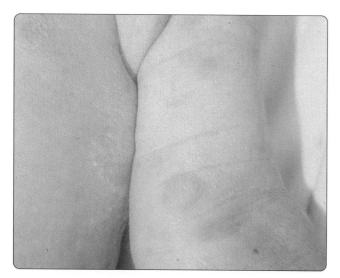

Fig 2.87 Congenital leukemia cutis. This newborn presented with a hemoglobin of 5.0 g/dL (3.1 mmol/L) and infiltrative, pale pink, annular plaques on the extremities.

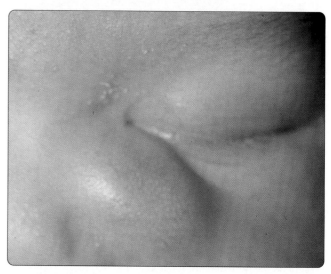

Fig 2.88 Rhabdomyo sarcoma. This rapidly growing congenital mass was part of an infiltrating rhabdomyosarcoma that involved the cheek, orbit, nose, and sinuses of this infant. This child was treated with surgical debulking of the mass and chemotherapy.

REACTIVE ERYTHEMAS

Reactive erythema refers to a group of disorders characterized by erythematous macules, plaques, and nodules, which vary in size, shape, and distribution. Unlike specific dermatoses, they represent reaction patterns in the skin triggered by a number of different endogenous and environmental factors. In infants, erythema multiforme, erythema nodosum, urticaria, and vasculitis occur after exposure to various infections and drugs. Just as in older children and adults, management of affected infants involves identification and elimination of the offending agent and supportive care. Several reactive erythemas, however, are peculiar to infancy.

Neonatal lupus erythematosus

Neonatal lupus erythematosus is the most common cause of congenital heart block. Although cutaneous lesions may not appear until several months of age, they are frequently present at birth. Affected infants demonstrate annular erythematous plaques with a central scale, telangiectasias, atrophy, and pigmentary changes (Fig 2.89). Lesions are typically in the range 0.5–3.0 cm in diameter and may spread from the scalp and face to the neck, upper trunk, and upper extremities. Although development of the cutaneous rash does not require sunlight, it may be triggered or exacerbated by sun exposure.

The cause of neonatal lupus is unknown. However, the presence of transplacentally acquired ssA (Ro) and ssB (La) antibodies is thought to play a primary role in the pathogenesis of the disorder. In adults, ssA and ssB antibodies are associated with Sjögren syndrome and a photosensitive variant of systemic lupus known as subacute cutaneous lupus erythematosus.

In addition to conduction defects and structural cardiac anomalies, affected infants may develop hepatosplenomegaly, anemia, leukopenia, thrombocytopenia, and lymphadenopathy. With the exception of cardiac involvement, neonatal lupus usually resolves spontaneously in 6–12 months, as transplacentally derived antibody wanes. The use of low- and medium-potency topical corticosteroids on intensely inflammatory cutaneous lesions for several weeks may reduce the risk of scarring. Subtle atrophy, telangiectasias, and pigmentary changes may persist indefinitely. Rarely, infants require systemic corticosteroids and supportive care. Parents are instructed to protect children with sunscreens and to ensure

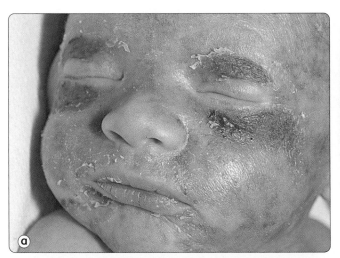

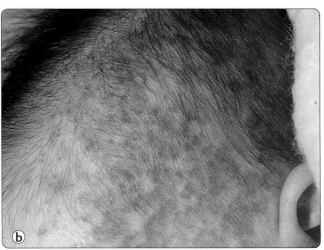

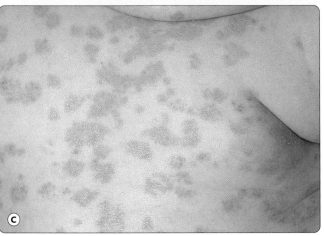

Fig 2.89 Neonatal lupus erythematosus. **(a)** This newborn presented with extensive cutaneous atrophy and telangiectasias of the face, hepatosplenomegaly, and thrombocytopenia. **(b,c)** At 1 month of age this infant developed an extensive eruption of annular red plaques with central atrophy. **(b)** Lesions first appeared on the scalp and face, and **(c)** subsequently spread to the neck and trunk.

that the infant avoids direct sun exposure for at least 4–6 months. Mothers who have no clinical signs of lupus also require careful follow-up, because they are at increased risk of developing overt disease.

Annular erythema of infancy

Annular erythema of infancy is an innocent gyrate erythema that presents during the first 6 months of life with red papules and plaques that enlarge in a centrifugal pattern (Fig 2.90). Lesions may develop a dusky center and exceed 10 cm in diameter over 1–3 weeks. Plaques periodically fade, only to recur for months to years. Although this reaction may be triggered by infections, drugs, and malignancy, evaluation for an underlying disease is usually unrevealing. Fortunately, infants generally continue to thrive and lesions eventually resolve without treatment.

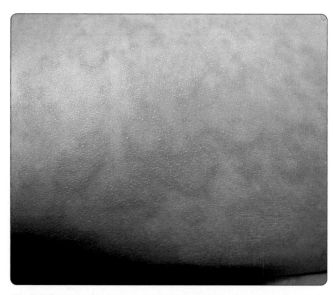

Fig 2.90 Annular erythema of infancy. This eruption persisted for months on the trunk and extremities of an otherwise healthy infant.

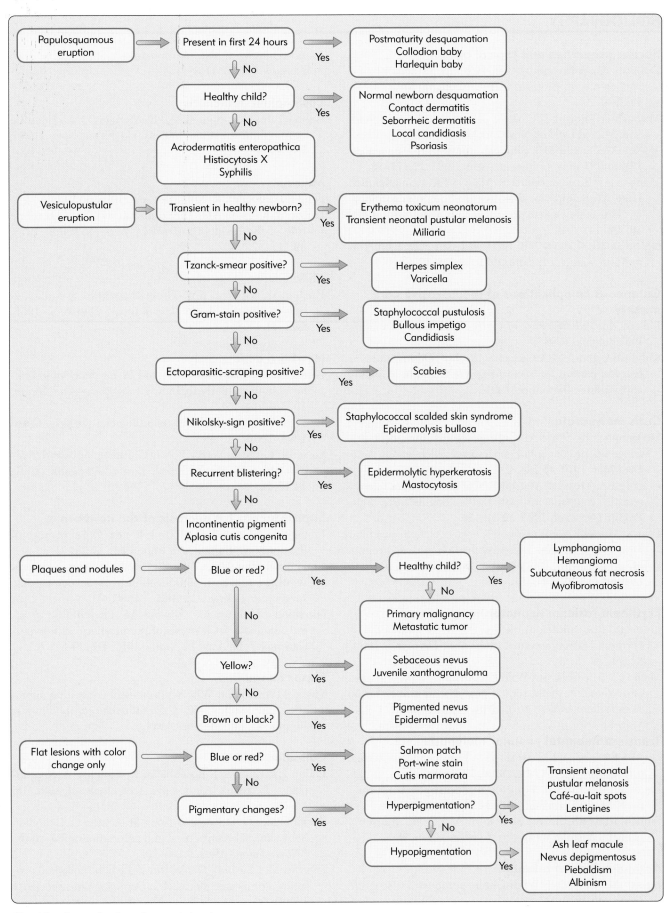

Algorithm for evaluation of neonatal rashes.

BIBLIOGRAPHY

Barrier properties and topical agents

Dollison EJ, Beckstrand J. Adhesive tape vs pectin-based barrier use in preterm infant. *Neonatal Netw.* 1995, 14:35–9.

Maibach HI, Boisits EK. *Neonatal skin structure and function.* Marcel Dekker, New York, 1982.

Malloy-McDonald MB. Skin care for high risk neonates. *J Wound Ostomy Continence Nurs.* 1995. 22:177–82.

Mancini AJ, Sookedo-Dorst S, Madison KC, Smoller BR, Lane AT. Semipermeable dressings: improved epidermal barrier function in preterm infants. *Pediatr Res.* 1994, 36:306–14.

Nachman RL, Esterly NB. Increased skin permeability in preterm infants. *J Pediatr.* 1971, 79:628–32.

Cutaneous complications of the intensive care nursery

Ballard RA. *Pediatric care of the ICN graduate.* Saunders, Philadelphia, 1988.

Cohen BA, Jones MD, Gleason CA, *et al. Dermatology in hospital care of the recovering NICU infant.* Williams and Wilkins, Baltimore, 1991.

Cutis marmorata

Fitzsimmons JS, Starks M. Cutis marmorata telangiectatica congenita or congenital generalized phlebectasia. *Arch Dis Child.* 1970, 45:724–6.

O'Toole EA, Deasy P, Watson R. Cutis marmorata telangiectatica congenita associated with a double aortic arch. *Pediatr Dermatol.* 1995, 12:348–50.

Pehr K, Moro ZB. Cutis marmorata telangiectatica congenita: long-term follow-up, review of the literature and report of a case with congenital hypothyroidism. *Pediatr Dermatol.* 1993, 10:6–11.

Erythema toxicum neonatorum

Freeman RG, Spiller R, Knox JM. Histopathology of erythema toxicum neonatorum. *Arch Dermatol.* 1960, 82:586–9.

Maffei FA, Michaels MG, Wald ER. An unusual presentation of erythema toxicum scrotal pustules present at birth. *Arch Pediatr Adolesc Med.* 1996, 150:649–50.

Transient neonatal pustular melanosis

Barr RJ, Globerman LM, Werber FA. Transient neonatal pustular melanosis. *Int J Dermatol.* 1979, 18:636–8.

Laude TA. Approach to dermatologic disorders in black children. *Semin Dermatol.* 1995, 14:15–20.

Ramamurthy RS, Reveri M, Esterly MB, *et al.* Transient neonatal pustular melanosis. *J Pediatr.* 1976, 88:831–5.

Acropustulosis of infancy

Jarratt M, Ramsdell W. Infantile acropustulosis. *Arch Dermatol.* 1979, 115:834–6.

Kahn G, Rywlin AM. Acropustulosis of infancy. *Arch Dermatol.* 1979, 115:831–4.

Eosinophilic folliculitis

Garcia-Patos V, Pujol RM, DeMoragas JM. Infantile eosinophilic pustular folliculitis. *Dermatology.* 1994, 189:33–8.

Miliaria

Feng E, Janniger CK. Miliaria. *Cutis.* 1995, 55:213–6.

Holzle E, Kligman AM. The pathogenesis of miliaria rubra: role of the resident microflora. *Br J Dermatol.* 1978, 99:117–37.

Milia

Epstein W, Kligman AM. The pathogenesis of milia and benign tumors of the skin. *J Invest Dermatol.* 1956, 26:1–11.

Newborn acne

Forest MG, Cathaird AM, Bertrand JA. Evidence of testicular activity in early infancy. *J Clin Endocrinol Metab.* 1973, 37:148–51.

Janniger CK. Neonatal and infantile acne vulgaris. *Cutis.* 1993, 52:16.

Jansen T, Burgdorf WHC, Plewig G. Pathogenesis and treatment of acne in childhood. *Pediatr Dermatol.* 1997, 14:17–22.

Subcutaneous fat necrosis of the newborn

Beneggi A, Adamoli P, Conforto F, Bonora G. Fat necrosis of the newborn. *Pediatr Med Chir.* 1995, 17:281–2.

Chuang SB, Chin HC, Chuang CC. Subcutaneous fat necrosis of the newborn complicating hypothermic cardiac surgery. *Br J Dermatol.* 1995, 132:805–10.

Norwood-Galloway A, Lebwohl M, Phelps RG, *et al.* Subcutaneous fat necrosis of the newborn with hypercalcemia. *J Am Acad Dermatol.* 1987, 16:435–9.

Minor anomalies

Steele MW, Golden WL. Syndromes of congenital anomalies. In: Kelley VC (ed.), *Practice of pediatrics.* Lippincott, Philadelphia, 1984.

Collodion baby

Baden HP, Kubilus J, Rosenbaum K, Fletcher A. Keratinization in the harlequin fetus. *Arch Dermatol.* 1982, 18: 14–18.

deDobbeleer G, Heenen M, Song M, Achten G. Collodion baby skin. Ultrastructural and autoradiographic study. *J Cutan Pathol.* 1982, 9:196–202.

Lareque M, Gharbi R, Daniel J, *et al.* Le bebe collodion evolution a propos de 29 cas. *Ann Dermatol Venereol.* 1976, 103:31–56.

Ichthyosis

Niemi KM, Kanerva L, Kuokkanen K, Ignatius J. Clinical, light and electron microscopic features of recessive congenital ichthyosis type I. *Br J Dermatol*. 1994, **130**:626–33.

Rand RE, Baden HP. The ichthyoses – a review. *J Am Acad Dermatol*. 1983, **8**:285–305.

Parmentier L, Blanchet-Bardon C, Nguyen S, Prud'homme JF, Dubertret L, Weissenbach J. Autosomal recessive lamellar ichthyosis: identification of a new mutation transglutaminase and evidence for genetic heterogeneity. *Hum Mol Genet*. 1995, **4**:1391–5.

Smith DL, Smith JG, Wong SW, De Shazo RD. Netherton syndrome: a syndrome of elevated IgE and characteristic skin and hair findings. *J Allergy Immunol*. 1995, **95**:116–23.

Diaper dermatitis

Jordan WE, Blaney TL. Factors influencing diaper dermatitis. In: Maibach HI, Boisits EK (eds), *Neonatal skin structure and function*. Marcel Dekker, New York, 1982, p. 217.

Neville EA, Finn OA. Psoriasiform napkin dermatitis – a follow-up study. *Br J Dermatol*. 1975, **92**:279–85.

Sires UI, Mallory SB. Diaper dermatitis: how to treat and prevent. *Postgrad Med*. 1995, **98**:79–86.

Stein H. Incidence of diaper rash when using cloth and disposable diapers. *J Pediatr*. 1982, **101**:721–3.

Seborrheic dermatitis

Skinner RB Jr, Noah PW, Taylor RM, *et al*. Double blind treatment of seborrheic dermatitis with 2% ketoconazole cream. *J Am Acad Dermatol*. 1985, **12**:852–6.

Yates VM, Kerr EI, Mackie RM. Early diagnosis of infantile seborrheic dermatitis and atopic dermatitis – clinical features. *Br J Dermatol*. 1983, **108**:633–45.

Histiocytosis X

Esterly NB, Maurer HS, Gonzales-Crussi F. Histiocytosis X: a seven year experience at a children's hospital. *J Am Acad Dermatol*. 1985, **13**:481–96.

Gianotte F, Caputo R. Histiocytic syndromes: a review. *J Am Acad Dermatol*. 1985, **13**:383–404.

Roper SS, Spraker MK. Cutaneous histiocytosis syndromes. *Pediatr Dermatol*. 1985, **3**:19–30.

Acrodermatitis enteropathica

Campo AG Jr, McDonald CJ. Treatment of acrodermatitis enteropathica with zinc sulfate. *Arch Dermatol*. 1976, **112**:687–9.

Danbolt N, Closs K. Acrodermatitis enteropathica. *Acta Dermatol Venereol (Stockh)*. 1942, **23**:127–69.

Ghali FE, Steinberg JB, Tunnessen WW Jr. Picture of the month: acrodermatitis enteropathica-like rash in cystic fibrosis. *Arch Pediatr Adolesc Med*. 1996, **150**:99–100.

Gonzalez JR, Botet MV, Sanchez JL. The histopathology of acrodermatitis enteropathica. *Am J Dermatopathol*. 1982, **4**:303–11.

Congenital syphilis

Dorfman DH, Glaser JH. Congenital syphilis presenting in infants after the newborn period. *N Engl J Med*. 1990, **323**:1299–301.

Mascola L, Pelosi R, Blount JH, *et al*. Congenital syphilis revisited. *Am J Dis Child*. 1985, **139**:575–80.

McIntosh K. Editorial: Congenital syphilis – breaking through the safety net. *N Engl J Med*. 1990, **323**:1339–40.

Rathbun KC. Congenital syphilis. *Sex Transm Dis*. 1983, **10**:93–9.

Herpes simplex

Jenista JA. Perinatal herpesvirus infections. *Semin Perinatol*. 1983, **7**:9–15.

Whitley R, Arvin A, Prober C, *et al*. A controlled trial comparing vidarabine with acyclovir in neonatal herpes simplex infection. *N Engl J Med*. 1991, **324**:444–9.

Whitley R, Arvin A, Prober C, *et al*. Predictors of morbidity and mortality in neonates with herpes simplex virus infections. *N Engl J Med*. 1991, **324**:450–4.

Varicella

Glickman FS, Albanese P, Kuhnlein E. Congenital varicella. *Cutis*. 1981, **28**:578–80.

Herrmann KL. Congenital and perinatal varicella. *Clin Obstet Gynecol*. 1982, **25**:605–9.

La Foret E, Lynch CL. Multiple congenital defects following maternal varicella. *N Engl J Med*. 1947, **236**:534–7.

Staphylococcal scalded skin syndrome

Elias PM, Fritsch P, Epstein EH Jr. Staphylococcal scalded skin syndrome (review). *Arch Dermatol*. 1977, **113**:207–19.

Gemmell CG. Staphylococcal scalded skin syndrome. *J Med Microbiol*. 1995, **43**:318–27.

Ginsburg CM. Staphylococcal toxin syndromes. *Pediatr Infect Dis*. 1983, **2**(Suppl.):23.

Lina G, Gillet Y, Vandenesch F, Jones ME, Floret D, Etienne J. Toxin involvement in staphylococcal scalded skin syndrome. *Clin Infect Dis*. 1997, **25**:1369–73.

Lyell A. Toxic epidermal necrolysis (the scalded skin syndrome): a reappraisal. *Br J Dermatol*. 1979, **100**:69–86.

Candidiasis

Chapel TA, Gagliardi C, Nichols W. Congenital cutaneous candidiasis. *J Am Acad Dermatol*. 1998, **6**:926–8.

Gibrey MD, Siegfried EC. Cutaneous congenital candidiasis: a case report (see comments). *Pediatr Dermatol*. 1995, **12**:359–63.

Johnson DE, Thompson TR, Ferrieri P. Congenital candidiasis. *Am J Dis Child*. 1981, **135**:273–5.

Scabies

Meinking TL, Taplin D, Hermida JL, Pardo R, Kerdel FA. The treatment of scabies with ivermectin. *N Engl J Med*. 1995, **333**:26–30.

Orkin M, Maibach HI. Scabies treatment: current considerations. *Curr Prob Dermatol*. 1996, **24**:151–6.

Taplin D, Meinking TL, Chen JA, Sanchez R. Comparison of crotamiton 10% cream (Eurax) and permethrin 5% cream (Elimite) for the treatment of scabies in children. *Pediatr Dermatol*. 1990, **7**:67–73.

Epidermolysis

Hintner H, Stingl G, Schuler G, *et al*. Immunofluorescence mapping of antigen determinants within the dermal–epidermal junction in mechanobullous diseases. *J Invest Dermatol*. 1981, **76**:113–18.

Lin AN. Management of patients with epidermolysis bullosa. *Dermatol Clin*. 1996, **14**:381–7.

Aplasia cutis congenita

Evers ME, Steijlen PM, Hamel BC. Aplasia cutis congenita and associated disorders: an update. *Clin Genet*. 1995, **47**:295–301.

Frieden IJ. Aplasia cutis congenita: a clinical review and proposal for classification. *J Am Acad Dermatol*. 1986, **14**:646–60.

Mastyocytosis

Caplan RM. The natural course of urticaria pigmentosa. *Arch Dermatol*. 1983, **87**:146–57.

Guzzo C, Lavker R, Roberts LJ, Fox K, Schechter N, Lazarus G. Urticaria pigmentosa: systemic evaluation and successful treatment with topical steroids. *Arch Dermatol*. 1991, **127**:191–6.

Simon RA. Treatment of mastocytosis. *N Engl J Med*. 1980, **302**:231–2.

Smith, ML, Orton PW, Chu HM, Weston W. Photochemotherapy of dominant, diffuse, cutaneous mastocytosis. *Pediatr Dermatol*. 1990, **7**:251–5.

Soter NA, Austen KF, Wasserman SL. Oral sodium cromoglycate in the treatment of systemic mastocytosis. *N Engl J Med*. 1979, **401**:465–9.

Incontinentia pigmenti

Carney RG. Incontinentia pigmenti, a world statistical analysis. *Arch Dermatol*. 1976, **112**:535–42.

Cohen BA. Incontinentia pigmenti. *Neurol Clin North Am*. 1987, **5**:361–77.

Francis JS, Sybert VP. Incontinentia pigmenti. *Semin Cutan Med Surg*. 1997, **16**:54–60.

Vascular nevi

Burns AJ, Kaplan LC, Mulliken JB. Is there an association between hemangiomas and syndromes with dysmorphic features? *Pediatrics*. 1991, **88**:1257–67.

Cohen BA. Management of vascular lesions in adolescents. *Adolesc Med*. 1990, **1**:385–400.

Enjolas O, Riche MC, Merland JJ, *et al*. Management of alarming hemangiomas in infancy: a review of 25 cases. *Pediatrics*. 1990, **85**:491–8.

Ezekowitz RAB, Mulliken JB, Folkman J. Interferon α-2a therapy for life-threatening hemangiomas of infancy. *N Engl J Med*. 1992, **326**:1456–63.

Margileth AM, Museles M. Current concepts in diagnosis and management of congenital cutaneous hemangiomas. *Pediatrics*. 1965, **36**:410–6.

Martinez-Perez DM, Fein N, Boon LM, Mulliken JB. Not all hemangiomas look like strawberries: uncommon presentation of the most common tumor of infancy, *Pediatrics*. 1995, **12**:1–6.

Reyes BA, Geronemus R. Treatment of port-wine stains during childhood with the flashlamp-pumped pulsed dye laser. *J Am Acad Dermatol*. 1990, **23**:1142–8.

Sadan N, Wolach B. Treatment of hemangiomas of infants with high dose prednisone, *J Pediatr*. 1996, **128**:141–6.

Tallman B, Tan O, Morelli JG, Piepenbrink J, Stafford B, *et al*. Location of port-wine stains and the likelihood of ophthalmic and/or central nervous system complications. *Pediatrics*. 1991, **87**:323–7.

Lymphangiomas

Hilliard RI, McKendry JBJ, Phillips MJ. Experience and reason – briefly recorded: congenital abnormalities of the lymphatic system: a new clinical classification. *Pediatrics*. 1990, **86**:988–94.

Levine C. Primary disorders of the lymphatic vessels: a unified concept. *J Pediatr Surg*. 1989, **24**:233–40.

Epidermal nevus

Rogers M. Epidermal nevus and the epidermal nevus syndromes: a review of 233 cases. *Pediatr Dermatol*. 1992, **9**:342–44.

Happle R. Epidermal nevus syndromes. *Semin Dermatol*. 1995, **14**:111–21.

Sebaceous nevus

Domingo J, Helwig EB. Malignant neoplasmas associated with nevus sebaceus of Jadassohn. *J Am Acad Dermatol*. 1979, **1**:545.

Morioka S. The natural history of nevus sebaceus. *J Cutan Pathol*. 1985, **12**:200–13.

Smooth muscle nevus

Bronson DM, Fretzin DF, Farrell LN. Congenital pilar and smooth muscle nevus. *J Am Acad Dermatol*. 1983, **8**:111–4.

Connective tissue nevus

Gantan RK, Kar HK, Jain RK, Bagga GR, Sharma SK, Bhardwaj M. Isolated collagenoma: a case report with a review of connective tissue nevi of the collagen type. *J Dermatol*. 1996, **23**:476–8.

Schorr WF, Opitz JM, Reyes CN. The connective tissue nevus–osteopoikilosis syndrome. *Arch Dermatol*. 1972, **106**:208–14.

Verbov J, Graham R. Buschke–Ollendorff syndrome – disseminated dermatofibrosis with osteopoikilosis. *Clin Exp Dermatol*. 1986, **11**:17–26.

Pigmented nevi

Everett MA. Histopathology of congenital pigmented nevi. *Am J Dermatopathol*. 1989, **11**:11–12.

Marghoob AA, Schoenbach P, Kopf AV, Orlow SJ, Nossa R, Bart RS. Large congenital melanocytic nevi and the risk for the development of malignant melanoma: a prospective study. *Arch Dermatol*. **132**:170–5.

Silvers DN, Helwig EB. Melanocytic nevi in neonates. *J Am Acad Dermatol*. 1981, **4**:166–75.

Swerdlow AJ, English JS, Qiao Z. The risk of melanoma in patients with congenital nevi: a cohort study. *J Am Acad Dermatol*. 1995, **32**:595–9.

Juvenile xanthogranuloma

Cohen BA, Hood A. Xanthogranuloma: report on clinical and histologic findings in 64 patients. *J Pediatr Dermatol*. 1989, **6**:262–6.

Sangueza OP, Salmon JK, White CR Jr, Beckstead JH. Juvenile xanthogranuloma: a clinical, histologic and immunohistochemical study. *J Cutan Pathol*. 1995, **122**:327–35.

Dermoid cyst

Kennard CD, Rasmussen JE. Congenital midline nasal masses: diagnosis and management. *J Dermatol Surg Oncol*. 1990, **16**:1025–36.

Smirniotopoulos JG, Chiechi MV. Teratomas, dermoids and epidermoids of the head and neck. *Radiographics*. 1995, **15**:1437–55.

Recurrent infantile digital fibroma

Burgert S, Jones DH. Recurring digital fibroma of childhood. *J Hand Surg (Br)*. 1996, **21**:400–2.

Falco NA, Upton J. Infantile digital fibroma. *J Hand Surg (Am)*. 1995, **20**:1014–20.

Infantile myofibromatosis

Spraker MK, Stack C, Esterly NB. Congenital generalized fibromatosis. *J Am Acad Dermatol*. 1984, **10**:365–71.

Variend S, Bax NM, van Gorp J. Are infantile myofibromatosis, congenital fibrosarcoma and congenital haemangiopericytoma histogenetically related? *Histopathology*. 1995, **26**:57–62.

Venecie PV, Bigel P, Desgruelles C, *et al*. Infantile myofibromatosis. *Br J Dermatol*. 1987, **117**:255–9.

Malignant tumors

Abdesalam AR, Heyn R, Tefft M, Hays D, Newton WA Jr, Beltangady M. Infants younger than 1 year of age with rhabdomyosarcoma. *Cancer*. 1986, **58**:2606–10.

Francis JS, Sybert VP, Benjamin DR. Congenital monocytic leukemia: report of a case with cutaneous involvement, and review of the literature. *J Pediatr Dermatol*. 1989, **6**:306–11.

Schneider KM, Becker GM, Krasna IH. Neonatal neuroblastoma. *Pediatrics*. 1965, **36**:359–66.

Xue H, Horwitz JR, Smith MB, *et al*. Malignant solid tumors in neonates: a 40 year review. *J Pediatr Surg*. 1995, **30**:543–5.

Neonatal lupus erythematosus

Buyon JP. Neonatal lupus syndromes. *Curr Opin Rheumatol*. 1994, **6**:523–9.

Lee LA, Weston WL. New findings in neonatal lupus syndrome. *Am J Dis Child*. 1984, **138**:233–6.

Watson RM, Lane AT, Barnett NK, *et al*. Neonatal lupus erythematosus. A clinical, serological and immunogenetic study with review of the literature. *Medicine (Baltimore)*. 1984, **63**:362–78.

Annular erythema of infancy

Helm TN, Bass J, Chang LW, Bergfeld WF. Persistent annular erythema of infancy. *Pediatr Dermatol*. 1993, **10**:46–8.

Peterson AQ Jr, Jarratt M. Annular erythema of infancy. *Arch Dermatol*. 1981, **117**:145–8.

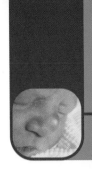

Chapter Three

Papulosquamous Eruptions

INTRODUCTION

Papulosquamous eruptions comprise a group of disorders characterized by the presence of superficial papules and scale. These conditions account for a large number of patients in both pediatric dermatology and pediatric primary-care practice. In disorders of keratinization (psoriasis, pityriasis rubra pilaris, keratosis follicularis, ichthyosis, hyperkeratosis of the palms and soles, and porokeratosis), cutaneous lesions develop as a result of genetically programmed retention or increased production of scale at the surface. In the inflammatory dermatoses (dermatitides, pityriasis rosea, pityriasis lichenoides, lichenoid dermatoses, and fungal infections), clinical findings result from epidermal response to dermal inflammation.

DISORDERS OF KERATINIZATION

Psoriasis

Psoriasis is a common disorder characterized by red, well demarcated plaques with a dry, thick, silvery scale (Fig 3.1). The condition affects 1–3% of Americans, of whom almost 20% develop the rash before the age of 20 years.

Psoriasis is a multifactorial disorder with both hereditary and environmental components. In more than one-third of patients, other family members are affected. A number of human leukocyte antigen (HLA) types have been associated with psoriasis in different populations.

Cutaneous lesions tend to locate on the scalp, the sacrum, and the extensor surfaces of the extremities. About 50% of children present with large plaques over the knees and

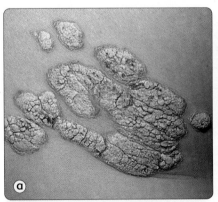
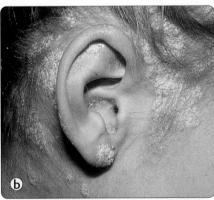
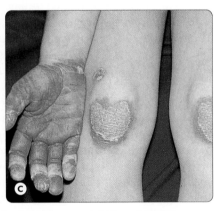
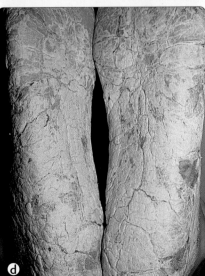
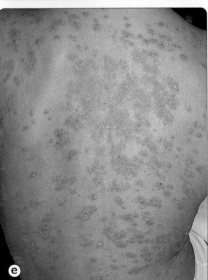

Fig 3.1 Psoriasis. **(a)** Typical erythematous plaques are topped by a silver scale on the trunk of an adolescent. **(b)** Thick tenacious scale extends from the forehead, neck, and ears onto the scalp of this 10-year-old girl. **(c)** Thick plaques on the palms, soles, elbows, and knees of this 8-year-old boy caused severe pain when he attempted to walk or use his hands. **(d)** Another boy with an impressive plantar keratoderma had difficulty walking. **(e)** Widespread guttate lesions erupted on the trunk and extremities of this child 1 week after a streptococcal pharyngitis.

elbows. Thickening and fissuring of the skin of the palms and soles may also be present (Fig 3.1c,d). In a third of children, many drop-like lesions (guttate psoriasis) are scattered over the body, including the face, trunk, and extremities (Fig 3.1e). In infancy, psoriasis may present as a persistent diaper dermatitis. In older children the eyelids, genitals, and periumbilical areas are commonly involved (Fig 3.2). Scalp disease may develop as an isolated finding, but is often seen with other variants (see Fig 3.1b). Itchy red plaques with thick, tenacious scale are often evident at the frontal hair line and around the ears. Nail changes include onycholysis (separation of the nail plate from the nail bed to produce 'oil drop changes'), nail pitting, yellowing, increased friability, and subungual hyperkeratosis (see Fig 8.38).

Of psoriasis patients, 8% suffer from psoriatic arthritis, one of the seronegative spondyloarthropathies. In half of these individuals arthritis develops before the skin rash. Examination of the joints characteristically demonstrates heat, pain, and swelling of multiple joints of the hands and feet, particularly the distal interphalangeal joints. The arthritis tends to be progressive with the development of flexure deformities and contractures. In addition to the typical lesions of plaque psoriasis, patients often demonstrate severe psoriatic involvement of the hands, nails and feet (Fig 3.3). The HLA B-27 antigen is usually positive.

Rarely, children develop erythrodermic psoriasis with acute widespread erythema and scaling or pustular psoriasis with generalized erythema and pustule formation (Fig 3.4). These variants are associated with high fevers, chills, arthralgias, myalgias, and severe cutaneous tenderness. Fluid and electrolyte losses and leukocytosis may be marked. Secondary bacterial infection and sepsis can occur.

Although the factors that initiate the rapid turnover in epidermal cells, which contributes to psoriatic plaques, are unknown, a hereditary predisposition is suspected, and upper respiratory tract and streptococcal infections are known to precipitate outbreaks. Psoriatic lesions are often induced in areas of local injury, such as scratches, surgical scars, or sunburn, a response termed the Koebner or isomorphic phenomenon (Fig 3.5). In areas of thick scale, tortuous capillary loops proliferate close to the surface. Gentle removal of the scale results in multiple, small bleeding points, referred to as the Auspitz sign (Fig 3.6).

The diagnosis is usually made by identifying the typical morphology and by the distribution of skin lesions. Confirmatory skin biopsy findings include regular thickening of the epidermal rete ridges, elongation and edema of the dermal papillae, thinning of the epidermis overlying tortuous dermal capillaries, absence of the granular layer, parakeratosis, spongiform pustules, and Munro microabscesses.

The course of psoriasis is chronic and unpredictable, marked by remissions and exacerbations. A number of different topical agents, which include lubricants, corticosteroids, tar, anthralen (dithranol), and keratolytics, are useful in managing cutaneous lesions. Topical tazarotene ointment (a member of the acetylenic class of retinoids), and new topical corticosteroids with ultra-high potency may also play

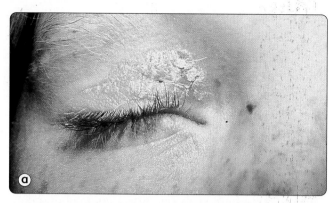

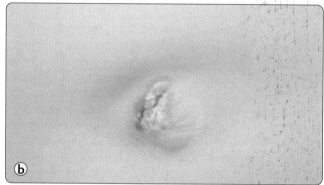

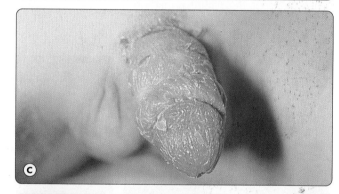

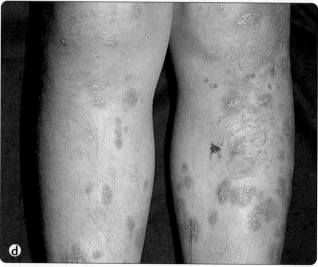

Fig 3.2 These lesions were present on **(a)** the eyelids, **(b)** periumbilical area, and **(c)** penis of this 8-year-old for 6 months before the diagnosis of psoriasis was considered. **(d)** He subsequently developed widespread plaques on the arms and legs.

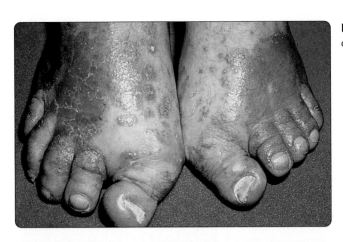

Fig 3.3 Psoriasis and psoriatic arthritis were debilitating in this adolescent girl.

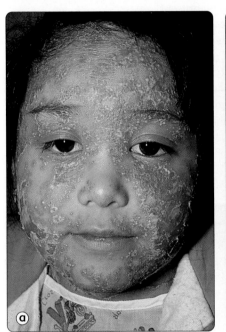

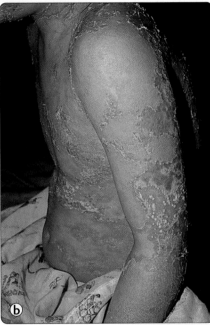

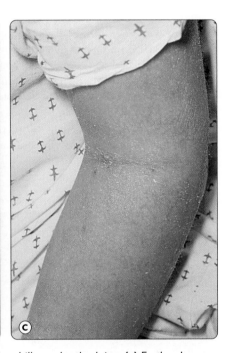

Fig 3.4 Pustular and erythrodermic psoriasis. **(a,b)** Generalized pustulation developed suddenly within psoriatic plaques on this 8-year-old child. Skin lesions were associated with fever, chills, and arthralgias. **(c)** Erythroderma appeared in another 8-year-old girl with psoriasis. She also complained of chills, pruritus, and fatigue.

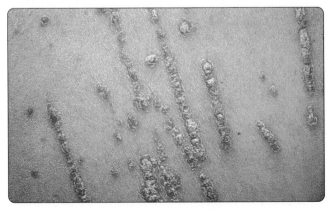

Fig 3.5 Koebner phenomenon in psoriasis. Pruritus was severe in this child who developed linear plaques in excoriations.

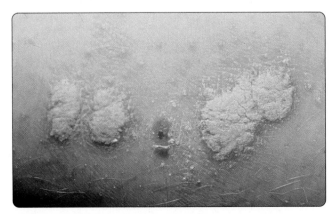

Fig 3.6 Auspitz sign. Removal of the thick scale from a psoriatic plaque produces small points of bleeding from underlying tortuous capillaries.

a role in the treatment of thick, localized plaques in some children. Chronic or recalcitrant disease and psoriatic arthritis may require ultraviolet (UV) light therapy (UVB = sun burn wavelengths and/or PUVA = psoralen photosensitizer plus UVA or long-wavelength ultraviolet light). Life-threatening erythrodermic and pustular psoriasis and psoriatic arthritis usually respond to oral retinoids and antimetabolites. However, the use of systemic agents requires close laboratory and clinical monitoring.

Pityriasis rubra pilaris

Pityriasis rubra pilaris (PRP) is an uncommon disorder of keratinization characterized by small follicular papules, widespread orange–red scaly plaques surrounded by islands of spared skin, and marked thickening of the skin on the palms and soles (Fig 3.7). Onset of disease occurs most commonly in prepubertal children and in adults over 50 years old, and has been associated with trauma and acute, self-limited illness. Most cases are sporadic and acquired, but a familial variant has been reported. Overall, 75% of cases resolve spontaneously within 3–4 years, but in familial disease persistence is the rule.

In childhood, the circumscribed variant, which accounts for a majority of the cases, begins with the development of coalescing hyperkeratotic papules on the elbows and knees and a palmoplantar keratoderma (Fig 3.8). Superficial, red, scaly plaques occasionally appear on the face and trunk. Less commonly, children develop a pattern that mimics the classic adult variety. The eruption begins with follicular, hyperkeratotic patches on the back, chest, and abdomen, which expand to involve interfollicular skin. Lesions on the scalp and other sebaceous areas develop simultaneously or soon thereafter and may disseminate. Even in widespread disease, islands of spared skin of normal appearance are characteristic. Discrete, hyperkeratotic papules may also remain present over the knuckles, wrists, elbows, and knees. In erythrodermic PRP, facial edema and scale may result in ectropion formation. Nail dystrophy with subungual hyperkeratoses may also be present.

The clinical presentation, particularly with keratoderma of the hands and feet and follicular papules, helps to differentiate PRP from psoriasis, seborrheic dermatitis, atopic dermatitis, and pityriasis rosea. A skin biopsy that demonstrates interfollicular orthohyperkeratosis and perifollicular parakeratosis is typical, but not diagnostic.

Although PRP is usually self-limited in childhood, severe, disabling disease may require systemic therapy with retinoids or methotrexate.

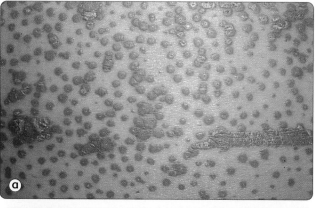

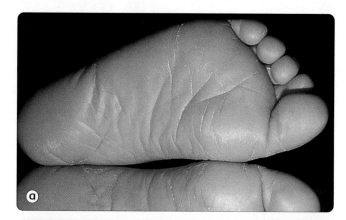

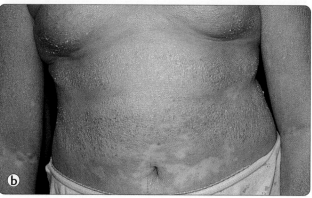

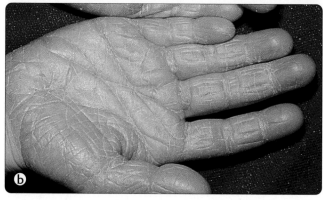

Fig 3.7 Pityriasis rubra pilaris. **(a)** Discrete hyperkeratotic follicular papules on the trunk and extremities of this 10-year-old girl progressed over several weeks to give confluent plaques.
(b) Note several discrete areas of sparing on the abdomen and arm flexures.

Fig 3.8 Pityriasis rubra pilaris. This child developed a salmon-colored keratoderma of the **(a)** soles and **(b)** palms.

Keratosis follicularis (Darier disease)

Keratosis follicularis is an autosomal-dominant disorder that typically presents in children from 8 to 15 years old and is characterized by hyperkeratotic follicular papules on the face, scalp, neck, and seborrheic areas of the trunk (Fig 3.9). Although the onset is usually insidious, a rapidly progressive course may follow an inciting event, such as intense sun exposure or a viral infection. Red, scaly papules coalesce to form widespread, thick, odoriferous, greasy plaques, particularly on the scalp, forehead, around the ears, shoulders, mid-chest, and mid-back. Flexures may also be involved, with moist vegetative plaques.

Other characteristic lesions include flat-topped, warty papules on the dorsum of the hands and tiny hyperkeratotic papules and pits on the palms and soles. Subtle pebbly papules on the oral mucosa may simulate leukoplakia. Nail dystrophy, with thickening or thinning of the nail plate, fracture of the distal nail plate, longitudinal white and red streaks, and subungual hyperkeratosis, may also be present.

Although the cause of Darier disease is unknown, the identification of various T-cell abnormalities by several investigators suggests an immunologic basis. The tendency of affected individuals to develop disseminated herpes simplex (Kaposi varicelliform eruption) and recurrent staphylococcal infections has been recognized for years.

The characteristic clinical picture permits easy differentiation of Darier disease from other papulosquamous disorders such as seborrheic dermatitis, PRP, and psoriasis. Classic histologic changes from skin biopsy, which include dyskeratosis (with the formation of corps ronds and corps grains), suprabasal acantholysis (leading to the formation of suprabasal clefts), and the formation of villi by upward proliferating dermal papillae, confirm the diagnosis.

Although Darier disease tends to persist throughout life, many patients experience episodic flares and remissions in disease activity. Topical vitamin A acid may be helpful in managing early lesions. However, its use is limited by a high

risk of irritation. Experience with oral retinoids has been promising, but prolonged use may be associated with unacceptable complications, which include hyperostosis, epiphyseal plate changes, increased skin fragility, and teratogenicity. Aggressive protection from the sun and treatment of secondary bacterial and viral infections also control exacerbations.

Ichthyoses

The ichthyoses are a heterogeneous group of scaling disorders characterized by retention hyperkeratosis (ichthyosis vulgaris, X-linked ichthyosis) or increased proliferation of epidermal cells (lamellar ichthyosis, epidermolytic hyperkeratosis). These diseases may be differentiated by clinical findings, histopathology, and biochemical markers, as outlined in Chapter 2.

Hyperkeratosis of the palms and soles

Hyperkeratosis includes a heterogeneous group of keratodermas characterized by focal or generalized thickening of the skin of the palms and/or soles and occasionally by more widespread cutaneous lesions associated with systemic disease (Fig 3.10). Unna–Thost, the most common variant, is inherited in an autosomal dominant pattern and presents in the first year of life with diffuse hyperkeratosis restricted to the palmar and plantar surfaces (Fig 3.11). Although lesions may be asymptomatic, hyperhidrosis may lead to maceration and the formation of painful fissuring, blisters, and bacterial superinfection. Unna–Thost must be differentiated from a number of unusual keratodermas associated with hyperkeratoses that extend to the dorsal surfaces of the hands and feet, elbows, knees, and other distant sites (Fig 3.12).

Focal keratoderma with discrete papules and plaques on the palms and soles also appears as an isolated phenomenon or in association with other cutaneous findings and systemic disease. A mild autosomal-dominant variant with pits and hyperkeratotic papules in the hand and foot creases occurs in 2–5% of blacks (Fig 3.13). Occasionally, this keratoderma is painful and requires surgical treatment.

Neurosensory deafness, carcinoma of the esophagus (Howel–Evans syndrome), and peripheral neuropathy (Charcot–Marie–Tooth disease) are rarely associated with palmoplantar keratoderma and may be excluded by auditory screening and a careful family history. Hyperkeratosis of the extremities that presents as part of a diffuse disorder of keratinization, such as psoriasis or PRP, is differentiated by a thorough examination of the integument.

Porokeratosis

Porokeratosis is a disorder of keratinization characterized by annular, sharply demarcated plaques with raised hyperkeratotic borders (Fig 3.14). Four variants are recognized, based on morphology and distribution of the lesions, time of onset, triggering factors, and mode of inheritance.

Porokeratosis of Mibelli

Subtle, reddish-brown, scaly papules that slowly enlarge to form irregularly shaped plaques with hypopigmented atrophic

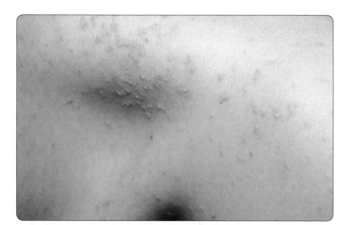

Fig 3.9 Keratosis follicularis. Hyperkeratotic follicular papules erupted progressively on the trunk and face of this 9-year-old girl. Some of the most prominent lesions are demonstrated on her shoulder.

Variants of palmoplantar keratoderma						
Type	Disorder	Genetics	Onset	Involvement	Hyperhidrosis	Associated findings
Diffuse palmoplantar keratoderma	Unna–Thost syndrome	Autosomal dominant (1/200–1/40,000; varies with ethnic group)	Infancy	Palms, soles	Severe	
	Keratoma hereditarium mutilans (Vohwinkel syndrome)	Autosomal dominant (rare)	Infancy	Honeycombe keratoderma; star-shaped plaques on hands, feet, elbows, knees	±	Digital constriction band; deafness; alopecia
	Mal de Meleda	Autosomal recessive	Infancy	Palms, soles, elbows, knees, including dorsal surfaces (transgridiens)	±	Flexion contractures; constriction bands; koilonychia
	Howel–Evans syndrome	Autosomal dominant	Adolescence	Soles, sometimes palms	±	Esophageal carcinoma; epidermal cysts; thin lateral eyebrows; follicular papules
	Papillon–Lefèvre syndrome	Autosomal recessive	Birth to 2–3 years	Soles more severe than palms, intense erythema, wrists, ankles, elbows, knees; follicular hyperkeratoses	±	Nail dystrophy; periodontitis; calcification of falx cerebri; mental retardation; arachnodactyly
	Olmsted syndrome	Autosomal recessive?	Infancy	Progressive, diffuse involvement of hands, feet, leads to flexion contractures, digital amputation	(Anhidrosis)	Periorificial hyperkeratosis
Focal palmoplantar keratoderma	Punctate palmoplantar keratoderma	Autosomal dominant (2–5% African–Caribbeans)	Childhood	Palms, soles	–	Variable
	Palmoplantar keratoderma striata	Autosomal dominant	Adolescence	Palms, fingers		Variable
	Tyrosinemia Type II (Richner–Hanhart syndrome)	Autosomal recessive	Infancy through adulthood	Fingertips, palms		Corneal ulcerations; mental retardation
	Porokeratosis	Autosomal dominant (rare)	Childhood through adulthood	Extremities, trunk	–	Squamous cell carcinoma

Fig 3.10 Variants of palmoplantar keratoderma.

centers and raised, grooved borders are typical of this condition, which invariably develops in childhood (Fig 3.14a,b). Plaques are usually unilateral, and vary in size from a few millimeters to several centimeters in diameter. One to three lesions are usually present. This rare, autosomal-dominant variant appears most commonly on the extremities, thighs, and perigenital skin, although any area that contains mucous membranes can be involved. Biopsies of the longitudinal furrow in the border demonstrate the diagnostic coronoid lamella, which consists of a parakeratotic column that fills a deep, epidermal invagination. Squamous cell carcinoma may arise within these slowly progressive lesions. Although excision or carbon dioxide laser surgery may be useful, recurrences have been reported.

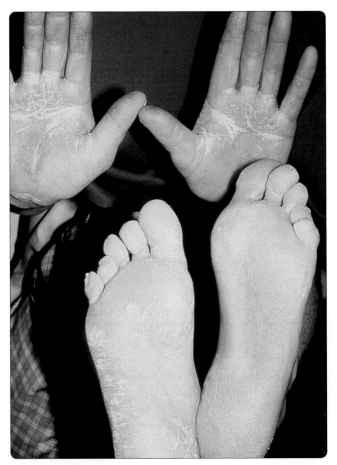

Fig 3.11 Progressive hyperkeratosis of the palms and soles began at 5 months of age in this 10-year-old child whose father and sister had similar findings.

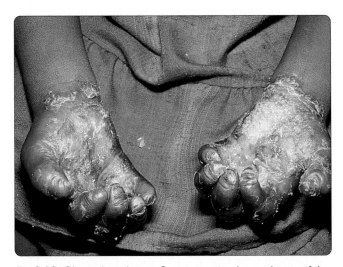

Fig 3.12 Olmsted syndrome. Severe scarring keratoderma of the palms and soles was associated with perioral and perigenital hyperkeratosis, hyperhidrosis, recurrent cutaneous infections, and poor growth in this 5-year-old girl. Treatment with oral retinoids resulted in some decrease in the palmar and plantar lesions.

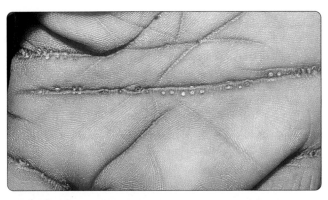

Fig 3.13 Focal keratoderma. Asymptomatic hyperkeratotic papules and pits on the hand creases of a black teenager.

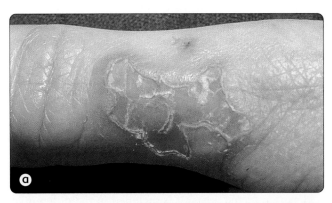

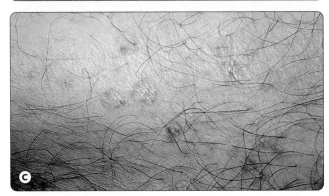

Fig 3.14 Porokeratosis. Porokeratosis of Mibelli on **(a)** the thumb and **(b)** upper thigh. **(c)** This adolescent with disseminated superficial actinic porokeratosis began to develop asymptomatic nummular patches on his legs after a sunburn when he was 16 years old. Note the hyperkeratotic borders, which demonstrated a coronoid lamella on skin biopsy. All lesions were slowly progressive.

Linear porokeratosis

This variant presents much like the Mibelli variant. However, plaques are linearly arranged on the distal extremities and trunk, where they demonstrate a zosteriform pattern. Onset is also in early childhood, but the mode of inheritance has not been established.

Disseminated superficial actinic porokeratosis

Disseminated superficial actinic porokeratosis is a common autosomal-dominant variant with delayed expression, found primarily in lightly pigmented individuals of Celtic extraction. Many small, 2–4 mm diameter hyperkeratotic papules appear symmetrically on sun-exposed surfaces of the extremities during the second and third decades of life (Fig 3.14c). These brown, red, or skin-colored lesions may coalesce to form irregular, circinate patterns. Progression of papules, which occurs particularly during the summer months, can be slowed by aggressive use of sun protection.

Punctate porokeratosis

Punctate porokeratosis affects the palms and soles and has been described as a distinct entity. However, it usually presents in association with the Mibelli or linear variant. Punctate porokeratosis may also occur as a widely disseminated form reminiscent of disseminated superficial actinic porokeratosis, but with involvement of both sun-exposed and sun-protected areas. It is included in the differential diagnosis of punctate keratoderma.

INFLAMMATORY DERMATOSES

Many of these disorders demonstrate changes of both acute (erythema, edema, vesiculation, crusts) and chronic (scaling, lichenification, hypopigmentation, hyperpigmentation) inflammation. Microscopically, dermatitis is recognized by the presence of intercellular edema (spongiosis), variable epidermal thickening (acanthosis), and the presence of dermal inflammatory cells, usually lymphocytes. Various dermatitic disorders may be differentiated by clinical features and specific histologic patterns.

A reasonable way to think of the dermatitides is as exogenous ('outside job') versus endogenous ('inside job') phenomena. Exogenous disorders include irritant and allergic contact dermatitis, and photodermatitis. Endogenous dermatitides include atopic dermatitis, dyshidrotic eczema, nummular dermatitis, and seborrheic dermatitis. Juvenile palmar and plantar dermatoses and perioral dermatitis are triggered by a combination of inside and outside factors. Pityriasis rosea and parapsoriasis present with distinctive dermatitic patterns, but their causes are unclear.

Contact dermatitis

Contact dermatitis refers to a group of conditions in which an inflammatory reaction in the skin is triggered by direct contact with environmental agents. In the most common form, irritant contact dermatitis, changes in the skin are induced by caustic agents such as acids, alkalis, hydrocarbons, and other primary irritants. Anyone exposed to these agents in a high enough concentration for a long enough period of time develops a reaction. The rash is usually acute (occurring within minutes), with itching or burning, well-demarcated erythema, edema, blister formation, and/or crust formation.

In contrast, allergic contact dermatitis is a T-cell mediated immune reaction to an antigen that comes into contact with the skin. Although it frequently presents with dramatic onset of erythema, vesiculation, and pruritus, the rash may become chronic with scaling, lichenification, and pigmentary changes (Fig 3.15). At times the allergen is obvious, such as poison ivy or nickel-containing jewelry. Often, however, some detective work is required to elicit the inciting agent. The initial reaction occurs after a period of sensitization of 7–14 days in susceptible individuals. Once sensitization has occurred, re-exposure to the allergen provides a more rapid reaction, sometimes within hours. This is a classic example of a Type IV delayed-hypersensitivity response.

The most common allergic contact dermatitis in the US is poison ivy or rhus dermatitis, which typically appears as linear streaks of erythematous papules and vesicles (Fig 3.16). However, with heavy exposure or in exquisitely sensitive individuals, the rash may appear in large patches. When lesions involve the skin of the face or genitals, impressive swelling can occur and obscure the primary eruption. Direct contact with the sap of the plant (poison ivy, poison oak, or poison sumac), whether from leaves, stems, or roots, produces the dermatitis (Fig 3.17). Indirect contact, such as with clothing or pets that have brushed against the plant, with logs or railroad ties on which the vine has been growing, or with smoke from a fire in which the plant is being burned, is another means of exposure. Areas of skin exposed to the highest concentration of rhus antigen develop the changes first. Other sites that have received lower doses react in succession, which gives the illusion of spreading. However, once on the skin, the allergen becomes fixed to epithelial cells within about 20 minutes and cannot be spread further. Thorough washing within minutes of exposure may prevent or reduce the eruption. Barrier creams (e.g. Ivy Guard®) applied before exposure may afford some protection.

Other common contact allergens include nickel, rubber, glues and/or dyes in shoes, ethylenediamine in topical lubricants, neomycin in topical antibiotics, and topical anesthetics. Several studies using standard patch-test techniques show that the prevalence of contact sensitivity in children to these common allergens is similar to the prevalence in adults.

Some allergens, known as photosensitizers, require sunlight to become activated. Photocontact dermatitis caused by drugs (e.g. tetracyclines, sulfonylureas, and thiazides) characteristically erupts in a symmetric distribution on the face, the 'V' of the neck, and the arms below the shirt sleeves. Topical photosensitizers (e.g. dyes, furocoumarins, halogenated salicylanilides, p-aminobenzoic acid) produce localized patches of dermatitis when applied to sun-exposed sites. These agents are found in cosmetics, sunscreens, dermatologic products, germicidal soaps, and woodland and house plants (see Chapter 7).

Occasionally, the local reaction in a contact dermatitis is so severe that the patient develops a widespread, secondary eczematous dermatitis. When the dermatitis appears at sites that have not been in contact with the offending agent, the reaction is referred to as 'autoeczematization' or an 'id' reaction.

A careful history usually reveals the source of contact dermatitis. In some patients, patch testing with a standardized tray of common antigens or the suspected antigen and several controls is necessary to confirm the diagnosis.

Although small areas of contact dermatitis are best treated topically, widespread reactions require and respond within 48 hours to a 2-to 3-week tapering course of systemic corticosteroid; these begin at 0.5–1.0mg/kg/day. Patients may

experience rebound of the rash when treated with a shorter course. Oral corticosteroids may also be indicated in severe local reactions that involve the eyelids, extensive parts of the face, the genitals, and/or the hands, where swelling and pruritus may become incapacitating.

Atopic dermatitis

Also known as eczema, this is a chronically recurrent, genetically influenced skin disorder of early infancy, childhood, and occasionally adult life. Although it was initially described in the nineteenth century, it was not until 1935 that Hill and

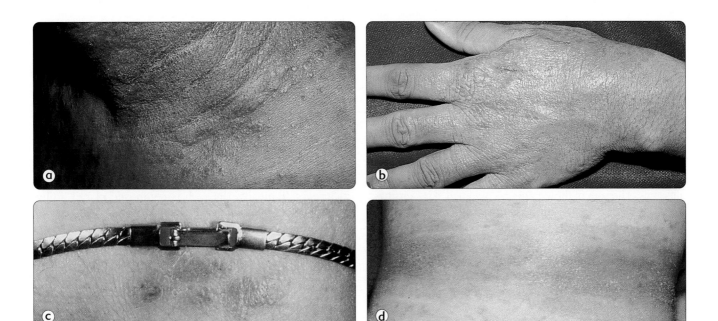

Fig 3.15 Allergic contact dermatitis. Allergic contact dermatitis as a result of the application of benzocaine demonstrates sharply demarcated, hyperpigmented, lichenified patches on **(a)** the neck and **(b)** the top of the hands. **(c)** The location of the rash helps to determine the cause of a contact dermatitis, such as in this girl with a nickel allergy. **(d)** This child became sensitized to the elastic waistbands of his underwear.

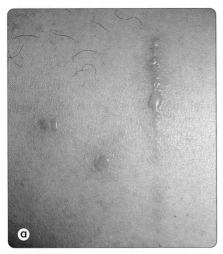
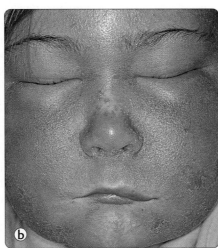
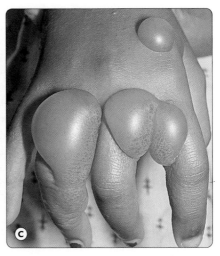

Fig 3.16 Poison ivy or rhus dermatitis. **(a)** Linear streaks of pruritic papules and vesicles are typical of contact dermatitis to a plant, as seen on the thigh of this 13-year-old boy. **(b)** A 10- year-old girl developed intense facial edema after brushing against poison ivy. **(c)** In highly sensitized children, large blisters can develop. This child was swinging from vines in the woods.

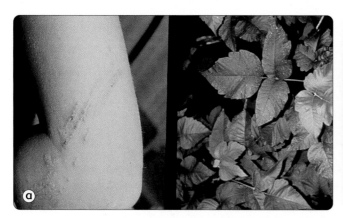

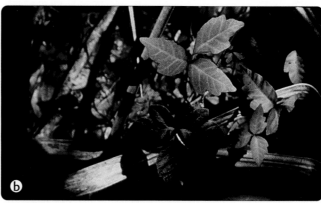

Fig 3.17 Plants that provoke dermatitis after direct contact with the sap. **(a)** Poison ivy has characteristic shiny leaves in groups of three; it may grow as a vine or low shrub or bush.

(b) Poison oak (courtesy of Dr Mary Jelks) also has leaves in groups of three, although the edges tend to be more scalloped than those of poison ivy.

Sultzberger first characterized the clinical entity. The term atopy, derived from the Greek word which means 'not confined to a single place', was introduced in 1923 by Coca and Cooke to describe a cohort of patients with asthma and allergic rhinitis who demonstrated immediate wheal and flare reactions upon skin testing with a variety of environmental allergens. The sera of these patients contained skin-sensitizing antibodies that were subsequently characterized as IgE immunoglobulins. It was later recognized that these atopic individuals also frequently manifested the itchy, eczematous dermatitis which was labeled atopic dermatitis.

Although data are not precise, recent surveys reveal that atopic dermatitis is rather common, with an incidence of 7/1000 individuals in the US. The prevalence is highest among children, affecting 3–5% of all children between 6 months and 10 years of age. Subtle findings may be present during the first few months of life, and nearly 60% of patients have an initial outbreak by their first birthday. Another third develop disease between 1 and 5 years. The onset of eczema in adolescence and adulthood is unusual and should alert the clinician to possibility of other diagnoses.

In families with a history of allergic rhinitis of asthma, nearly one-third of the children are expected to develop skin lesions of atopic dermatitis. Inversely, in patients with atopic dermatitis, one-third are expected to have a personal history of allergic rhinitis or asthma, with two-thirds showing a family history of these disorders. Half of those who manifest the dermatologic condition in infancy or childhood ultimately develop allergic respiratory symptoms. Atopic dermatitis does not appear to be linked to the histocompatability locus antigen, as has been described in allergic rhinitis. Rather, it seems to be inherited as an autosomal trait with multifactorial influences.

The term eczema, which means 'boil over', is used by many physicians when referring to atopic dermatitis. However, most dermatologists use the word eczematous as a morphologic term to describe the clinical findings in various sorts of acute (erythema, scaling, vesicles, and crusts) and chronic (scaling, lichenification, and pigmentary changes) dermatitis. Both acute and chronic dermatitis may be present in atopic patients at different sites at the same time and the same site at different times during the course of the disease.

The distribution and morphology of skin lesions in atopic dermatitis are diagnostic, and the clinical findings show a characteristic pattern of evolution (Fig 3.18). The infantile phase begins between 1 and 6 months of age and lasts about 2–3 years. Typically, the rash is composed of red, itchy papules and plaques, many of which ooze and crust. Lesions are symmetrically distributed over the cheeks, forehead, scalp, trunk, and the extensor surfaces of the extremities (Fig 3.19). The diaper area is usually spared.

The childhood phase of atopic dermatitis occurs between 4 and 10 years of age. Circumscribed, erythematous, scaly, lichenified plaques are symmetrically distributed on the wrists, ankles, and flexural surfaces of the arms and legs (Fig 3.20). The ear creases and back of the neck are also commonly involved. These areas develop frequent secondary infections, probably as a result of the introduction of organisms by intense scratching. Although the eruption may become chronic and rarely generalized, remissions may occur at any time. Most children experience improvement during the warm, humid summer months and exacerbations during the fall and winter.

Of children with atopic dermatitis, 75% improve by 10–14 years of age; the remaining individuals may go on to develop chronic adult disease. Major areas of involvement include the flexural creases of the arms, neck, and legs. Chronic dermatitis may be restricted to the hands or feet, but some patients develop recurrent, widespread lesions.

Nummular eczematous dermatitis
Although nummular eczematous dermatitis was initially described as distinct from atopic dermatitis, clinicians frequently use this term to describe the discrete, coin-shaped, red patches seen on many patients with atopic dermatitis (Fig 3.21). Lesions typically appear as tiny papules and vesicles, which form confluent patches on the arms and legs. Nummular lesions may be extremely pruritic, and they are difficult to treat, particularly during the winter months when the incidence seems to peak.

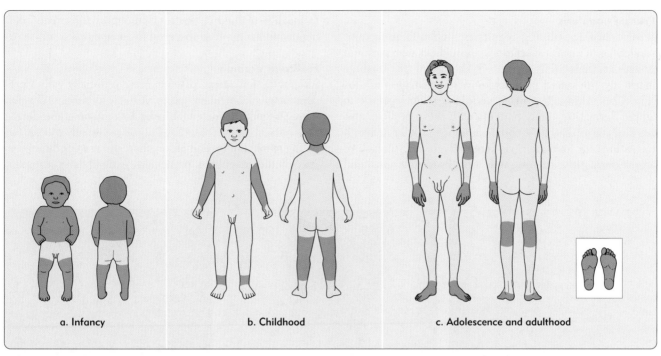

a. Infancy   b. Childhood   c. Adolescence and adulthood

Fig 3.18 Characteristic distribution of lesions of atopic dermatitis in infancy, childhood, and adulthood. **(a)** In infancy, widespread lesions may be generalized, sparing only the diaper area. The head and neck, as well as the flexural and extensor surfaces of the distal extremities, are often severely involved. **(b)** In older childhood, lesions tend to involve the flexural surfaces of the upper and lower extremities, as well as the neck. With severe flares of disease activity, the rash may become more generalized. **(c)** In adults, the lesions are usually restricted to the flexural creases. In some patients, however, involvement of the palms and soles may become particularly prominent.

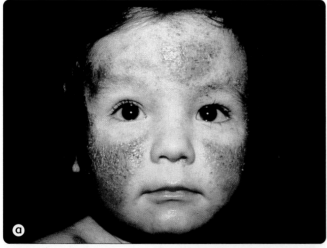

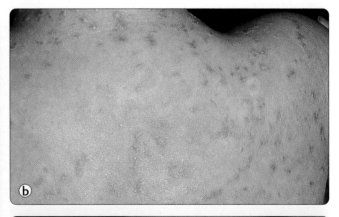

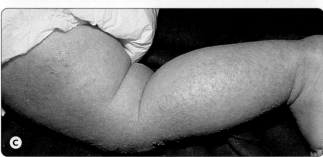

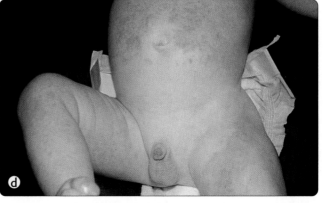

Fig 3.19 Infantile eczema. **(a)** This infant has an acute, weeping dermatitis on the cheeks and forehead. Involvement of **(b)** the trunk and **(c)** the extremities with erythema, scaling, and crusting is evident. Note the severe involvement of the extensor surfaces of the leg and sparing of the leg crease. **(d)** Usually the diaper area is the only portion of the skin surface that is spared.

Prurigo nodularis

While chronic rubbing results in lichenification, and scratching in linear excoriations, individuals who pick and gouge at their itchy, irritated skin tend to produce markedly thickened papules known as prurigo nodules (Fig 3.22). Although prurigo nodularis is not specific to atopic dermatitis, many patients with these nodules also have an atopic diathesis, which manifests as allergic rhinitis, asthma, or food allergy. Frequently, other stigmata of atopic dermatitis are present as well. Prurigo lesions tend to localize to the extremities, although widespread cutaneous involvement is observed in some cases.

Follicular eczema

Although a few atopic patients present initially with a predominance of follicular papules, virtually all patients develop these 2–4 mm diameter follicular lesions sometime during their clinical course (Fig 3.23). Lesions are usually widespread on the trunk, but careful observation also reveals their presence on the extremities, particularly early in flares of disease

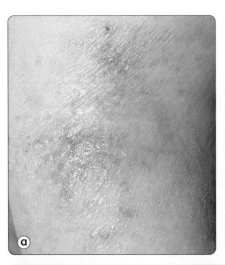
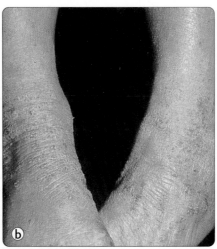
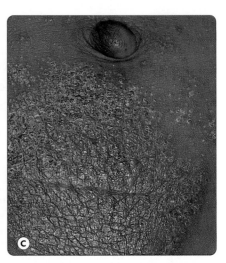
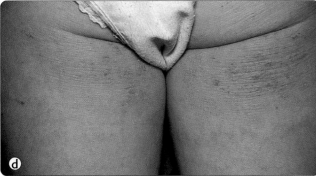

Fig 3.20 Childhood eczema with lesions on **(a)** the arm, **(b)** the ankles, **(c)** the suprapubic area and **(d)** the buttock creases.

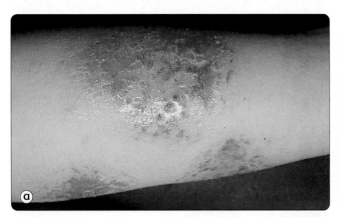
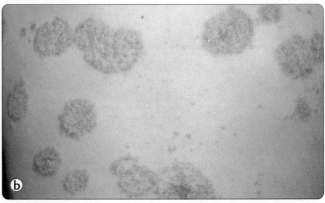

Fig 3.21 Nummular eczema. **(a)** A 14-year-old girl demonstrated the acute exudative round patches of nummular eczema. **(b)** The term nummular eczema is also used to describe the chronic circular patches on the extremities and trunks of atopic patients, exemplified by the patches on the back of this 5-year-old boy.

activity. In children with chronic disease, discrete papules may be obscured by excoriations and lichenification, particularly in the flexural creases.

Ichthyosis vulgaris

Hyperlinearity of the palms and soles typical of ichthyosis vulgaris is a common finding in patients with atopic dermatitis (Fig 3.24). Retained polygonal scales are usually evident on the distal lower extremities (see Fig 2.34), but they may also show a generalized distribution. Xerosis associated with ichthyosis may contribute to the pruritus present in atopic dermatitis.

Keratosis pilaris

Although keratosis pilaris is often an isolated finding, it is commonly associated with atopic dermatitis and/or ichthyosis vulgaris. Keratosis pilaris results from localized perifollicular retention of scales, which clinically is characterized by horny follicular papules and erythema on the upper arms, medial thighs, and cheeks (Fig 3.25).

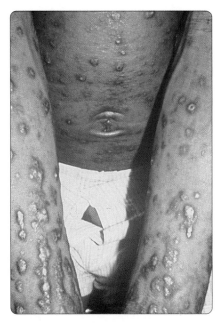

Fig 3.22 Prurigo nodularis. Widespread lichenified nodules involve the trunk and extremities of an adolescent boy with severe atopic dermatitis. Nodules may be particularly resistant to therapy.

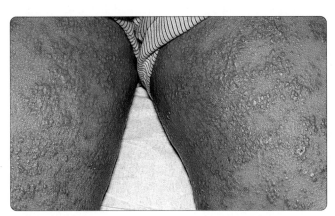

Fig 3.23 Follicular eczema. In some patients, follicular papules may be the only manifestation of atopic dermatitis. These lesions also occur in many atopic patients during the course of their disease, as in this adolescent with follicular papules on his thighs and legs.

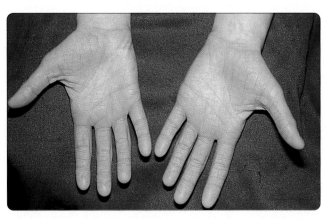

Fig 3.24 Ichthyosis vulgaris. Hyperlinearity of the palms and soles was marked in this patient with atopic dermatitis and ichthyosis vulgaris.

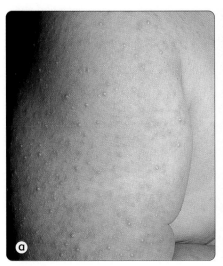

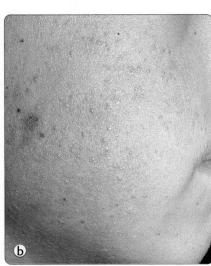

Fig 3.25 Keratosis pilaris. Asymptomatic sandpaper-like follicular papules were symmetrically distributed on the cheeks, upper arms, and upper thighs of **(a)** this toddler and **(b)** adolescent boy .

Infraorbital folds

Often referred to as Dennie sign or Morgan lines, extra infraorbital folds are suggestive of atopy (Fig 3.26). In many patients, these represent current or past local inflammation produced by persistent scratching and rubbing of the tissues. Although not specific for atopic dermatitis, it may be a useful finding when seen in association with other typical physical signs.

Pigmentary changes

Postinflammatory hypopigmentation and hyperpigmentation occur commonly in atopic patients, especially in the setting of chronic disease (Fig 3.27). Although pigmentary changes my be quite prominent, this is not always the case; subtle and poorly demarcated areas of hypopigmentation in atopic subjects are referred to as pityriasis alba (Fig 3.28). Changes are most marked in darkly pigmented individuals or lighter-skinned patients after tanning. The extremities and face are the areas most commonly involved. Although some post-inflammatory pigmentary changes persist indefinitely, fading of hyperpigmentation and repigmentation of lightened areas usually occur during prolonged remissions.

Hand (and foot) dermatitis

Involvement of the hands and feet is common at all ages and may be the only manifestation of atopic dermatitis in adolescents and adults. The rash is commonly triggered by contact irritants. Clinical findings include dry, scaly patches on the palms and soles and frequent fissuring of the palms, soles, and digits. The term 'dyshidrotic eczema' is reserved for patients with atopic dermatitis who develop intensely pruritic, deep-seated, inflammatory vesicles on the sides of the palms, soles, and/or digits (Fig 3.29). This is actually an inaccurate name, because histopathology of these lesions demonstrates spongiotic vesicles, typical of an acute dermatitis, and normal sweat glands. Involvement of the

paronychial skin may result in separation of the nail from the underlying nail bed (onycholysis) as well as in yellowing and pitting of the nail plate (Fig 3.30).

Secondary bacterial infection is the most frequent complication of atopic dermatitis. Since it may also trigger an acute exacerbation of clinical disease, early recognition and treatment are mandatory. Crusted, exudative patches suggest superinfection (Fig 3.31). Although Group A β-hemolytic streptococci are occasionally found in these infected areas, investigators now report a predominance of *Staphylococcus aureus*.

Eczema herpeticum

Primary *Herpes simplex* may produce widespread cutaneous and, on rare occasions, disseminated visceral disease in patients with atopic dermatitis. The acute development of multiple, grouped, 2–3 mm diameter vesicles or crusts associated with high fever and worsening pruritus suggests the diagnosis of eczema herpeticum (Fig 3.32). Tzanck smears and viral cultures confirm the diagnosis and acyclovir is started immediately.

A number of other organisms, which include human papillomaviruses (warts), the virus that causes molluscum contagiosum, and dermatophytes, such as *Trichophyton rubrum*, may produce chronic, recalcitrant infections in atopic patients.

The cause of atopic dermatitis remains elusive. An immunologic etiology is suggested by the chronic elevation of IgE seen in a majority of patients and the association with rare immunodeficiency states. Some investigators have proposed a primary role for an aberrant response to histamine and other mediators of inflammation in the skin. A number of other immunologic parameters have been studied in patients with atopic dermatitis. However, laboratory findings vary from patient to patient, and in the same patient at different times in the course of disease.

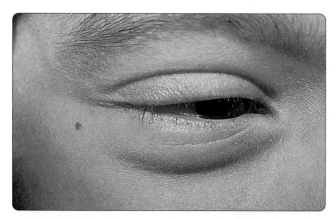

Fig 3.26 Dennie's sign or Morgan line. Eyelid edema and lichenification from chronic rubbing resulted in the development of a double infraorbital fold. Although not specific to atopic dermatitis, this feature suggests such a diagnosis when seen in association with other, more pathognomonic findings.

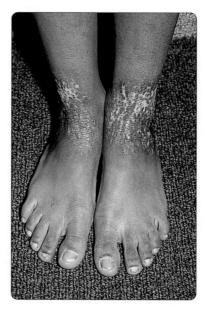

Fig 3.27
Postinflammatory hypopigmentation and hyperpigmentation are marked on the ankles of this 9-year-old girl with severe, chronic atopic dermatitis.

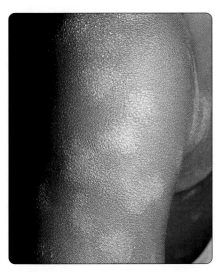

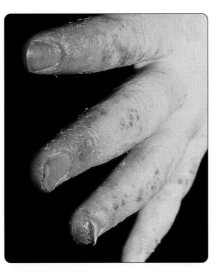

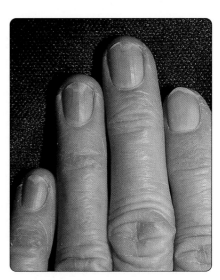

Fig 3.28 Pityriasis alba. In some atopic patients, subtle inflammation may result in poorly demarcated areas of hypopigmentation, known as pityriasis alba. Lesions are most prominent in darkly pigmented individuals.

Fig 3.29 Dyshidrosis. Chronic cracking, oozing, and scaling develop after the tiny pruritic vesicles have been scratched.

Fig 3.30 Nail dystrophy. Nail changes, including onycholysis and pitting, can occur when chronic dermatitis affects the fingertips, as in this adolescent.

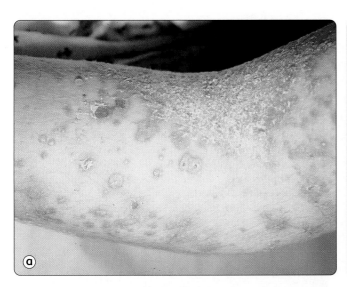

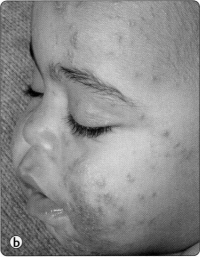

Fig 3.31 Secondary bacterial infection in atopic dermatitis. **(a)** Bullous impetigo developed in the flexural creases of an 8-year-old-child with severe atopic dermatitis. **(b)** This toddler with atopic dermatitis required multiple courses of oral antibiotics for recurrent impetigo of the face.

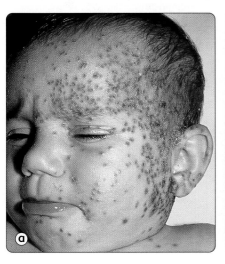

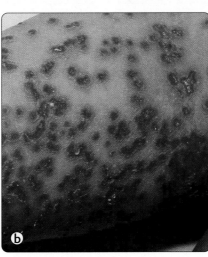

Fig 3.32 Herpes simplex. Eczema herpeticum, the primary cutaneous manifestation of *Herpes simplex virus* infection in atopic patients, spread rapidly over **(a)** the trunk and face, and **(b)** the extremities of this 10-month-old girl. Note the uniform, clustered 2–3 mm diameter vesicles and punched-out vesicles and erosions. A Tzanck smear at the bedside showed multinucleated giant cells, and a positive viral culture confirmed the diagnosis 12 hours later.

Pathophysiologically, many external factors, which include dry skin, soaps, wool fabrics, foods, infectious agents, and environmental antigens, may act in concert to produce pruritus in susceptible individuals. The resultant scratching leads to acute and chronic changes diagnostic of atopic dermatitis (Fig 3.33).

Although the histopathology of affected skin is characteristic (scale, acanthosis, spongiosis, lymphocytic dermal inflammation), skin biopsies are not diagnostic. Atopic dermatitis is a clinical diagnosis. Characteristic pruritic cutaneous findings in a patient with a family history of atopy suggest the disorder. To aid in diagnosis, several investigators have proposed a number of primary and secondary criteria (Fig 3.34).

A number of conditions may mimic the clinical findings of atopic dermatitis. It can be differentiated from infantile seborrheic dermatitis by the distribution of lesions, since atopic dermatitis spares moist, intertriginous areas such as the axilla and perineum, where seborrhea is prominent. Exposure history and distribution help differentiate contact dermatitis, as do the discreteness of lesions, pattern, and lack of symptoms in pityriasis rosea. Thick, silvery scale and the Koebner phenomenon help differentiate psoriasis, and central clearing with an active, scaly, vesiculopustular border helps to differentiate tinea corporis. The eruption in histiocytosis X is usually hemorrhagic and accompanied by chronic draining ears, hepatosplenomegaly, and other systemic findings. An acral distribution of lesions, lack of pruritus, and associated viral symptoms suggest Gianotti–Crosti syndrome.

Therapeutic measures are individualized according to the morphology of the skin lesions, distribution of the rash, and age of the patient. Infants, for instance, may benefit from aggressive efforts to protect their skin from environmental irritants and scratching. Loose-fitting cotton clothing with long sleeves and foot coverings may be optimal.

Although bathing and the use of soaps was once believed to exacerbate atopic dermatitis, increasing evidence contradicts this view. Daily swimming or baths in the summer and

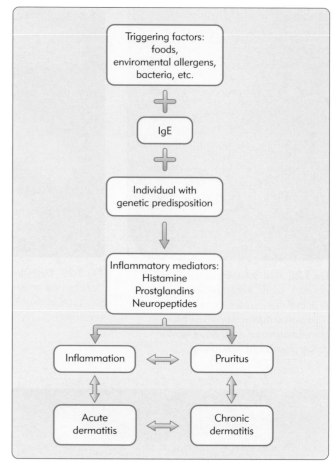

Fig 3.33 The processes by which external factors, including foods, bacteria, and environmental allergens, trigger the release of cutaneous inflammatory factors, resulting in pruritus and inflammation of the skin of susceptible individuals. Secondary manipulation of the skin (i.e. rubbing and excoriation) produces many of the symptoms of acute and chronic dermatitis. Dermatitic changes in the skin result in further pruritus, which potentiates an escalating cycle of increasing clinical findings, particularly during flare periods.

Fig 3.34 Diagnostic criteria for atopic dermatitis. (Adapted from Hanifin JM, Lobitz WC, New concepts of atopic dermatitis. *Arch Dermatol.* 1977, **113**:663.)

Diagnostic criteria for atopic dermatitis		
Major criteria (all required for diagnosis)	**Common findings (at least two)**	**Associated findings (at least four)**
Pruritus	Personal or family history of atopy	Ichthyosis, xerosis, hyperlinear palms
Typical morphology and distribution of rash	Immediate skin-test reactivity	Pityriasis alba
	White dermographism	Facial pallor, infraorbital darkening
	Anterior subcapsular cataracts	Dennie–Morgan folds
		Keratoconus
		Hand dermatitis
		Repeated cutaneous infections

on alternating days in winter, followed by liberal application of lubricants, help to cleanse and hydrate the skin. Emollients are tailored to the patient to increase compliance. In general, greasy, occlusive preparations are safest and most effective. However, some patients may prefer less occlusive agents. Mild soaps may help to reduce bacterial colonization and the risk of secondary infection. Their use should be restricted to areas in which bacteria are most likely to thrive, such as the groin, axilla, and umbilicus.

Low- and medium-potency topical corticosteroids are particularly useful during periods of increased disease activity. Twice-daily applications are restricted to the worst areas and tapered as soon as possible. The skin is monitored for signs of corticosteroid overuse, which include atrophy, loss of pigment, and telangiectasias. High-potency products are reserved for special instances in which severe disease is limited to small patches of thick skin, such as on the hands and feet.

When eczema is severe, antihistamines may relieve pruritus. They are particularly useful at bedtime, when itching is the most severe, and their sedative effects may help. However, antihistamines must be used with caution in infants and toddlers, who may develop paradoxic excitation. Tachyphylaxis to a given agent may develop after prolonged therapy, and it may be necessary to change the class of antihistamine prescribed.

Secondary bacterial infections are frequently associated with exacerbation, and may cause an acute flare of atopic dermatitis. This complication initiates prompt intervention. Oral antibiotics, such as erythromycin, or, alternatively, cephalosporins and semisynthetic penicillins, are indicated when infection is evident. If the infection is widespread, parenteral antibiotics may be necessary. Localized patches of impetiginization may be managed with topical antibiotics, such as bacitracin and mupirocin. In severe disseminated infections, appropriate cultures are obtained prior to initiating antibiotic therapy.

Infection unresponsive to antibacterials raises the specter of eczema herpeticum. Patients with disseminated primary cutaneous *Herpes simplex* infection also present with acute worsening of their dermatitis and, not infrequently, fever, adenopathy, irritability, and decreased appetite. These children require aggressive, symptomatic treatment and immediate parenteral antiviral therapy (acyclovir 15mg/kg/day in three divided doses). Unfortunately, oral acyclovir is not well absorbed in children. However, several new antiviral medications, famcyclovir and valacyclovir hydrochloride, are readily bioavailable when taken orally. Hopefully, liquid formulations of these drugs and approval for use in children will come soon.

During acute flares with vesicle and crust formation, application of tepid tap-water compresses three times a day for 15–20 minutes, topical lubricants such as petrolatum, Eucerin® cream, Aquaphor®, and Acid Mantle® cream, and oral antibiotics should result in rapid improvement. In chronic disease, liberal use of emollients, judicious use of low- and medium-potency topical corticosteroid ointments

twice daily, antihistamines, and avoidance of environmental irritants may bring symptomatic relief. Most patients with chronic atopic dermatitis are troubled by the effect of the rash on their physical appearance. Therefore, emotional support and psychologic counseling may be helpful adjuncts in the care of these patients.

Seborrheic dermatitis

Seborrheic dermatitis is characterized by a symmetric, red, scaling eruption, which occurs predominantly on hair-bearing and intertriginous areas, which include the scalp, eyebrows, eyelashes, perinasal, presternal, and postauricular areas, and the neck, axilla, and groin. In affected infants, scalp lesions consist of a greasy, salmon-colored, scaly dermatitis called cradle cap (see Fig 2.38). A severe type may be more generalized. In adolescents, the dermatitis may manifest as dandruff or flaking of the eyebrows, postauricular areas, nasolabial folds, and/or flexural areas. When the patches on the face are well defined, they may form a petaloid pattern (Fig 3.35).

Although the pathogenesis of seborrheic dermatitis is unknown, *Pityrosporum* and *Candida* species have been implicated as causative agents. A role for neurologic dysfunction is suggested by the increased incidence and severity in neurologically impaired individuals. Immunodeficiency states, particularly acquired immunodeficiency syndrome, may also be associated with severe clinical manifestations.

The dermatitis of seborrhea is usually subtle and non-pruritic. Most cases respond to low-potency topical corticosteroids and may clear spontaneously. Antiseborrheic shampoos that contain pyrithione zinc, selenium, or salicylic acid may help. Ketoconazole shampoo and cream have also been approved for the treatment of seborrhea.

In infants and young children, atopic dermatitis may be confused with seborrheic dermatitis. However, atopic dermatitis in infants invariably spares moist sites, such as the diaper area and axilla, and produces intense pruritus. The

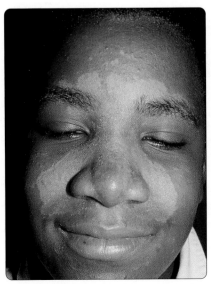

Fig 3.35
Seborrheic dermatitis. This boy developed scaly, red, hypopigmented patches on the face in a petaloid pattern.

distribution of rash in histiocytosis X may resemble seborrheic dermatitis. However, the presence of purpura, poor growth, diarrhea, and other systemic complaints would be unusual for uncomplicated seborrheic dermatitis. Erosive patches in a seborrheic distribution associated with poor growth, diarrhea, irritability, and hair loss suggest the diagnosis of acrodermatitis enteropathica. Finally, persistent diaper dermatitis and cradle cap may be difficult to differentiate from psoriasis without a skin biopsy.

Juvenile palmar–plantar dermatosis

Also known as sweaty sock syndrome, juvenile palmar–plantar dermatosis is seen commonly in toddlers and children of school age. Chronic pink, scaly patches with cracking and fissuring begin in the fall or winter on the anterior plantar surfaces of the feet and great toes (Fig 3.36). Occasionally, patches spread to the other toes and hands. Although the cause is unknown, excessive sweating and/or the repeated cycle of wetting of the skin during the day while shoes are worn and drying of the skin at night may trigger the condition. Consequently, treatment consists of lubrication and covering the feet at night. Topical corticosteroids may be necessary in severe cases. The eruption tends to subside in the summer, and resolution in adolescence is common. Children with atopic dermatitis may be particularly prone to develop this dermatosis.

Contact dermatitis differs from sweaty sock syndrome by the tendency for involvement of the dorsum of the hands and feet. Tinea pedis usually presents on the instep and interdigital web spaces. Chronic atopic dermatitis may be difficult to differentiate from sweaty sock syndrome unless other stigmata of atopy are present.

Perioral dermatitis

In the simplest form, perioral dermatitis represents a contact dermatitis from repeated wetting and drying of the skin associated with persistent lip-licking or thumb-sucking, especially during the winter months. Elements of both acute and chronic dermatitis closely encircle the mouth and may involve the vermilion border (Fig 3.37).

Some children develop asymptomatic red papules, pustules, and nodules on either a normal appearing or red, scaly base on the chin and nasolabial folds (Fig 3.38a). Lesions may extend to the cheeks, eyelids, and forehead. Although initially reported in association with the use of fluorinated topical corticosteroids on the face, this type of perioral dermatitis occurs more frequently in children with no history of topical agents. It has also been described most commonly in black school-age boys (Fig 3.38b). Interestingly, histopathology demonstrates features of dermatitis, folliculitis, and occasionally granulomatous inflammation consistent with rosacea or sarcoidosis. However, affected children are otherwise healthy, and the rash improves with oral antibiotics such as erythromycin and tetracycline (for children over 12 years old). Topical antibiotics, benzoyl peroxide, vitamin A acid, and other keratolytics may also be useful. Topical corticosteroids are used with extreme caution because of the risk of precipitating a superimposed folliculitis, telangiectasias, and atrophy, particularly with long-term exposure.

Pityriasis rosea

Pityriasis rosea is an innocent, self-limited disorder that can occur at any age, but is more common in school-age children and young adults. A prodrome of malaise, headache, and mild constitutional symptoms occasionally precedes the rash. In about half of the cases the eruption begins with the appearance of a 'herald patch' (Fig 3.39a). This 3–5 cm diameter, isolated, oval, scaly, pink patch may appear anywhere on the body surface, although it occurs most commonly on the trunk and thighs. Central clearing produces a lesion that commonly simulates tinea corporis. Within 1–2 weeks numerous smaller lesions appear on the body, usually concentrated on the trunk and proximal extremities (Fig 3.39b–d). These begin as small, round papules, which enlarge to form 1–2 cm diameter oval patches with dusky centers and scaly borders. The long axes of the patches often run parallel to the skin lines over the

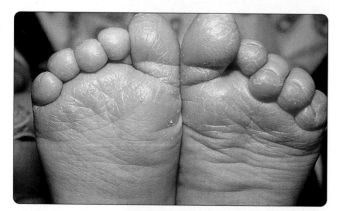

Fig 3.36 Sweaty sock syndrome was evident in this child with symmetric, scaly, fissured patches on the anterior soles and bottom of the toes. The rash resolved with aggressive use of lubricants alone.

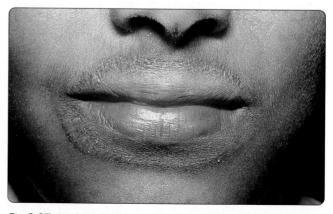

Fig 3.37 Lip licker's contact dermatitis recurred every winter in this teenage boy. Involvement was always restricted to the lips and contiguous skin.

thorax and back, to create a 'Christmas-tree' pattern. Occasionally, pityriasis rosea spreads to involve much of the skin surface, including the face and distal extremities. Inflammation may be so intense that some blistering and hemorrhage become clinically apparent. The rash reaches a peak in several weeks and slowly fades over 6–12 weeks.

Ultraviolet light may hasten the disappearance of the eruption. However, postinflammatory hyperpigmentation, particularly in dark-complected individuals, may persist for months. Although the cause is unknown, the peak incidence in late winter and low recurrence rate favor an infectious, probably viral, etiology.

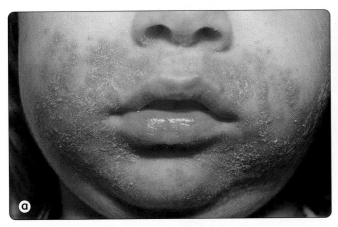

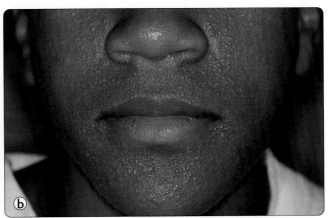

Fig 3.38 Perioral dermatitis with bright-red papules, pustules, and scale erupted on the cheeks, chin, and upper lip of this 4-year-old boy. **(a)** Lesions subsequently appeared around the nose and eyes. The rash vanished after 2 weeks of treatment with oral erythromycin and noncomedogenic moisturizers. **(b)** The perioral dermatitis in this adolescent failed to respond to topical and oral agents, but resolved without treatment in 6 months.

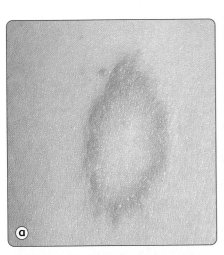

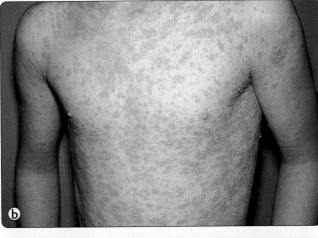

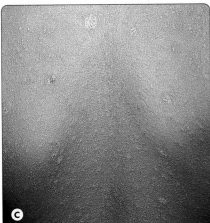

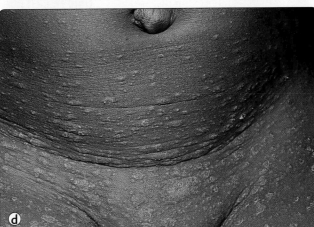

Fig 3.39 Pityriasis rosea. **(a)** The large herald patch on the chest of this 10-year-old girl shows central clearing, which mimics tinea corporis.
(b) Numerous oval lesions on the chest of a white teenager.
(c) Note the Christmas-tree pattern on the back of a black adolescent.
(d) Small, papular lesions, as well as larger scaly patches, were most prominent on the abdomen and thighs of this 5-year-old girl.

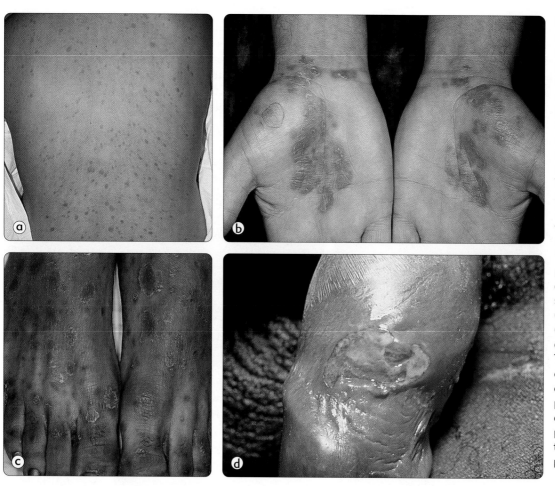

Fig 3.40 The rash of secondary syphilis may mimic pityriasis rosea. **(a)** A truncal rash in a Christmas-tree pattern on this adolescent resolved after treatment with intramuscular penicillin. Her Venereal Disease Research Laboratories titer was 1:2056. Hyperkeratotic 'copper penny' papules, which are distinctive for syphilis, are seen on **(b)** the palms and **(c)** tops of the feet of adolescents. These also resolved quickly with antibiotics. **(d)** A painless chancre developed on the penile shaft of a teenage boy with primary syphilis.

Other eruptions that can resemble pityriasis rosea include guttate psoriasis, viral exanthems, drug rashes, and secondary syphilis (Fig 3.40A–D). The herald patch may suggest tinea, but fungus can be excluded by a negative potassium hydroxide (KOH) preparation and fungal culture.

Pityriasis lichenoides

Pityriasis lichenoides includes a group of self-limiting disorders with a spectrum of clinical presentations from the acute, papulonecrotic eruption of pityriasis lichenoides et varioliformis acuta (PLEVA, Mucha–Habermann disease) to the chronic dermatitic papules of pityriasis lichenoides chronica (PLC). Although most common in older children and young adults, pityriasis lichenoides may occasionally occur in infants and young children, with a slight predominance in boys.

Acute forms usually begin with the sudden onset of 2–4 mm diameter red macules and papules, which evolve over several days into vesicular, necrotic, and eroded lesions (Fig 3.41). Healing occurs within several weeks with postinflammatory pigmentary changes and occasionally chicken pox-like scars. Although the rash is usually asymptomatic and has a predilection for the trunk, pruritus may be intense and lesions may spread to involve the neck, face, and extremities, which include the palms and soles. Fever and other mild constitutional symptoms may precede or accompany the acute phase. The eruption appears in successive crops, which settle down over weeks to months. Relapses and remissions occur episodically, but after several months most patients develop the more subtle lesions of PLC.

In PLC, which may also appear *de novo*, the typical rash consists of round 2 mm to 1 cm diameter reddish-brown papules which develop a shiny brown scale adherent at the center (Fig 3.42). Episodic crops of papules heal over several weeks, with pigmentary changes but no evidence of scarring. In fact, postinflammatory pigmentary changes may be the first findings to bring attention to the rash (Fig 3.43). Although the eruption is self-limiting and usually heals without scarring, it may evolve for 5–10 years.

The histopathology of skin biopsies is distinctive, but not diagnostic. In the mild form, minimal dermatitic changes are seen, with spongiosis and parakeratosis. A mild, chronic, perivascular infiltrate is found in the dermis associated with some hemorrhage and pigment incontinence. In acute disease the inflammation may be intense and extend down into the deep dermis and up into the epidermis. Dyskeratosis is usually marked and necrosis of the epidermis may occur, with the formation of erosions. Endothelial cell swelling is marked, and vascular necrosis may occur. Hemorrhage is seen in the dermis and epidermis.

Although most children do well without treatment, phototherapy with UVB, PUVA, or natural sunlight may be useful in persistently symptomatic individuals. There may also be a role for oral antibiotics, such as erythromycin or tetracycline, in difficult patients. However, the use of systemic corticosteroids and methotrexate does not seem warranted.

At the onset, PLEVA may be mistaken for varicella. However, the lack of symptoms or mucous membrane lesions and the subsequent chronic course help to exclude chicken pox. Lymphomatoid papulosis is a chronic, benign, self-limiting disorder that is often clinically indistinguishable from PLEVA. However, the histopathology is characterized by an atypical lymphohistiocytic infiltrate, suggestive of lymphoma.

In some children and adults a lymphomatoid papulosis-like eruption rarely occurs as a presenting picture for systemic lymphoma. Cutaneous vasculitis, impetigo, insect bites, and scabies are also considered during the acute phase.

The only differentiation between PLC and pityriasis rosea is the extremely protracted course. In pityriasis alba the borders of the patches are indistinct and other stigmata of atopy are usually present. Patch-stage mycosis fungoides, a cutaneous T-cell lymphoma, may begin with subtle, scaly, hypopigmented or hyperpigmented patches that mimic PLC (Fig 3.44). Consequently, any child with a long-standing rash suggestive of PLC must have a skin biopsy to exclude lymphoma. Parents are counseled regarding the chronic but innocent course of this disorder.

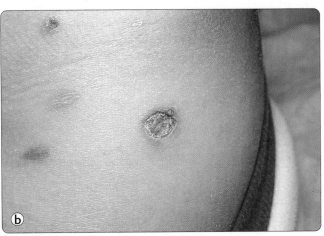

Fig 3.41 Pityriasis lichenoides et varioliformis acuta.
(a) Asymptomatic hemorrhagic papules erupted in a pityriasis rosea-like pattern on the trunk and proximal extremities of this

15-year-old boy. (b) Recurrent papulonecrotic lesions continued to evolve on the trunk of this 5-year-old for over a year.

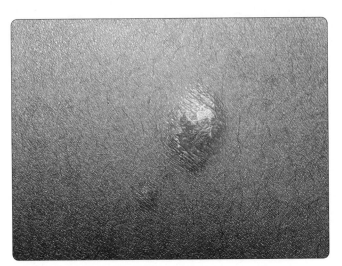

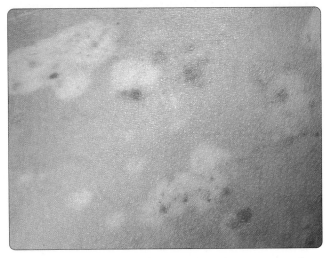

Fig 3.42 Pityriasis lichenoides chronica. A few diffusely scattered, shiny, hyperpigmented papules continued to appear for years in this 11-year-old boy. Note the central adherent scale.

Fig 3.43 Postinflammatory hyperpigmentation was severe in this child with generalized pityriasis lichenoides et varioliformis acuta. Fortunately, the pigmentary changes healed over several months as his disease evolved into the more indolent pityriasis lichenoides chronica.

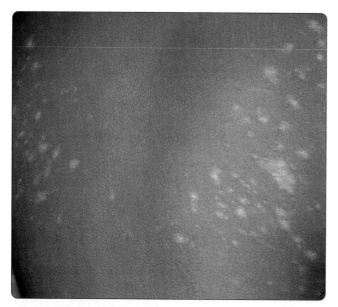

Fig 3.44 A 10-year-old child had asymptomatic, hypopigmented, minimally scaly oval patches on his trunk for several years. A skin biopsy demonstrated atypical, dermal, lymphocytic inflammation with extension into the epidermis characteristic of cutaneous T-cell lymphoma.

LICHENOID DERMATOSES

Lichen planus

Lichen planus (LP) is a distinctive dermatosis characterized by pruritic, purple, polygonal papules (the '4-p sign') which involve the flexures of the arms and legs, mucous membranes, genitals, nails, and scalp (Fig 3.45). The eruption in LP typically demonstrates the Koebner or isomorphic phenomenon, in which cutaneous lesions appear or extend in areas of trauma (scratches, excoriations, burns, scars). Only 2% of cases present before 20 years of age; however, patients with the familial variant develop LP in childhood. Although the cause of LP is unknown, complement and immunoglobulin depositions along the basement membrane zone suggest an immunologic mechanism.

Typically, itchy, violaceous 3–6 mm diameter papules appear abruptly on the wrists, ankles, and/or genitals. Lesions may spread over the forearms, shins, and lower back. Rarely, widespread rash covers much of the body surface. In areas of involvement contiguous, shiny-topped papules may form a white, lacy, reticulated network known as Wickham striae. Their visibility may be enhanced by the application of a small quantity of mineral oil and examination with side lighting and

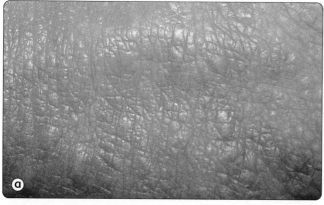

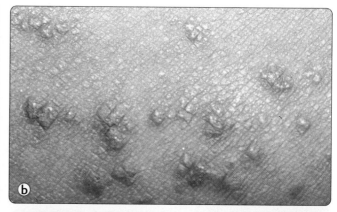

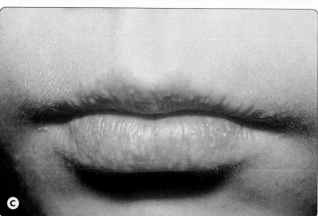

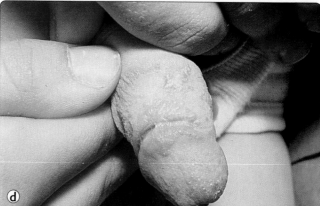

Fig 3.45 Lichen planus. **(a)** Violaceous, polygonal papules almost to confluence appeared over several weeks on the dorsum of the hands and feet, ankles, and wrists of this 16-year-old boy. **(b)** Lesions are somewhat hyperpigmented on the forearm of this black adolescent. **(c, d)** White papules formed Wickham's striae on the lips of this child, who also had typical papules on the penis.

a hand lens. Confluent lesions may form annular or linear plaques. Intense, dermal inflammation may be associated with the development of vesiculobullous lesions, and hypertrophic, verrucous plaques may evolve, particularly on the shins, in chronic disease (Fig 3.46).

Wickham striae may also be present on the buccal mucosa, gingivae, lips, and tongue. Mucous membrane findings, which are present in two-thirds of patients with LP, also include erythema, white papules that resemble leukoplakia, vesicles, erosions, and deep, painful ulcerations.

Also, LP may present with follicular papules, particularly in the scalp where cicatricial alopecia may be progressive. Nail involvement, seen in about 10% of patients, includes brittleness, thinning, fragmentation, longitudinal ridging or striations, and partial or complete shedding of the nail. Pterygium formation, atrophy, subungual hyperkeratosis, and lifting of the distal nail plate may also occur (see Fig 8.40). Rarely, nail disease appears without cutaneous involvement.

Skin biopsies characteristically demonstrate hyperkeratosis, focal thickening of the granular layer, irregular acanthosis, and a band-like infiltrate of lymphocytes and histiocytes in the dermis, close to the epidermis and associated with damage to the basal cell layer.

Graft versus host disease and a number of medications have also been implicated in the development of a lichenoid rash indistinguishable from that of LP. The presence of eosinophils in the dermal infiltrate suggests the possibility of a drug reaction. Prurigo nodules in eczema may be associated with other stigmata of atopic dermatitis, and the lesions of discoid lupus erythematosus usually demonstrate atrophy. Nail disease must be differentiated from other causes of nail dystrophy, and oral LP may mimic viral infection, primary blistering dermatoses, erythema multiforme, and leukoplakia.

Although many cases resolve within 1–2 years, some eruptions persist for 10–20 years. Localized lesions often respond well to topical corticosteroids. Oral LP may be resistant to treatment, and some success has been achieved with topical retinoic acid, intralesional corticosteroids, oral retinoids, oral corticosteroids, and swish-and-spit cyclosporin. Although quite painful, intralesional corticosteroids are also useful in the treatment of nail disease. Patients with generalized LP have been treated with systemic corticosteroids and retinoids. However, therapeutic benefits must be weighed against the long-term consequences of these medications. In fact, PUVA may provide a relatively safe alternative for disseminated disease.

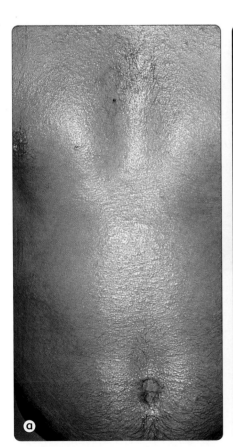

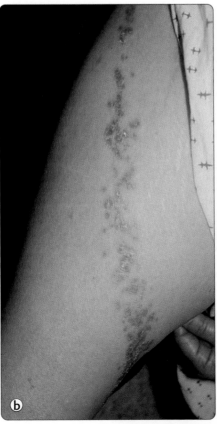

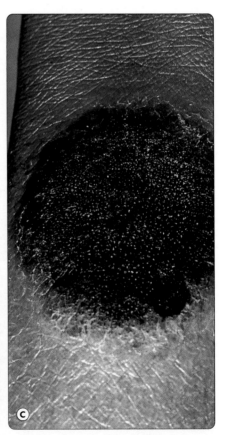

Fig 3.46 Lichen planus variants. **(a)** Diffuse, eruptive lichen planus responded to treatment with psoralen–ultraviolet A. Over 90% of this boy's body was involved with confluent papules on the trunk and extremities. **(b)** This asymptomatic, linear plaque progressed slowly for over a year. **(c)** Extremely pruritic, hypertrophic plaques were present on the shins of this 18-year-old girl.

Lichen nitidus

Lichen nitidus, an uncommon, chronic, asymptomatic eruption, is characterized by flat-topped, flesh-colored 2–3 mm diameter papules that demonstrate the isomorphic phenomenon (Fig 3.47). Although many practitioners consider lichen nitidus to be a variant of LP, the peak incidence in children between 7 and 13 years, the uniformly tiny lesions (which do not have a tendency to coalesce), and the lack of pruritus establish this disorder as a distinct entity. The rash progresses slowly over months to years, with a predilection for the arms, abdomen, and genitals. The majority of patients are male.

Skin biopsies demonstrate findings reminiscent of LP, but are restricted to only one or a few papillae. The overlying horny layer exhibits parakeratosis, and at the lateral margin of the lesion the rete ridges extend downward to form a claw around the underlying infiltrate.

Papular or follicular eczema may be differentiated from lichen nitidus by the presence of pruritus and other markers of atopy. Keratosis pilaris appears in characteristic locations and is inherited as an autosomal-dominant trait. Examination of flat warts with side lighting and magnification usually reveals a rough surface, unlike the smooth, shiny surface of papules in lichen nitidus. However, both lichen nitidus and flat warts develop Koebner phenomenon, and a skin biopsy may be necessary to differentiate them.

Lichen striatus

Lichen striatus is a linear, lichenoid eruption that appears most commonly in children of school age. Flat-topped papules arise suddenly in streaks and swirls, usually on the extremities, upper back, or neck. However, any area, including the palms, soles, nails, genitals, and face, may become involved (Fig 3.48). Lesions usually develop some overlying dusty scale and mild erythema. Hypopigmentation may bring attention to the eruption, especially in dark-skinned children.

Lichen striatus usually fades without treatment in 1–2 years. Lubricants and topical corticosteroids may be useful to decrease scale and inflammation in cosmetically important areas.

This condition can be mistaken for linear epidermal nevi, linear LP, linear porokeratosis, flat warts, linear psoriasis, and linear ichthyotic eruptions. When the clinical course is confusing, a skin biopsy helps to differentiate these disorders. Lichen striatus usually demonstrates dermatitic changes in the epidermis, with a lymphocytic perivascular infiltrate in the superficial and mid dermis that frequently extends into the deep dermis.

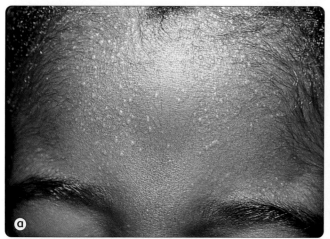

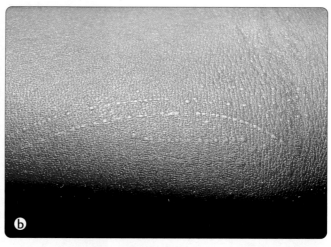

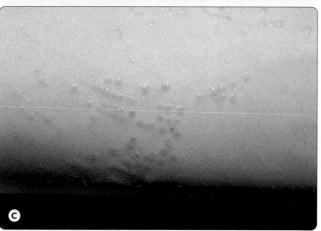

Fig 3.47 Lichen nitidus. **(a)** Asymptomatic, uniform, 2–3 mm diameter, shiny papules began on the face and spread to the trunk and extremities of this 6-year-old boy. **(b)** Note Koebner's phenomenon on the arm, where papules developed in an incidental excoriation. **(c)** Koebner's phenomenon is also evident in this lightly pigmented girl with minimally inflammatory papules on her arms.

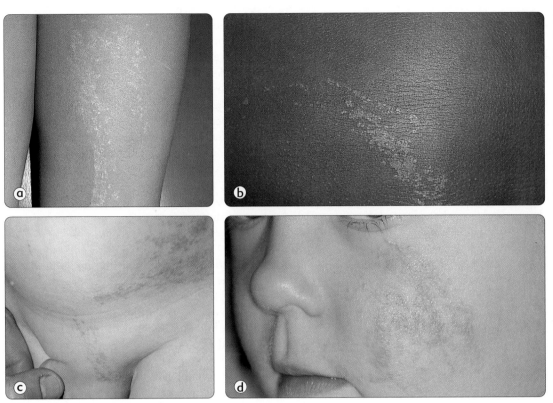

Fig 3.48 Lichen striatus. Asymptomatic, linear, scaly papules appeared on (**a**) the leg, (**b**) abdomen, (**c**) abdomen and scrotum, and (**d**) face of young children. In each case histology demonstrated findings typical of lichen striatus. After a variable period of progression (6–24 months) these lesions resolved without treatment.

FUNGAL INFECTIONS

Tinea

Two types of fungal organisms, dermatophytes and yeasts, produce clinical cutaneous disease. Dermatophytes include tinea or ringworm fungi, which infect skin, nails, and hair (see Chapter 9). Although *Candida* and *Pityrosporum* yeast infections usually involve the skin, *Candida* can infect mucous membranes and rarely disseminates to viscera, particularly in immunocompromised patients.

Tinea corporis

This is a superficial fungal infection of nonhairy or glabrous skin. It has been called tinea (Latin for intestinal worm) or 'ringworm' because of its characteristic configuration, which consists of pruritic annular plaques with central clearing or scale and an active, indurated, and/or vesiculopustular, worm-like border (Fig 3.49). Lesions, which may be single or multiple, typically begin as red papules or pustules that expand over days to weeks to form 1–5 cm diameter plaques. Tinea corporis can be found in any age group and is usually acquired from an infected domestic animal (*Microsporum canis*) or through direct human contact (*Trichophyton*, *Microsporum*, and *Epidermophyton* species).

Clinically, tinea may be differentiated from atopic dermatitis by its propensity for autoinoculation from the primary patches to other sites on the patient's skin, by spread to close contacts, and by the central clearing noted in many lesions. Moreover, the rash of atopic dermatitis

tends to be symmetric, chronic, and recurrent in a flexural distribution. Unlike tinea, patches of nummular eczema are self-limited and do no clear centrally. The herald patch of pityriasis rosea is often mistaken for tinea. However, scrapings obtained for KOH preparation are negative, and subsequent development of the generalized rash with its characteristic truncal distribution is distinctive. The clinical patterns, associated findings, and chronicity help differentiate psoriasis and seborrhea from tinea. Granuloma annulare produces a characteristic ringed plaque. However, on palpation, the lesions are firm and do not have epidermal changes (scales, vesicles, pustules). Granuloma annulare is also asymptomatic.

The diagnosis of tinea is confirmed by KOH examination of the skin (see Fig 1.7). The first step is to obtain material by scraping the loose scales, vesicles, and pustules at the margin of a lesion. These are mounted on the center of a glass slide and one or two drops of 20% KOH are added. Next, a glass coverslip is applied and gently pressed down with a finger tip or the eraser end of a pencil to crush the scales. The slide can then be heated gently, taking care not to boil the KOH solution and, again, the coverslip is pressed down. The slide is placed under a microscope, with the condenser and light at low levels to maximize contrast, and with the objective at low power. On focusing up and down, true hyphae are seen as long, greenish, hyaline, branching, often septate rods of uniform width that cross the borders of epidermal cells. Cotton fibers, cell borders, or other artifacts may be falsely interpreted as positive findings.

Tinea infections on glabrous skin respond readily to topical antifungal creams (imidazoles such as clotrimazole, econazole, miconazole, ketoconazole, sulconazole, oxiconazole; the allylamines naftifine and terbinafine; ciclopirax olamine; tolnaftate). When lesions are multiple and widespread, oral therapy with griseofulvin is indicated.

Tinea pedis

Commonly referred to as athlete's foot, tinea pedis is a fungal infection of the feet with a predilection for web space involvement (Fig 3.50). It is common in adolescence, but somewhat less so in prepubertal children. The infecting organisms are probably acquired from contaminated showers, bathrooms, and locker room and gym floors, and their growth is fostered by the warm, moist environment of shoes.

In some cases scaling and fissuring predominate; in others, vesiculopustular lesions, erythema, and maceration are found. The infection starts and may remain between and along the sides of the toes. However, lesions can extend over the dorsum of the foot and can involve the plantar surface as well, particularly the instep and the ball of the foot. Patients complain of burning and itching, which are frequently intense. Although the rash occasionally involves both feet and the hands, asymmetric involvement with sparing of one hand or foot is typical of tinea.

Diagnosis is suspected on clinical grounds and confirmed by KOH preparation of skin scrapings. The mainstays of treatment include topical antifungal creams or powders and measures to reduce foot moisture. Many individuals do better during the summer months while wearing sandals. For those

with severe inflammatory lesions, oral antifungal agents may be required, and secondary bacterial infections, particularly with Gram-negative organisms, may be a problem.

Tinea pedis is differentiated from contact dermatitis of the feet by the tendency of the latter to involve the dorsum of the feet and to spare the interdigital web spaces. In dyshidrotic eczema, KOH preparations and fungal cultures are negative. Psoriasis and PRP are differentiated from tinea by their symmetric moccasin-glove distribution and other characteristic stigmata.

Yeast

Candida and *Pityrosporum* account for the majority of yeast-related cutaneous disease.

Candidiasis

Candida colonize the gastroinstestinal tract and skin shortly after birth and may produced localized (thrush and diaper dermatitis), as well as disseminated cutaneous and systemic infection in the newborn. Recurrent and persistent infection in infancy may be associated with the use of antibiotics. However, it should also raise the suspicion of heritable or acquired immunodeficiency (Fig 3.51a,b). Candidal paronychia is also a common problem in otherwise healthy toddlers who suck on fingers and toes (Fig 3.51c). Yellowing, pitting, and other signs of nail dystrophy associated with *Candida* in this setting usually resolve without therapy; however, they may benefit from the application of topical antifungal creams. Pèrleche, manifested as erythema, maceration, and fissuring of the corners of the mouth, occurs commonly in diabetics

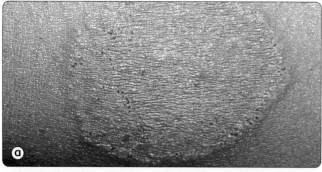

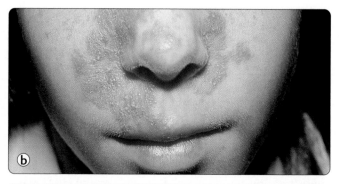

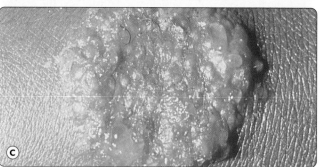

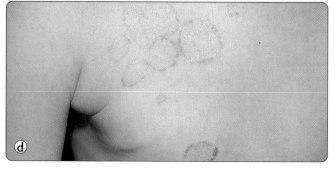

Fig 3.49 Tinea corporis. The characteristic annular lesions show many variations in appearance. **(a)** This lesion has a raised active border and shows some central clearing and scale. **(b)** Sharply circumscribed tinea faciei demonstrates erythema, scale, and pustule formation throughout the expanding patch. **(c)** An inflammatory tinea or kerion on the arm has marked edema and vesiculation. **(d)** Multiple expanding lesions spread quickly in a toddler who acquired infection from the family kitten.

and lip lickers, and may become secondarily infected by *Candida*. Topical antifungals, as well as aggressive use of lubricants, may be necessary to eradicate the condition.

Tinea versicolor

Tinea versicolor is a common dermatosis characterized by multiple, small, oval scaly patches that measure 1–3 cm in diameter, usually located in a guttate or raindrop pattern on the upper chest, back, and proximal portions of the upper extremities of adolescents and young adults (Fig 3.52a,b). However, all ages may be affected, including infants (Fig

3.52c). Facial lesions are seen occasionally and may be the only area of involvement in breast-feeding babies, who acquire the organism from their mothers.

The rash is usually asymptomatic, although some patients complain of mild pruritus. Typically, the cosmetic appearance is more bothersome. Lesions may be light tan, reddish, or white in color, giving rise to the term versicolor. Patches tend to appear hyperpigmented in light-pigmented patients and hypopigmented in dark-pigmented patients. In some individuals a folliculitis characterized by 2–3 mm diameter red papules and pustules develops on the chest, back, and occasionally the face.

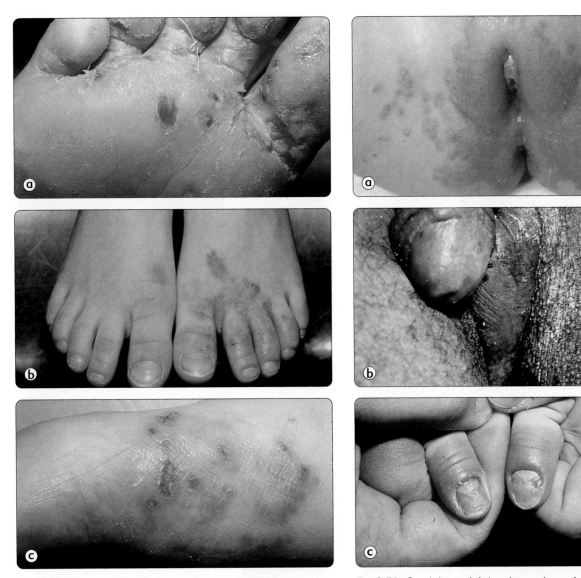

Fig 3.50 Tinea pedis. (a) Macerated, eroded, and crusted patches extend from the toe web spaces to the plantar surfaces of the toes and foot. (b) Dry, scaly, red patches extend from the web spaces to the top of the toes and foot. (c) The instep and medial surface of the foot is another commonly involved area. All of these children were under 5 years of age and had at least one parent with chronic or recurrent tinea pedis.

Fig 3.51 Candidiasis. (a) A red, papular rash with pustules at the periphery erupted on the anogenital area of this child who was on chronic antibiotics for recurrent ear infections.
(b) A teenage diabetic on antibiotics developed a painful, red, macerated eruption dotted with pustules on the scrotum, penis, and groin. (c) A chronic paronychia with erythema at the base of the nail, loss of the cuticle, and dystrophic changes of the nail developed in a 2-year-old thumb sucker. Scrapings from all three patients grew *Candida* species.

Tinea versicolor is caused by a dimorphous form of *Pityrosporum* which commonly colonizes the skin by 4–6 months of age. Warm, moist climates, pregnancy, immunodeficiency states, and genetic factors predispose to the development of clinical lesions.

The diagnosis of tinea versicolor can generally be made on the basis of the clinical appearance of lesions and their distribution. It can be confirmed by a KOH preparation of the surface scale, which demonstrates short pseudohyphae and yeast forms that resemble spaghetti and meatballs. Although the pathogenesis of the color change is not fully understood, the fungus is known to produce a substance that interferes with tyrosinase activity and subsequent melanin synthesis.

The differential diagnosis of tinea versicolor includes postinflammatory hypopigmentation and vitiligo. The history, distribution, and distinct borders help to differentiate tinea versicolor from postinflammatory hypopigmentation, and the presence of fine, superficial scaling and some residual pigmentation helps to exclude vitiligo.

Topical desquamating agents, such as selenium sulfide and propylene glycol, produce rapid clearing of tinea versicolor. Localized lesions may be treated effectively with topical antifungal creams, while recalcitrant cases respond to oral ketoconazole. Patients must be counseled about the high risk of recurrence and reminded that pigmentary changes may take months to clear, even after eradication of the fungus.

Confluent and reticulated papillomatosis of Gougerot and Carteaud

Gougerot–Carteaud syndrome is an uncommon eruption that comprises brown or slate-gray papules, which often become confluent on the seborrheic areas of the chest and back, particularly in black adolescents and young adults (Fig 3.53). Reticulated patches may extend over much of the back, shoulders, chest, and abdomen. Although the cause is not known, many investigators attribute the rash to *Pityrosporum* infection. Unfortunately, the rash is usually refractory to treatment. However, some patients improve spontaneously, and others respond to traditional therapy for tinea versicolor.

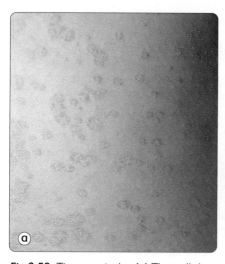
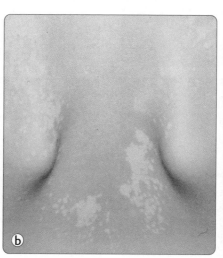
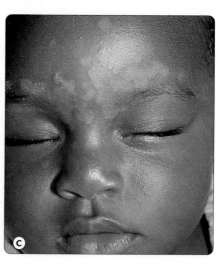

Fig 3.52 Tinea versicolor. **(a)** The well-demarcated, scaly papules appear darker than surrounding skin on the back of a white adolescent. **(b)** Sun-exposed papules on the back of this child failed to tan, resulting in a hypopigmented rash. **(c)** A 4-month-old black girl developed hypopigmented, scaly papules on her face. Her mother had widespread lesions on the chest and back.

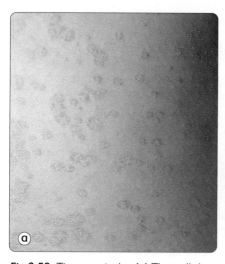
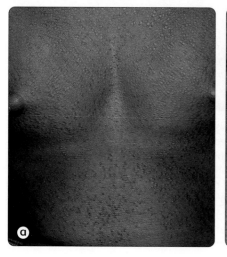
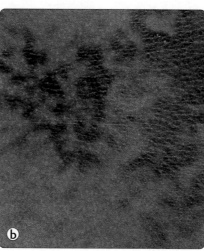

Fig 3.53 Confluent and reticulated papillomatosis. **(a)** Asymptomatic, hyperpigmented papules disseminated over the trunk of this healthy black adolescent. Multiple scrapings for tinea versicolor were negative, and he failed therapy with topical keratolytics. **(b)** At a visit several months later the papules on his upper trunk were confluent and reticulated. The rash disappeared 2 years later without treatment.

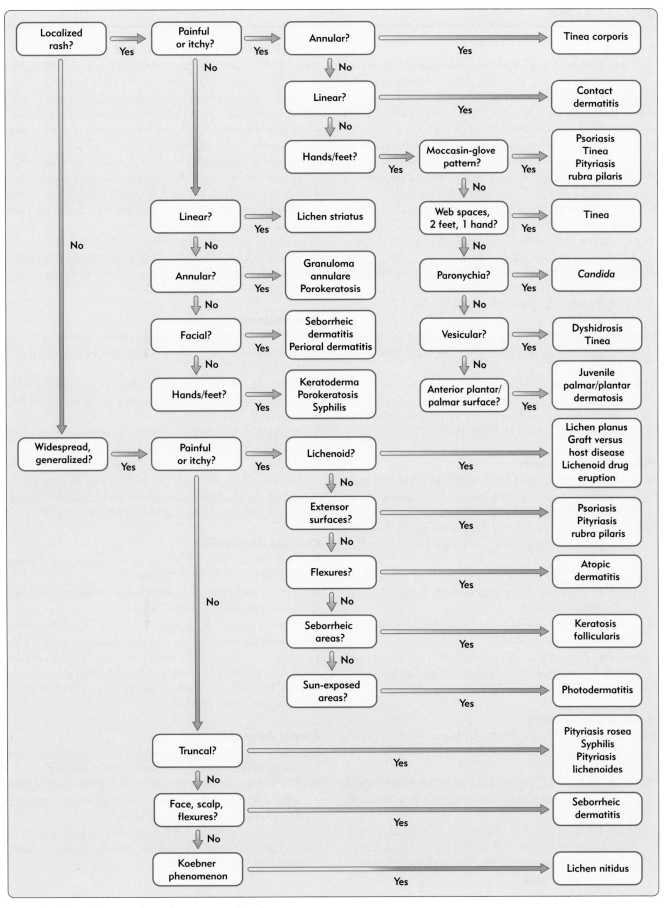

Algorithm for evaluation of papulosquamous disorders.

BIBLIOGRAPHY

Psoriasis

Beylot C, Puisant A, *et al*. Particular clinical features of psoriasis in infants and children. *Acta Dermatol Venereol (Stockh)*. 1979, **87**(Suppl.):95–7.

Farber EM, Nall ML. The natural history of psoriasis in 5600 patients. *Dermatologica*. 1974, **148**:1–18.

Holgate MC. The age-of-onset of psoriasis and the relationship to parental psoriasis. *Br J Dermatol*. 1975, **92**:443–8.

Judge MR, McDonald A, Bloit MM. Pustular psoriasis in childhood. *Clin Exp Dermatol*. 1993, **189**:97–9.

Karman B, Dhar S, Handa S, Kano I. Methotrexate in childhood psoriasis. *Pediatr Dermatol*. 1994, **11**:1271–3.

Koo J, Nguyen Q, Ganebla C. Advances in psoriasis therapy. *Adv Dermatol*. 1997, **12**:47–72.

National Psoriasis Foundation Bulletin, Suite 210, 6443 SW Beaverton Hwy, Portland, Oregon 97221.

Nyfors A, Lemholt K. Psoriasis in children. *Br J Dermatol*. 1975, **92**:437–42.

Oranje AP, Marcoux D, Svenson A, *et al*. Topical calcipotriol in childhood psoriasis. *J Am Acad Dermatol*. 1997, **32**(2 Pt 1):203–8.

Stern RS, Nicholas T. Therapy with orally administered methoxsalen and ultraviolet A radiation during childhood increases the risk of basal cell carcinoma. The PUVA follow-up study. *J Pediatr*. 1996, **129**:915–7.

Pityriasis rubra pilaris

Braun-Falco O, Ryckmanns F, Schmoeckel C, *et al*. Pityriasis rubra pilaris: a clinicopathological and therapeutic study. *Arch Dermatol Res*. 1983, **275**:287–95.

Cohen PR, Prystowsky JH. Pityriasis rubra pilaris. A review of diagnosis and treatment. *J Am Acad Dermatol*. 1989, **20**:801–7.

Darmstadt GL, Tunnessen WW. Picture of the month. Juvenile pityriasis rubra pilaris. *Arch Pediatr Adolesc Med*. 1995, **149**:923–4.

Huntley CC. Pityriasis rubra pilaris. *Am J Dis Child*. 1971, **122**:22–3.

Snahidullah H, Aldridge RD. Changing forms of juvenile pityriasis rubra pilaris, a case report. *Clin Exp Dermatol*. 1994, **19**:354–6.

Keratosis follicularis

Beck AL Jr, Finochio AF, White JP. Darier disease: a kindred with a large number of cases. *Br J Dermatol*. 1977, **97**:335–9.

Harris A, Burge SM, Dykes PJ, Finlay AY. Handicap in Darier disease and Hailey–Hailey disease. *Br J Dermatol*. 1996, **35**:685–94.

Svendsen IB, Albrechtseb B. The prevalence of dyskeratosis follicularis (Darier disease) in Denmark. An investigation of the hereditary in 22 families. *Acta Derm Venereol (Stockh)*. 1959, **39**:356.

Hyperkeratosis of the palms and soles

Kress DW, Seraly MP, Falo L, Dan B, Jegasothy BV, Cohen B. Olmsted syndrome, case report and identification of a keratin abnormality. *Arch Dermatol*. 1996, **132**:297–300.

Mascaro JM, Torros H. A child with unusual palms and soles, epidermolytic palmoplantar keratoderma of Vorner. *Arch Dermatol*. 1996, **132**:1509–12.

Ortega M, Quintana J, Camacho F. Keratosis punctata of the palmar creases. *J Am Acad Dermatol*. 1985, **13**:381–2.

Poulin Y, Perry HO, Muller SA. Olmsted syndrome – congenital palmoplantar and periorificial keratoderma. *J Am Acad Dermatol*. 1984, **10**:600–10.

Schnyder U. Inherited keratodermas of palms and soles. In: Fitzpatrick TB, Eisen AZ, Wolff K, Freedberg IM, Austen KF (eds). *Dermatology in general medicine*. McGraw-Hill, New York, 1993, pp.557–64.

Porokeratosis

Cox GF, Jarratt M. Linear porokeratosis and other linear cutaneous eruptions of childhood. *Am J Dis Child*. 1979, **133**:1258–9.

Ibbotson SH. Disseminated superficial porokeratosis: what is the association with ultraviolet radiation? *Clin Exp Dermatol*. 1996, **21**:48–50.

Madojana RM, Katz R, Rodman OG. Porokeratosis plantaris discreta. *J Am Acad Dermatol*. 1984, **10**:679–82.

Mikhail GR, Wertheimer FW. Clinical variants of porokeratosis (Mibelli). *Arch Dermatol*. 1968, **98**:124–31.

Sasson M, Krain AD. Porokeratosis and cutaneous malignancy, a review. *Dermatol Surg*. 1996, **22**:339–42.

Contact dermatitis

Beltrani VS, Beltrani VP. Contact dermatitis. *Ann Allergy Asthma Immunol*. 1997, **78**:160–73.

Rudzki E, Rebandel P. Contact dermatitis in children. *Contact Dermatitis*. 1996, **34**:66–7.

Wantke F, Hemmer W, Jarisch R, Gotz M. Patch test reactions in children, adults and the elderly, a comparative study in patients with suspected allergic contact dermatitis. *Contact Dermatitis*. 1996, **34**:316–19.

Weston WL. Allergic contact dermatitis in children. *Am J Dis Child*. 1984, **138**:932–6.

Atopic dermatitis

American Academy of Dermatology. Guidelines for atopic dermatitis. *J Am Acad Dermatol*. 1992, **26**:485–8.

Besnier E. Première note et observations préliminaires pour servir d'introduction a l'études des pruripos diathesiques. *Ann Dermatol Syph*. 1892, **23**:634–7.

Kim KH, Hwang JH, Park KC. Periauricular eczematization in childhood atopic dermatitis. *Pediatr Dermatol*. 1996, **13**:78–80.

Leung DY. Atopic dermatitism immunology and treatment with immune modulators. *Clin Exp Immunol*. 1997, **107**(Suppl. 1):25–30.

Oranje AP. Development of childhood eczema and its classification. *Pediatr Allergy Immunol*. 1995, **6**(Suppl. 7):31–5.

Resnick SD, Hornung R, Konrad TR. A comparison of dermatologists and generalists, management of childhood atopic dermatitis. *Arch Dermatol*. 1996, **132**:1047–52.

Rothe MJ, Grant-Kels JM. Atopic dermatitis, an update. *J Am Acad Dermatol*. 1996, **35**:1–13.

Seborrheic dermatitis

Broberg A. Pityrosporum ovale in healthy children, infantile seborrheic dermatitis and atopic dermatitis. *Arch Dermatol Venereol (Stockh)*. 1995, **191**(Suppl.):1–47.

Mimouni K, Mukamel M, Zehaira A, Mimouni M. Progress of infantile seborrheic dermatitis. *J Pediatr*. 1995, **127**:744–6.

Skinner RB, Noah PW, Taylor RM, Zanolli MD, West S, Guin JD. Doubleblind treatment of seborrheic dermatitis with 2% ketoconazole cream. *J Am Acad Dermatol*. 1985, **12**:852–6.

Yates VM, Kerr RE, Frier K, *et al*. Early diagnosis of infantile seborrheic dermatitis and atopic dermatitis: clinical features. *Br J Dermatol*. 1983, **108**:633–8.

Juvenile palmar–plantar dermatosis

Moorthy TT, Rajan VS. Juvenile plantar dermatosis in Singapore. *Int J Dermatol*. 1984, **23**:476.

Steck WD. Juvenile plantar dermatosis: the 'wet and dry foot syndrome.' *Cleve Clin Q*. 1983, **50**:145–9.

Perioral dermatitis

Hogan DJ. Perioral dermatitis. *Curr Prob Dermatol*. 1995, **22**:98–104.

Knautz MA, Lesher JL. Childhood granulomatous periorificial dermatitis. *Pediatr Dermatol*. 1996, **13**:131–4.

Marks R, Black MM. Perioral dermatitis. A histopathological study of 26 cases. *Br J Dermatol*. 1971, **84**:242.

Miller SR, Shalita AR. Topical metronidazole gel (0.75%) for the treatment of perioral dermatitis in children. *J Am Acad Dermatol*. 1994, **31**(5 Pt 2):847–8.

Pityriasis rosea

Allen RA, Janniger CK, Schwartz RA. Pityriasis rosea. *Cutis*. 1995, **56**:198–202.

Cavanaugh RM. Pityriasis rosea in children. *Clin Pediatr*. 1983, **22**:200.

Chuang Tsu-Yi, Ilstrup DM, Perry HO, Kurland LT. Pityriasis rosea in Rochester, Minnesota 1969–1978. *J Am Acad Dermatol*. 1982, **7**:80–9.

Parsons JM. Pityriasis rosea update. *J Am Acad Dermatol*. 1986, **15**:159–67.

Pityriasis lichenoides

Lambert WC, Everett MA. The nosology of parapsoriasis. *J Am Acad Dermatol*. 1981, **5**:373.

Hood AF, Mark EJ. Histopathologic diagnosis of pityriasis lichenoides et varioliformis acuta and its clinical correlation. *Arch Dermatol*. 1982, **118**:478.

Truhan AP, Hebert AA, Esterly NB. Pityriasis lichenoides in children: therapeutic response to erythromycin. *J Am Acad Dermatol*. 1986, **15**:66–70.

Tsuji T, Kasamatsu M, Yokota M, Morita A, Schwartz RA. Mucha–Haberman disease and its febrile ulceronecrotic variant. *Cutis*. 1996, **58**:123–31.

Lichen planus

Boyd AS, Neldner KH. Lichen planus (CME review). *J Am Acad Dermatol*. 1991, **25**:593–619.

Brice SL, Barr RJ, Rattet JP. Childhood lichen planus – a question of therapy. *J Am Acad Dermatol*. 1980, **3**:370.

Ragaz A, Ackerman AB. Evolution maturation, and regression of lesions of lichen planus. *Am J Dermatopathol*. 1981, **3**:5–25.

Rivers JK, Jackson R, Orozaga M. Who was Wickham and what are his striae? *Int J Dermatol*. 1986, **25**:611–3.

Sanchez-Perez J, DeCastro M, Buezo G, Fernandez-Herrera J, Garcia-Diez A. Lichen planus and hepatitis C virus: prevalence and clinical presentation of patients with lichen planus and hepatitis C virus infection. *Br J Dermatol*. 1996, **343**:715–9.

Silverman RA, Rhodes AR. Twenty-nail dystrophy of childhood: a sign of localized lichen planus. *Pediatr Dermatol*. 1984, **1**:207.

Lichen nitidus

Lapins NA, Willoughby C, Helwid EB. Lichen nitidus: a study of 43 cases. *Cutis*. 1978, **21**:634.

Sysa-Jedrzejowska A, Wozniacka A, Robak E, Waszczyska E. Generalized lichen nitidus, a case report. *Cutis*. 1996, **58**:170–2.

Lichen striatus

Charles CR, Johnson BL, Robinson TA. Lichen striatus. *J Cutan Pathol*. 1974, **1**:265–74.

Gianotti R, Restano L, Grindt R, Berti E, Alessi E, Caputo R. Lichen striatus – a chameleon: an histopathological and immunohistochemical study of 41 cases. *J Cutan Pathol*. 1995, **22**:18–22.

Herd RM, McLaren KM, Aldridge RD. Linear lichen planus and lichen planus – opposite ends of a spectrum. *Clin Exp Dermatol*. 1993, **18**:335–7.

Taieb A, Youbi AE, Grosshaus E, Maleville J. Lichen striatus. A Blaschko linear acquired inflammatory skin eruption. *J Am Acad Dermatol*. 1991, **25**:637–42.

Fungal infections

Elewski BE. Cutaneous mycoses in children. *Br J Dermatol.* 1996, **134**(Suppl. 46):7–11.

McLean T, Levy H, Lue YA. Ecology of dermatophyte infections in South Bronx, New York, 1969–1981. *J Am Acad Dermatol.* 1987, **16**:336–40.

Rosenthal JR. Pediatric fungal infections from head to toe: what's new? *Curr Opin Pediatr.* 1994, **6**:35–41.

Savin R. Diagnosis and treatment of tinea versicolor. *J Fam Pract.* 1996, **43**:127–32.

Confluent and reticulated papillomatosis of Gougerot and Carteaud

Hamilton D, Tavafoghi V, Shafer JC. Confluent and reticulated papillomatosis of Gougerot and Carteaud. Its relation to other papillomatoses. *J Am Acad Dermatol.* 1980, **2**:401.

Nordby CA, Mitchell AJ. Confluent and reticulated papillomatosis responsive to selenium sulfide. *Int J Dermatol.* 1986, **25**:194–9.

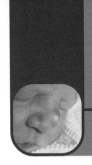

Chapter Four

Vesiculopustular Eruptions

INTRODUCTION

Vesiculopustular eruptions range from benign, self-limited conditions to life-threatening diseases. Early diagnosis, especially in the young or immunocompromised child, is mandatory.

An understanding of the structures that account for normal epidermal and basement membrane zone adhesion provides clues to the clinical diagnosis and pathogenesis of blistering diseases (Fig 4.1). Epidermal cells are held together by desmosome–tonofilament complexes. Electron-dense tonofilaments insert into desmosomes in the keratinocyte plasma membrane and project toward the nucleus. Intercellular bridges extend between keratinocytes and are associated with a sticky, glycoprotein-rich, intercellular, cement substance. In the basement membrane zone tonofilaments insert into hemidesmosomes, which are attached to the lamina densa by anchoring filaments that traverse an electron-lucent layer known as the lamina lucida. The electron-dense lamina densa is, in turn, affixed to the dermis by anchoring fibrils. Elastic microfibril bundles, which arise in the upper dermis, also insert into the lamina densa.

A number of proteins that play a role in the structural integrity of the skin have been identified in the basement membrane zone. Bullous pemphigoid (BP) antigen appears on the bottom of the basal cell plasma membrane and within the lamina lucida. Laminin is present within the lamina lucida, and Type IV collagen has been isolated to the lamina densa. Epidermolysis bullosa acquisita (EBA) antigen has recently been found in the dermis, just beneath the lamina densa. Fluorescein-tagged antibodies directed against these proteins may be used to identify the site of blister formation in disorders that involve the dermal–epidermal junction.

In general, flaccid bullae arise within the epidermis, and tense lesions involve the dermis. Specific diagnoses, however, rely on identification of clinical patterns, histopathology, and immunofluorescent findings. A few rapid diagnostic techniques also aid in developing a differential diagnosis.

VIRAL INFECTIONS

Herpes simplex virus

Herpes simplex virus (HSV) is a common cause of oral lesions in toddlers and children of school age. Primary herpetic gingivostomatitis begins with extensive perioral vesicles and pustules, and intraoral vesicles and erosions (Fig 4.2). The gingivae become edematous, red, friable, and bleed easily. Epithelial debris and exudates may form a membrane on the mucosal surfaces. The eruption is usually accompanied by fever, irritability, and cervical adenopathy. Lesions may also be scattered on the face and upper trunk. In infants and toddlers, lesions are frequently autoinoculated onto the hands. Patients are observed for dehydration as symptoms abate over 7–10 days.

Herpetic gingivostomatitis can be differentiated from enteroviral infections, which usually produce vesicles, ulcerations, and petechiae on the hard palate and spare the gingivae. Although aphthae may be very painful, they are usually isolated lesions that lack the diffuse inflammation associated with herpes.

Primary herpes simplex infections may involve any cutaneous or mucous membrane surface and generally result from direct inoculation of previously injured sites. Lesions consist of herpetiform or clustered red papules, which evolve into vesicles and, not infrequently, pustules in 24–48 hours (Figs 4.2 and 4.3). During the following 5–7 days vesicles rupture and crust over. Desquamation and healing is complete in 10–14 days. Primary herpes infections on the fingers are called herpetic whitlows (Fig 4.3b). Just as in herpetic gingivostomatitis, primary infections at other sites may be associated with painful local adenopathy and flu-like symptoms.

In children most infections are caused by HSV Type 1, whereas HSV Type 2 is most commonly found in genital infections in adolescents and adults (Fig 4.4). However, it can also be found in nongenital areas, and Type 1 virus may be spread from mouth to hand to genital sites. Although sexual contact must be considered in any child who develops genital herpes, nonvenereal sources are probably most common. Vesicles are usually restricted to the perineum and genital skin, and quickly ulcerate. Erythema and edema may result in severe dysuria and urinary retention.

In immunocompromised children or patients with certain skin conditions, such as atopic dermatitis, seborrheic dermatitis, and immunologic blistering disorders, herpes simplex may disseminate over the entire skin surface (eczema herpeticum or Kaposi varicelliform eruption; see Fig 3.32) and to the lungs, viscera, and central nervous system. Also, HSV may also produce life-threatening disease in the nursery.

Following the initial episode, HSV enters a dormant state. A number of endogenous and environmental factors may trigger reactivation of the virus, such as a *Streptococcus* infection of the throat, an upper respiratory infection, sunburn, and surgery (Fig 4.5). Lesions usually occur near the site of the primary eruption, mucous membranes are not usually involved, systemic symptoms are absent, and the rash heals in less than a week. Although recurrences are unpredictable, disease-free periods tend to increase with time, even in individuals who initially experience frequent recurrences.

A clinical suspicion of herpes simplex can be confirmed quickly by performing a Tzanck smear in the emergency room or at the bedside. Viral cultures in reliable laboratories turn positive in 12–36 hours. In some centers, polymerase chain reaction studies, immunofluorescent staining of blister fluid debris on glass slides, or electron microscopy is used for rapid confirmation.

The Tzanck smear is obtained by removing the roof of a blister with a scalpel or scissors and scraping its base to obtain the moist, cloudy debris (see Fig 1.10). This is spread onto a glass slide with the scalpel blade, desiccated with 95% ethanol, and stained with Giemsa or Wright

Cutaneous anatomy	Site of blister formation	Disorder
	Upper epidermis	Staphylococcal scalded-skin syndrome
	Mid-epidermis	Dermatitis Friction blister Pemphigus foliaceus
	Lower epidermis	Herpes simplex Varicella-zoster Pemphigus vulgaris Epidermolytic epidermolysis bullosa Bullous pemphigoid
	Basement membrane zone	Chronic bullous disease of childhood Dermatitis herpetiformis Junctional epidermolysis bullosa
	Dermis	Epidermolysis bullosa acquisita Dermolytic epidermolysis bullosa Toxic epidermal necrolysis Burn

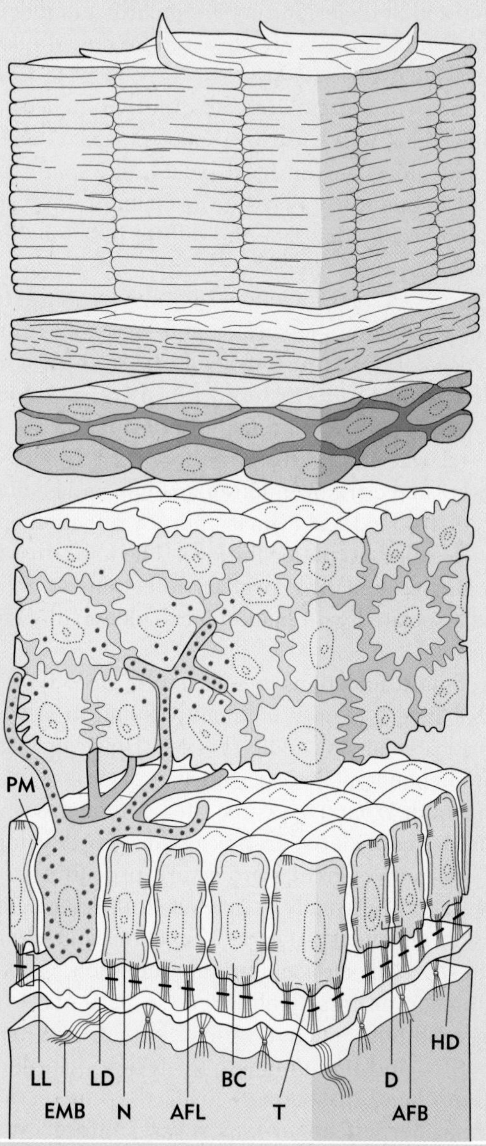

AFB = Anchoring fibril
AFL = Anchoring filament
BC = Basal cel
D = Desmosome

EMB = Elastic microfibril bundle
HD = Hemidesmosome
LD = Lamina densa

LL = Lamina lucida of basal cell
N = Basal cell nucleus
PM = Plasma membrane
T = Tonofilament

Fig 4.1 Anatomy of vesiculopustular dermatoses.

stain. The diagnostic finding in viral blisters is the multi-nucleated giant cell, which is a syncytium of epidermal cells with multiple, overlapping nuclei; hence, it is much larger than other inflammatory cells. Unfortunately, a

positive Tzanck smear cannot be used to differentiate one blistering viral eruption from another, and a viral culture should be obtained when the clinical situation dictates.

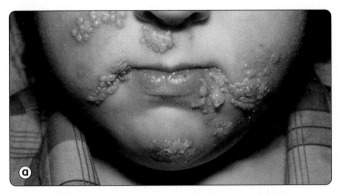

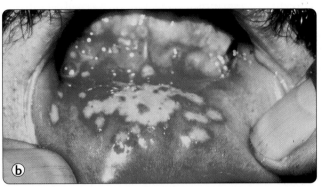

Fig 4.2 Herpetic gingivostomatitis. **(a)** This 6-year-old boy developed extensive perioral vesicles and mucous membrane erosions with his first bout of herpes simplex. **(b)** A 19-year-old experienced severe pain from widespread gingival and buccal mucosal vesicles and erosions during the peak of his primary herpes infection.

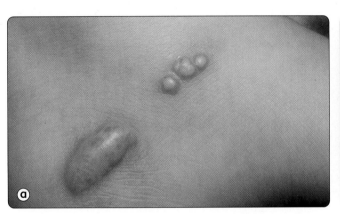

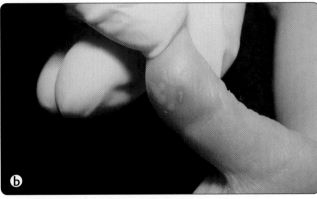

Fig 4.3 Primary herpes simplex infections. **(a)** Over 24 hours herpetic vesicles evolved into pustules on the foot of a 5-year-old boy. In one area near the heel several vesicles fused to form a multiloculated bulla. **(b)** Herpetic whitlow developed by autoinoculation from oral lesions in this 4-year-old boy. Oral and finger lesions resolved without treatment in 2 weeks.

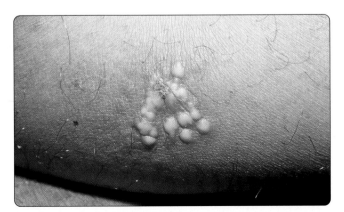

Fig 4.4 Clustered pustules appeared on the posterior thigh of a teenager with recurrent herpes simplex Type 2 infection.

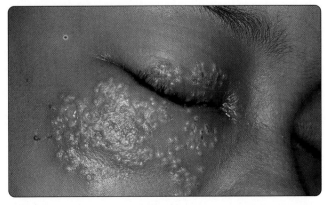

Fig 4.5 Recurrent herpes simplex erupted around the eye of this 11-year-old boy. The cornea was not involved, and vesicles crusted over in less than a week.

In general, management of herpes infections is symptomatic with cool compresses, lubricants, and oral analgesics. Topical acyclovir is of little use in the treatment of uncomplicated infections in normal hosts. Immunocompromised children with primary or recurrent herpes simplex infections and patients with severe primary herpetic gingivostomatitis or genital herpes usually improve quickly with parenteral acyclovir (5 mg/kg every 8 hours). Several new, orally administered drugs, which include valacyclovir hydrochloride and famciclovir achieve consistent blood levels. Although they are not yet approved for use in children, these medications should provide a safe, effective alternative to parenteral acyclovir for children with serious herpetic infections. In recurrent disease, initiation of oral acyclovir with the prodromal tingling in the skin before the appearance of blisters may abort the episode. In selected children with frequent, multiple, widespread recurrent eruptions long-term, suppressive therapy may be necessary.

Herpes simplex infections are usually differentiated from other blistering eruptions by the typical clustering of lesions, the clinical course, a positive Tzanck smear, and characteristic skin-biopsy findings. Impetigo may mimic herpes. However, bullae tend to be relatively large, with a central crust and peripheral extension, and a Gram stain demonstrates Gram-positive cocci. Blistering distal dactylitis, which is caused by Group A β-hemolytic streptococci, may be mistaken for a herpetic whitlow (Fig 4.6). In streptococcal infection, the lesions on the finger tips usually coalesce to form one or several 5–10 mm diameter blisters, and Gram stains and cultures demonstrate the causative bacterium. Occasionally, the eruption of herpes simplex may form a dermatomal pattern. In this situation a viral culture is required to exclude herpes zoster.

Varicella (chickenpox)

Varicella is a mild, self-limited infection in most children. However, disseminated disease is a problem in the neonate and immunosuppressed child. Early administration of varicella-zoster immune globulin to immunocompromised children exposed to varicella may be preventive, and antiviral therapy in patients with disseminated lesions may be lifesaving. The introduction of varicella vaccine into the primary immunization series should reduce the incidence of varicella and the risk of complications.

After exposure to varicella, the incubation period varies in the range 7–21 days. Fever, sore throat, decreased appetite, and malaise precede the skin lesions by several days. Early cutaneous findings vary from a few scattered, pruritic, red papules to generalized papules that evolve in 24 hours to vesicles on a bright red base (dew drops on a rose petal, Fig 4.7). Central umbilication of blisters follows rapidly, and crusting and desquamation occurs within 10 days. New papules and vesicles continue to appear for 3–4 days. Vesicles may also be identified on mucous membranes, particularly the buccal mucosa and gingivae. Although the blisters are intraepidermal and usually heal

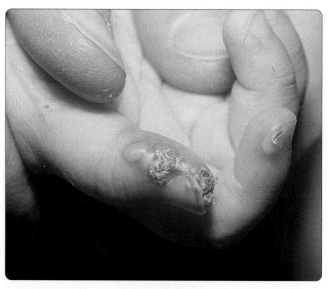

Fig 4.6 Blistering distal dactylitis developed on the right thumb and index finger of a 5-year-old girl. Cultures from her throat and thumb grew Group A β-hemolytic streptococci. The infection responded quickly to oral amoxicillin.

without scarring, some develop deep inflammation or become secondarily infected and heal with pitted or hypertrophic scars (Fig 4.8a).

Pruritus may be intense and responds to cool compresses, calamine lotion, and antihistamines. Secondary infection is usually caused by staphylococci, and is treated with oral antibiotics such as dicloxacillin, cephalexin, or erythromycin (Fig 4.8b). When cellulitis or other deep, soft-tissue infection complicates chickenpox, hospitalization and parenteral therapy may be required. An increase in Group A β-hemolytic streptococcal fasciitis has been reported in association with recent varicella epidemics (Fig 4.8c). Rarely, progressive purpura and necrosis of large areas of skin heralds the onset of disseminated intravascular coagulation (Fig 4.8d). This phenomenon, referred to as purpura fulminans, occurs in fewer than 1 in 20,000 cases of varicella.

Administration of systemic corticosteroids, even in normal children, is contraindicated during varicella infection and may result in severe blistering, disseminated viral infection, and increased risk of complications. As a consequence, it is important to differentiate chickenpox from contact dermatitis, insect bites, and mononucleosis or other viral infections. The Tzanck smear may be particularly useful early in the course of disease, when only a few skin lesions are present.

Herpes zoster

Herpes zoster or shingles represents a reactivation of the dormant varicella virus from the sensory root ganglia. The most commonly involved sites include the head and neck and the thoracic sensory nerves (Fig 4.9). After a variable prodrome, which may include mild constitutional

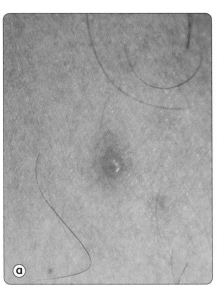

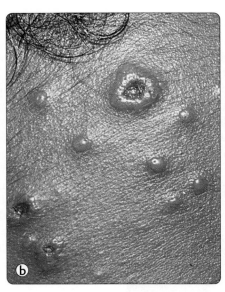

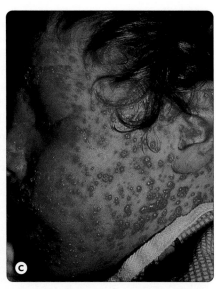

Fig 4.7 Chickenpox. **(a)** A dew drop on a rose petal is the characteristic primary lesion in chickenpox. **(b)** Lesions in various stages of development, including red papules, vesicles, umbilicated vesicles, and crusts developed in close proximity on the forehead of a toddler with varicella. **(c)** Severe varicella with blisters almost to confluence erupted within 24 hours over much of the skin surface of this 6-year-old boy who was on high-dose systemic corticosteroids for inflammatory bowel disease.

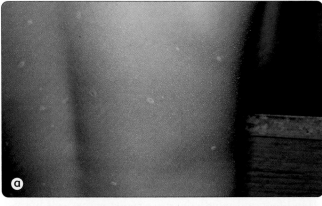

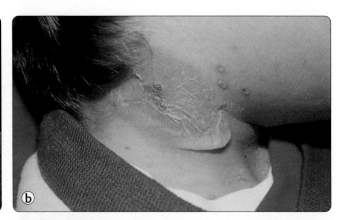

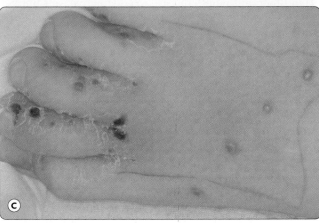

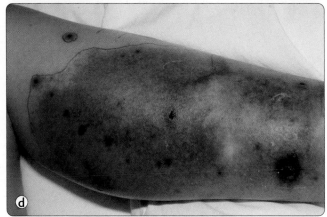

Fig 4.8 Complications of varicella. **(a)** Multiple hypopigmented scars developed on the trunk of this 10-year-old boy several weeks after chickenpox. **(b)** Bullous impetigo spread quickly by scratching in a 4-year-old boy with chickenpox. Note the pus at the bottom of the large bulla. **(c)** While this child was recovering from varicella, several lesions on the top of her foot became infected with Group A β-hemolytic streptococci. The rapidly spreading area of erythema responded quickly to high-dose parenteral penicillin. **(d)** A 7-year-old girl with healing chickenpox developed purpura fulminans, with expanding bruises on her legs. Laboratory studies were consistent with disseminated intravascular coagulation, which resolved on heparin therapy. Note the resolving chickenpox vesicles on her leg.

symptoms and localized itching and burning, linear, clustered, red papulovesicles appear in a unilateral linear pattern in one or several dermatomes. In some children, the eruption may be completely asymptomatic. Over 3–5 days the rash reaches its full extent, and during the ensuing 1–2 weeks vesicles and erosions develop umbilicated crusts and desquamate, much like in chickenpox.

Although 6–10 lesions may appear outside the primary dermatomes in normal individuals, the development of widespread cutaneous lesions suggests the possibility of an immunodeficiency state and an increased risk of visceral

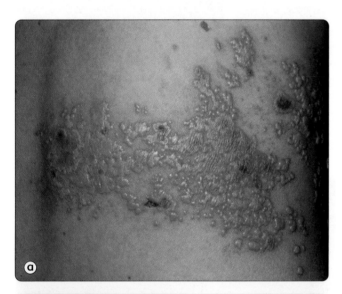

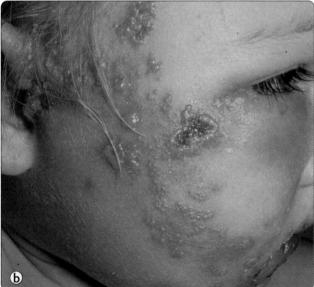

Fig 4.9 Herpes zoster infection. **(a)** Herpes zoster involved the right, mid-thoracic dermatomes in an otherwise healthy 10-year-old girl with a history of chickenpox when 2 years old.
(b) Periorbital cellulitis was initially considered in this toddler with impressive edema and erythema of the right eye. The diagnosis of shingles became apparent 1 day later, when the characteristic dermatomal vesiculopustular rash appeared. Both children had uneventful recoveries without treatment.

involvement. Children with lymphoreticular malignancies are over 100 times as likely to develop zoster as healthy children. However, most cases of childhood zoster occur in normal hosts.

Normal children who develop chickenpox during the first 2 months of life may also be prone to zoster. In these patients, protective antibody titers tend to be low and skin-test reactions are diminished, which suggests a blunted, immunologic response to varicella in early infancy. This phenomenon may result from transient, maternal antibody protection, which wanes during the first 4 months of life.

The presence of a dermatomal bullous eruption is virtually diagnostic for herpes zoster. However, herpes simplex occasionally presents in a dermatomal pattern. Moreover, zoster may be confused with herpes simplex early in the course, when only a few clustered vesicles are present and the dermatomal organization is not yet apparent.

Management of shingles is usually limited to supportive measures similar to those for chickenpox. In disseminated disease administration of parenteral acyclovir may be life-saving. Normal individuals who develop eye involvement also benefit from antiviral therapy and are followed closely by an ophthalmologist. The high risk of zoster in patients undergoing bone marrow transplantation or other elective immunosuppression may require antiviral prophylaxis in these children.

Although systemic corticosteroids may be administered to reduce the risk of postherpetic neuralgia in adults over 60 years of age, this treatment has not been shown to be beneficial in young adults or children. Moreover, the incidence of this problem in childhood is extremely low. Children with shingles must be isolated from individuals who are susceptible to chickenpox because of the risk of acquiring infection from direct contact with skin lesions.

Hand-foot-and-mouth disease

Hand-foot-and-mouth disease is a distinctive, self-limited viral eruption caused most frequently by *Coxsackie virus A16*. The disease is highly infectious and, like other enteroviruses, peak incidence occurs in the late summer and fall. After exposure, the incubation period is 4–6 days. A 1–2 day prodrome of fever, anorexia, and sore throat are followed by the development of 3–6 mm diameter elongated, gray, thin-walled vesicles on a red or noninflamed base. As the name suggests, lesions appear most commonly on the palms, soles, and sides of the hands and feet, but red papules and vesicles may also erupt on the buttocks, trunk, face, arms, and legs (Fig 4.10a, b). The enanthema is characterized by vesicles that rapidly ulcerate to leave sharply marginated erosions on a red base on the tongue, buccal mucosa, and posterior pharynx (Fig 4.10c). Although cutaneous and mucosal lesions may be completely asymptomatic, pruritus and burning can be severe. Systemic symptoms, which include fever, diarrhea, sore throat, and cervical adenopathy, may be absent or mild, and treatment is supportive. The eruption usually clears in less than a week.

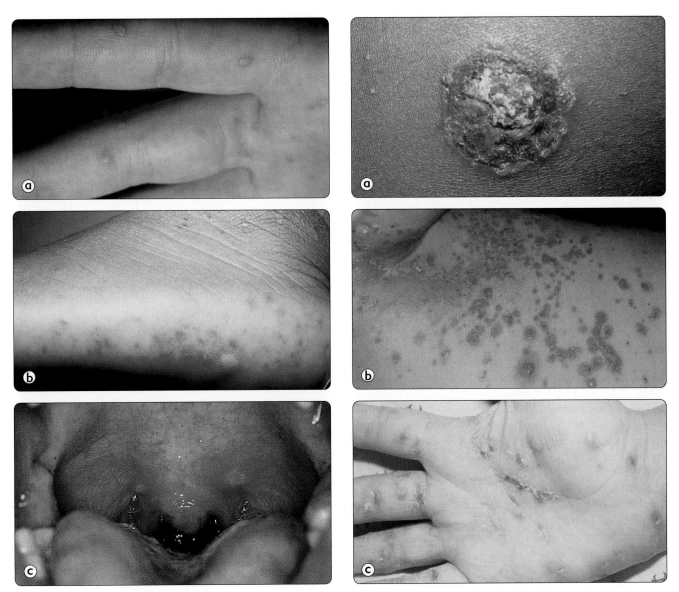

Fig. 4.10 Hand-foot-and-mouth disease. Characteristic elongated vesicles on a red base are shown on **(a)** the palmar surface of the fingers and **(b)** plantar surface of the foot of children with Coxsackie hand-foot-and-mouth disease. **(c)** The enanthema, consisting of shallow yellow ulcers surrounded by red halos, may be found on the labial or buccal mucosa, the tongue, soft palate, soft palate, uvula, and anterior tonsilar pillars. When the enanthema occurs in the absence of a rash, the disorder is known as herpangina.

Fig 4.11 Bullous impetigo. **(a)** A large doughnut-shaped blister with a central crust and smaller satellite lesions suggests the diagnosis of bullous impetigo. **(b)** Widespread blisters in this toddler responded quickly to oral cephalexin. **(c)** Painful impetiginized pustules obscured the primary diagnosis of scabies in this teenager. A careful examination, however, revealed burrows on her palms and soles, and she was treated with oral cephalexin and topical 5% permethrin cream.

BACTERIAL INFECTIONS

Impetigo

Expanding, honey-colored, crusted patches or bullae with a central crust suggest the diagnosis of impetigo (Fig 4.11, also see Fig 3.31). In older children in temperate climates, lesions appear most commonly on exposed skin during the summer months. Although Group A β-hemolytic streptococci were the predominant organisms 25–30 years ago, *Staphylococcus aureus* alone or in combination with streptococci is recovered from a majority of cultures. As a consequence, antistaphylococcal antibiotics are now the drugs of choice for treatment.

Impetigo is often a self-limiting process. However, complications, which include cellulitis and disseminated infection, as well as spread to family members and classmates, can be limited by antibiotic therapy. Topical antibiotics such as bacitracin, polymixin B, neomycin, and mupirocin can be used in localized disease. Widespread lesions are treated with oral agents such as dicloxacillin, cephalexin, amoxicillin–

clavulanate, and erythromycin. Unfortunately, up to 40% of staphylococcal isolates are reported to be resistant to erythromycin in a number of surveys in the US. Consequently, the practitioner must select antibiotic coverage based on the resistance patterns in their respective communities.

Staphylococcal scalded-skin syndrome

Staphylococcal scalded-skin syndrome (SSSS) occurs almost exclusively in infants and toddlers (Fig 4.12, also see Fig 2.47). It has, however, been reported with increasing frequency in older children and adults, particularly in debilitated patients with decreased renal function. This process is considered in any child who develops a generalized, tender erythema associated with Nikolsky sign. When Nikolsky sign is present, a minimal shearing force produced by finger pressure induces a skin slough or blister formation.

Although SSSS is usually self-limiting in healthy children, immunocompromised patients may develop complications related to their primary staphylococcal infection. Most SSSS is associated with a primary cutaneous infection. However, the soluble toxin that causes the rash may be produced by an occult infection, such as osteomyelitis, septic arthritis, pneumonia, or meningitis. Healthy children respond to oral anti-staphylococcal antibiotics. Infants, severely ill older children, and patients with occult infection require appropriate culturing and parenteral therapy. Parents are also counseled about the generalized desquamation that develops 10–14 days after the acute infection.

Staphylococcal folliculitis

Staphylococcal folliculitis is a common problem in older children and adults. Red papules and pustules on an inflamed base erupt in a follicular pattern, most frequently on the buttocks, thighs, back, and upper arms (Fig 4.13).

Occasionally, superficial follicular pustules evolve into painful, deep-seated furuncles or spread to neighboring follicles and soft tissue to create an abscess or carbuncle. Abscesses and resultant cellulitis may be associated with fever, malaise, and sepsis.

Localized folliculitis may improve with topical antibiotics. However, widespread lesions respond best to systemic therapy. Additionally, abscesses are incised and drained, and cellulitis may require parenteral antibiotics.

Children with chronic folliculitis often have predisposing dermatoses such as keratosis pilaris. Children with Down syndrome are particularly prone to folliculitis on the trunk and proximal extremities. Long-term use of antiseptic soaps, topical antibiotics (e.g. clindamycin, tetracycline, erythromycin) and peeling agents (e.g. benzoyl peroxide, retinoic acid, salicylic acid) may reduce the risk of recurrent infection. Certain hydrating lotions and creams that are also designed to remove scale (e.g. Carmol® and Ureacin® with urea, LactiCare® and LacHydrin® with lactic acid) may be beneficial. Patients are also instructed to avoid tight clothing, and occlusive moisturizers. In toddlers, folliculitis may improve after toilet training. Older children with enuresis should also be encouraged to remove wet clothing as soon as possible.

IMMUNOBULLOUS DERMATOSES

Although there is clinical overlap among the various immunologically mediated vesiculobullous dermatoses, they can be differentiated on the basis of specific clinical patterns, histopathology, immunopathology, and response to therapy. In pemphigus, blisters form within the epidermis. Chronic bullous dermatosis of childhood or linear IgA dermatosis, BP, dermatitis herpetiformis (DH), and EBA are characterized by subepidermal blisters.

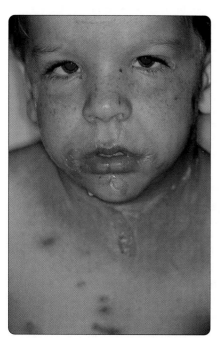

Fig 4.12 Staphylococcal scalded-skin syndrome. A healthy 4-year-old boy developed fever, periorificial crusting, and generalized, tender red skin. Nikolsky sign was present, and *Staphylococcus aureus* was cultured from his nares.

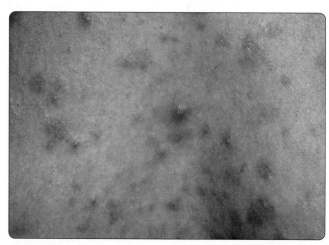

Fig. 4.13 Staphylococcal folliculitis recurred chronically on the buttocks of a 13-year-old boy with Down syndrome. Note the red papules and pustules around the gluteal cleft. He improved considerably with the use of topical benzoyl peroxide and mupirocin ointment, but he still required intermittent oral antibiotic therapy.

Intraepidermal disorders

Childhood pemphigus refers to a group of rare, chronic, potentially life-threatening immunobullous disorders characterized by flaccid intraepidermal bullae that erupt on normal-appearing or erythematous skin. Clinically and histologically, pemphigus can be divided into two types: pemphigus vulgaris and pemphigus foliaceus.

Pemphigus vulgaris

In pemphigus vulgaris (PV), intraoral erosions or scalp blisters precede more widespread lesions in half the patients for months. Eventually, vesicles and bullae develop on the trunk, scalp, face, and extremities in a seborrheic distribution (Fig 4.14a–c). By progressive extension, large areas of the body surface may become involved. Blisters heal insidiously without scarring, unless they become secondarily infected. Of these patients, 95% have intraoral involvement that may extend into the posterior pharynx and larynx. Pruritus, pain, and burning of the skin and mucous membranes may be severe, which results in decreased oral intake and marked weight loss. Nikolsky sign is usually present, and downward pressure on previously formed blisters may cause extension at the periphery (Asbaugh–Hansen sign). Pemphigus may also occur transiently in the newborn as a result of transplacental passage of the pemphigus antibody from the mother to the baby.

Although the pathogenesis of PV is not completely understood, an IgG antibody directed against epidermal intercellular cement substance has been identified in the skin, serum, and blister fluid of these patients. When the purified IgG obtained from blister fluid is injected into the peritoneal cavity of neonatal nude mice, it produces widespread blistering, which demonstrates acantholysis. Complement, IgA, and IgM have also been identified in blister fluid, but their roles in the development of bullae are not clear.

Biopsies of fresh, intact vesicles with perilesional skin demonstrate intercellular edema and disappearance of intercellular bridges in the lower portion of the epidermis at the periphery. Separation of epidermal cells from one another leads to the formation of suprabasilar clefts and then frank blister formation, with the basal cells left hanging onto the basement membrane. Rounded up acantholytic keratinocytes may be found within the bullae and are easily demonstrated on Tzanck smears.

In virtually 100% of patients, fluorescein-labeled IgG can be demonstrated to bind to the epidermal intercellular space in the patient's normal-appearing and perilesional skin (Fig 4.14d). This finding is referred to as positive direct

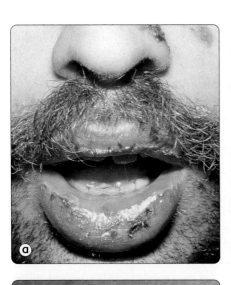
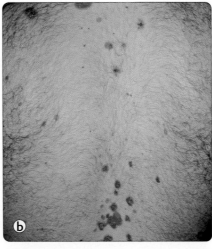
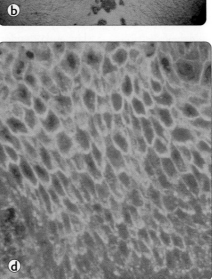

Fig. 4.14 Pemphigus vulgaris. A 20-year-old man developed superficial hemorrhagic blisters on **(a)** his face and lips, and **(b)** his trunk in a seborrheic distribution. Histopathology and immunofluorescence demonstrated findings typical for pemphigus vulgaris. **(c)** Note the flaccid blisters on a minimally inflamed base. **(d)** Anti-IgG antibody marks the epidermal intercellular cement substance on direct immunofluorescence.

immunofluorescence (DIF). Deposits of C3, IgA, or IgM are also identified in nearly half of the patients. For study of indirect immunofluorescence (IIF), unfixed frozen sections of various epithelium, such as monkey esophagus or normal human skin, are used. The patient's serum is applied to the specimen followed by fluorescein-labeled antihuman IgG at various dilutions. When the study is positive, fluorescence is seen in the intercellular spaces of the test specimen. The antibody titer refers to the highest dilution at which fluorescence is still noted. Although DIF is very sensitive, even early in the course of disease, IIF is less useful, particularly before lesions become widespread.

Early PV restricted to the mouth must be differentiated histologically from other disorders that involve the oral mucosa, such as erosive lichen planus and aphthosis. Once cutaneous lesions appear, the typical clinical pattern, histology, and immunofluorescence differentiate PV from other immunobullous disorders.

Before the introduction of corticosteroids, patients often succumbed to sepsis. Management of fluid and electrolyte losses and supportive skin care may require admission to a burn unit. High-dose prednisone (2–5mg/kg/day) may be lifesaving. After the eruption has been brought under control, corticosteroids may usually be tapered over 9–12 months to acceptable maintenance levels. Some patients may require corticosteroid-sparing immunosuppressive agents such as methotrexate, cyclophosphamide, or azathioprine, depending on their response to the corticosteroid taper.

Pemphigus foliaceus

Pemphigus foliaceus (PF) is a more superficial and less aggressive immunobullous disorder. Although it occurs most commonly in middle age, in children this variant is more common than PV. Although PF tends to be sporadic and most cases have been reported in North America and Europe, an endemic variant known as fogo selvagem occurs primarily in children and adolescents in Brazil. Clinically and histologically, PF is indistinguishable from Brazilian pemphigus. Some medications, such as penicillamine have also been reported to trigger a PF-like eruption.

Much like PV, PF begins with crops of vesicles, flaccid bullae, and erosions on an erythematous base in a seborrheic distribution. However, since the blisters arise high in the epidermis, they quickly crust over. Nikolsky sign is usually positive, but mucous membranes are invariably spared. When lesions become generalized, vesicles may be obscured by crust and scale, which gives the patient the appearance of an exfoliative erythroderma (Fig 4.15). Even with widespread rash, patients tend to appear clinically well, and the course is often self-limiting.

Histopathology demonstrates acantholysis and bullae formation, much like in PV. However, the action occurs in the upper half of the epidermis, sometimes restricted to the area immediately beneath the stratum corneum. The intercellular space in the upper half of the epidermis shows IgG staining with DIF, and the IIF is also usually positive. Chronic lesions typically show acanthosis, eosinophilic spongiosis, and eosinophilic dermal inflammation.

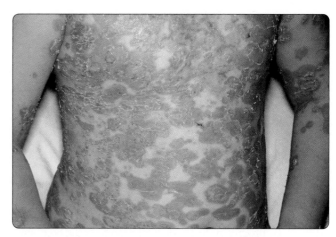

Fig 4.15 Pemphigus foliaceus. A 10-year-old girl with generalized, slightly itchy, scaly, and crusted patches was referred for evaluation of possible pemphigus foliaceus. Although a skin biopsy was suggestive of pemphigus, a skin culture grew *Staphylococcus aureus*, and the rash resolved after 7 days of oral dicloxacillin.

Patients with mild disease may respond to moderate- or high-potency topical corticosteroids. In many cases, systemic corticosteroids may be required for a while, and some investigators have reported success with antimalarials (hydroxychloroquine and chloroquine) and sulfonamides (sulfapyridine and dapsone).

Subepidermal disorders

Chronic bullous dermatosis of childhood (CBDC) is probably the most common subepidermal immunobullous disease in children. It is also known as linear IgA dermatosis, which describes the characteristic immunofluorescent finding in perilesional skin.

Although tense 1.0–2.0 cm diameter bullae typically appear in preschool children on the lower trunk, buttocks, legs, and top of the feet, children of any age may be affected (Fig 4.16). Widespread lesions may involve any site on the body surface including the face, scalp, upper trunk, hands, and arms. Lesions erupt on red as well as normal-appearing skin, and often form rings composed of sausage-shaped bullae around a central crust or healing blister. Linear or annular vesicles on an inflamed base may suggest a 'string of pearls'. (Fig 4.17) Mucous membranes are not usually involved, Nikolsky sign is not present, and burning and pruritus are variable. Some children are completely asymptomatic.

Histopathology is indistinguishable from that of BP, which demonstrates a subepidermal blister with a dermal infiltrate of neutrophils and eosinophils. Occasionally, eosinophils form microabscesses at the tips of the dermal papillae reminiscent of DH. However, DIF shows linear deposits of IgA at the dermal–epidermal junction and is diagnostic (Fig 4.18). Investigators have also shown that the site of deposition is within the lamina lucida, with accentuation near the basal cell membrane around hemidesmosomes. Circulating IgA antibodies are present in 50–75% of patients.

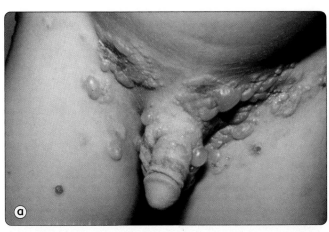

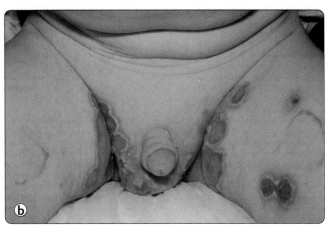

Fig. 4.16 Chronic bullous dermatosis of childhood. Two 3-year-old boys presented with chronic, recurrent blisters in the diaper area. **(a)** Fresh, tense bullae spread along the inguinal creases onto the thighs and penis. **(b)** Ruptured bullae left annular and scalloped erosions.

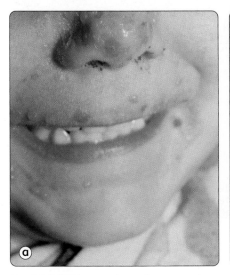

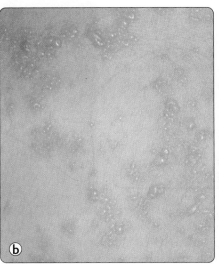

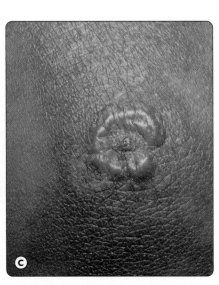

Fig 4.17 Widespread vesicles erupted over several days in a 5-year-old girl with chronic bullous dermatosis of childhood. Blisters were densest on **(a)** the face and **(b)** trunk. **(c)** Characteristic annular blisters spread over the trunk and extremities of this 4-year-old boy. The bullous dermatosis in both children responded quickly to 25 mg/day of dapsone.

Although CBDC is often self-limiting with spontaneous resolution over 3–5 years, occasional cases persist after adolescence. Many children are exquisitely sensitive to small doses of dapsone (0.5–1.0 mg/kg/day). Blisters often respond within 1–3 days of initiating therapy, and medication may be tapered to low maintenance doses (12.5–25 mg/day or less). Resistant cases may require systemic corticosteroids, at least until the eruption comes under control. All patients on dapsone must be monitored for clinical and laboratory signs of hemolysis, methemoglobinemia, and neurologic complications.

It is important that CBDC be differentiated from a less common immunobullous dermatosis, juvenile BP, in which the bullae are often large (>2.0 cm in diameter) and mucous membranes are frequently involved (Fig 4.19). Skin biopsies in BP also demonstrate subepidermal bullae with an eosinophilic dermal infiltrate. However, linear depositions

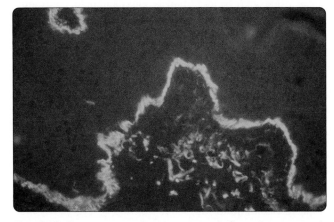

Fig. 4.18 Direct immunofluorescence in bullous dermatosis of childhood shows diagnostic linear IgA deposition along the dermal–epidermal junction.

of IgG and C3 at the dermal–epidermal junction in the lamina lucida are diagnostic for BP. An unusual cicatricial variant of BP involves primarily the mucous membranes and occurs only rarely in childhood.

Symmetric, extremely pruritic, clustered, 3–4 mm diameter vesicles on extensor surfaces of the extremities, lower trunk, and buttocks may suggest DH (Fig 4.20). In DH, the lesions arise on both red and normal-appearing skin and may occasionally exceed 1.0 cm in diameter. The skin biopsy of perilesional skin reveals characteristic, granular IgA deposits in the basement membrane zone and prominent neurophilic microabscesses at the dermal papillary tips. The high incidence of human leukocyte antigen (HLA) B8 antigens also defines DH, as does a gluten-sensitive entero-pathy and a rapid response to dapsone.

The target lesions of erythema multiforme (EM), particularly when blistering is present, may be confused with those of CBDC. However, the acute clinical course, histopathology, and negative immunofluorescence readily differentiate EM. Early in its course, CBDC is often misdiagnosed as bullous impetigo. Moreover, bullae of CBDC that are secondarily infected respond to antibiotic therapy. However, the persistence of blistering despite antibiotic therapy, the widespread distribution of the eruption, and negative Gram stains and cultures suggest a noninfectious etiology.

Recurrent *Herpes simplex virus* infection and the possibility of sexual abuse can also be excluded by the characteristic skin biopsy findings (Fig 4.21).

MECHANOBULLOUS DISORDERS

Friction blisters

Friction blisters occur frequently on the soles, palms, and palmar surfaces of the fingers after vigorous exercise or other repetitive activities which cause shearing of thick areas of epidermis that are firmly attached to underlying tissue (Fig 4.22a). In patients with chronic localized or generalized edema, particularly in the setting of malnutrition, minor trauma may result in blister formation. Similar blisters can result from rubbing and sucking (Fig 4.22b). Histologically, these lesions may be identified as noninflammatory, intraepidermal blisters, which are usually located just beneath the granular layer. Although blisters heal quickly in healthy individuals, impetiginization and cellulitis are frequent complications in compromised hosts.

Epidermolysis bullosa

Epidermolysis bullosa is a heterogeneous group of mechanobullous disorders differentiated by clinical findings, depth of blister formation, biochemical markers, and inheritance patterns (see Fig 2.50). In most of these conditions, vesiculobullous lesions appear at birth or in early infancy. Several variants, however, do not present until adolescence or adult life.

In recurrent epidermolysis bullosa of the hands and feet, or Weber–Cockayne syndrome (an autosomal-dominant epidermolytic variant), blisters may first appear on the soles

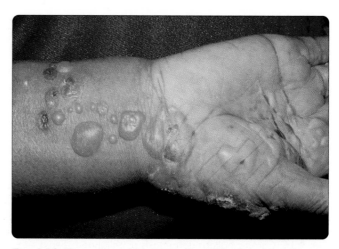

Fig. 4.19 Tense, large blisters developed insidiously on the extremities and trunk of a patient with bullous pemphigoid.

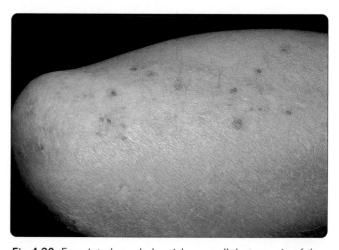

Fig 4.20 Excoriated, eroded vesicles are all that remain of the primary lesions of dermatitis herpetiformis in this teenager. Similar lesions were symmetrically distributed on the anterior thighs, knees, buttocks, back, and abdomen. Intact vesicles are only occasionally seen in dermatitis herpetiformis because of the intense pruritus and resultant scratching.

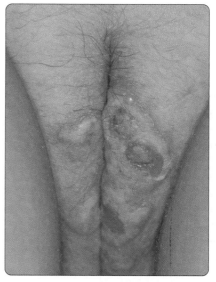

Fig 4.21 This adolescent girl with a 9-month history of genital blisters and erosions failed to improve with topical antibiotics, antifungal creams, lubricants, or oral acyclovir. Sexual abuse was suspected until a skin biopsy, which demonstrated the classic findings of chronic bullous dermatosis of childhood, was performed.

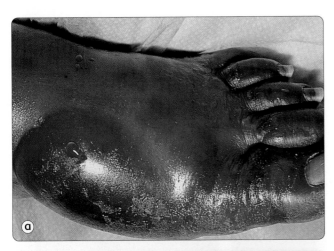

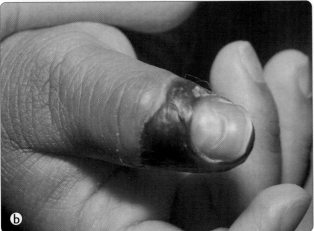

Fig 4.22 (a) Friction blisters. Large, hemorrhagic blisters developed in areas of minor trauma on the trunk and extremities of a cachectic, chronically ill child during an episode of acute renal failure. Blistering healed as renal function returned to normal and cutaneous edema resolved. A skin biopsy demonstrated intraepidermal blisters without inflammation. **(b)** Sucking blisters. Recurrent hemorrhagic blisters appeared on the thumb of a 10-year-old thumb sucker. These blisters can arise within the epidermis or basement membrane zone.

during rigorous physical activity such as track-and-field sports and military boot camp. Vesicles and bullae are usually restricted to the distal extremities, and particularly the palms and soles. Healing occurs without scar formation, and the nails and mucous membranes are not affected. Histopathology demonstrates a suprabasilar split in the epidermis, and electron microscopy shows cytolysis within the basal cell layer. Although these findings are also typical of friction blisters in normal individuals, clumping of tonofilaments in basal cell keratinocytes is specific for Weber–Cockayne syndrome.

Recurrent blistering of the palms and soles, particularly during warm weather when blistering is more common, suggest the disorder. A positive family history clinches the diagnosis. Blistering may be reduced by using extra cushioning in shoes and avoiding unnecessary trauma to the hands and feet, particularly during warm weather. Cool tap-water

compresses may help symptomatically, and topical antibiotics reduce the risk of secondary infection. The use of topical antiperspirants, such as 10–20% aluminum hydroxide, 10% formaldehyde, or 10% glutaraldehyde, may decrease the blistering as well as associated hyperhidrosis of the palms and soles. Some patients have also benefited from applications of tincture of benzoin or mastisol.

Epidermolysis bullosa acquisita

An acquired mechanobullous dermatosis, EBA may clinically resemble hereditary epidermolysis bullosa. However, onset of skin fragility and blister formation is widespread and does not usually occur until adolescence. Actually, EBA is an immunobullous dermatosis which is frequently associated with an underlying systemic disorder such as inflammatory bowel disease. Although skin biopsies show a subepidermal blister indistinguishable from CBDC and BP, immunoelectron microscopy reveals characteristic deposition of IgG and complement in the upper dermis beneath or contiguous with the lamina densa. Patients usually respond to systemic corticosteroids. However, in patients with bowel disease, cutaneous lesions may improve with aggressive management of gastrointesinal symptoms.

DERMATITIS

In acute dermatitides inflammation and associated edema may be so intense that vesiculation occurs (see Fig 3.16). Blisters erupt frequently in acute contact irritant and allergic dermatitis, as well as in atopic dermatitis, seborrhea, and insect-bite reactions (Fig 4.23). Whenever blistering develops in this setting, secondary infection with *Staphylococcus* or Herpes simplex virus is also considered.

A Tzanck smear and Gram stain exclude bacterial and viral infection. Skin biopsies demonstrate variable acanthosis or thickening of the epidermis, exocytosis or an influx of lymphocytes into the epidermis, and spongiosis or intercellular edema. It is the intense edema that eventually breaks apart desmosomal attachments and results in spongiotic blister formation. Immunofluorescence studies should be negative.

Blistering from dermatitic reactions can usually be differentiated clinically from thermal burns, cold injury, and ischemic insults to the skin that result in subepidermal blisters.

ERYTHEMA MULTIFORME

A distinctive, acute hypersensitivity syndrome, EM may be caused by a number of drugs as well as viruses, bacterial infections, foods, and immunizations. It may also arise in association with connective disorders and malignancy. Medications and infectious diseases are the most common triggering factors in children.

Erythema multiforme minor

In the classic eruption, originally described by Ferdinand von Hebra in 1860, the rash is symmetric and may occur on

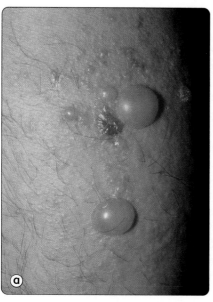
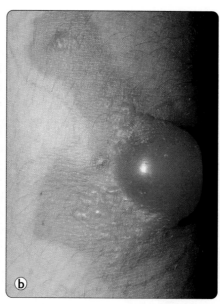
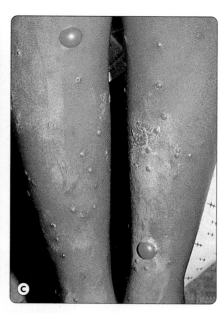

Fig 4.23 Dermatitic blisters. **(a)** Acute poison ivy dermatitis resulted in blisters on the arm of a 9-year-old boy. Note the surrounding erythema, edema, and papules typical of an allergic contact dermatitis. **(b)** Vesicles and a large bulla erupted on an extremely well demarcated red base on the arm of a teenager who admitted to applying acid to create the lesions. **(c)** This child's lower legs are studded with numerous, thick-walled vesicles and bullae, which formed in response to flea bites.

any part of the body, although it usually appears on the dorsum of the hands and feet and the extensor surfaces of the arms and legs (Fig 4.24a). Involvement of the palms and soles is common. The initial lesions are dusky, red macules or edematous papules that evolve into target lesions with multiple, concentric rings of color change. The annular configuration occurs as the central inflammatory process spreads peripherally and leaves behind a depressed, damaged epidermis. When epidermal injury is severe, full-thickness necrosis results in central bulla formation. The eruption continues in crops that last 1–3 weeks. In most children with this so-called minor variant, mucous membrane involvement is minimal (Fig 4.24b), the disease is self-limiting, and systemic manifestations are limited to low-grade fever, malaise, and myalgia.

Stevens–Johnson syndrome
Less commonly, EM presents as one of the major variants with variable amounts of epidermal involvement and large areas of mucous membrane necrosis and shedding. Stevens–Johnson syndrome (SJS) and toxic epidermal necrolysis (TEN) are thought to represent the most severe end of the spectrum of EM. In SJS, constitutional symptoms are severe and include high fever, cough, sore throat, vomiting, diarrhea,

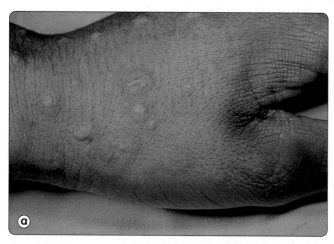
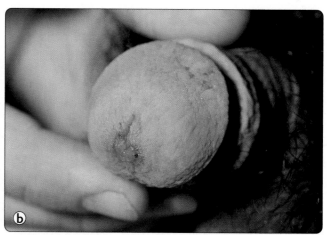

Fig. 4.24 Erythema multiforme. **(a)** Typical target lesions erupted on the arms and legs of this 9-year-old boy with recurrent erythema multiforme associated with herpes simplex infection. He had only minimal mucous membrane involvement. **(b)** An adolescent with erythema multiforme minor developed painful erosions around the urethra.

chest pain, and arthralgias. After a prodrome lasting 1–14 days, but usually 1–3 days, abrupt onset of symmetric erythematous macules occurs on the head and neck, and spreads to the trunk and extremities (Fig 4.25). Blister formation occurs within hours and is often hemorrhagic, extensive, and confluent. Mucous membrane involvement, particularly of the eyes, nose, and mouth, is widespread and severe. It consists of the formation of fragile, thin-walled bullae that rupture with minimal trauma, to leave ulcerations that are rapidly covered by exudate. Keratitis may result in ocular infection and synechiae formation. The urogenital and perirectal areas are also involved. Loss of the epidermal barrier results in fluid and electrolyte imbalances and a high risk of secondary bacterial infection. Mortality ranges between 5 and 25%.

Although the skin biopsy findings vary in EM minor and SJS, several histologic findings are characteristic of both disorders. A perivascular mononuclear cell infiltrate with some eosinophils is present in the papillary dermis. Variable hydropic degeneration of the basal cell layer is associated with the formation of colloid bodies and, in severe cases, with subepidermal blister formation. Dyskeratosis may be mild or widespread, with discrete satellite cell necrosis to almost total necrosis of the epidermis.

In the event of drug-induced EM, it is imperative that the clinician identify the inciting agent. Failure to do so may result in a persistent reaction and severe recurrent disease on re-exposure to the medication. Herpes simplex infections are also associated with repeated episodes of EM, usually the minor variant. Unfortunately, some children with HSV-induced recurrent EM develop oral erosions severe enough to require parenteral rehydration.

During acute episodes, careful cleaning and protection of bullous lesions is imperative to reduce the risk of infection. Patients with Stevens–Johnson syndrome may require intensive supportive care in a burn unit.

Toxic epidermal necrolysis

Although originally described in adults, TEN has been reported in children, especially in association with drug-hypersensitivity reactions. Patients usually begin with fever, sore throat, malaise, and a generalized, sunburn-like erythema, followed by sloughing of large areas of skin (Fig 4.26). The entire skin surface, as well as conjunctivae, urethra,

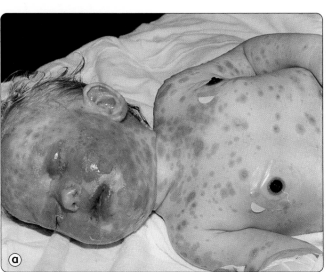
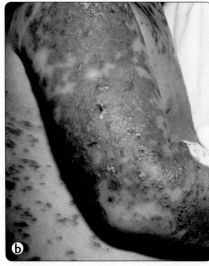
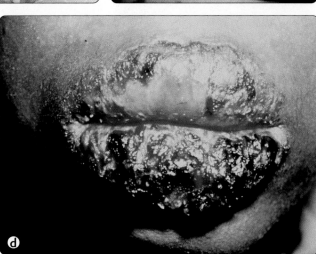

Fig. 4.25 Stevens–Johnson syndrome. **(a)** Widespread blistering and erosions developed on the skin and mucous membranes of this 3-year-old girl with Stevens–Johnson syndrome. **(b)** Widespread areas of necrotic blisters and ulcerations can heal **(c)** with marked permanent hyperpigmentation in dark-pigmented individuals. **(d)** Hemorrhagic crusts on the lips are characteristic of Stevens–Johnson syndrome.

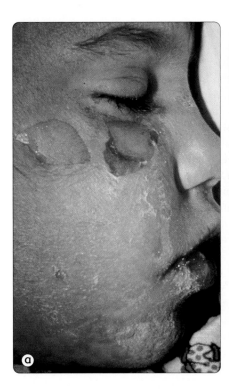

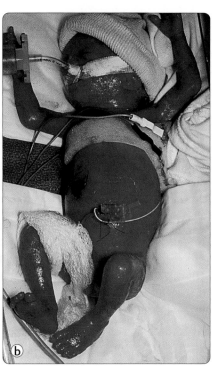

Fig. 4.26 Toxic epidermal necrolysis. **(a)** After 7 days of a course of oral co-trimoxazole for otitis media, this 8-year-old girl developed high fever, and generalized erythema and edema followed by sloughing of large sheets of skin. Mucous membranes were severely involved. Note Nikolsky sign on her upper cheek, induced by accidental minor trauma. **(b)** At 10 days of age this tiny premature infant developed toxic epidermal necrolysis while on multiple antibiotics. Denuded areas of skin occurred over bony prominences and around tape and monitor sites.

rectum, oral and nasal mucosa, larynx, and tracheobronchial mucosa, may become involved. Although Nikolsky sign is present and the erythema is reminiscent of SSSS, the site of cleavage in TEN is at the dermal–epidermal junction, which results in full epidermal necrosis. Many investigators equate TEN with the most fulminant presentation of Stevens–Johnson syndrome because the inciting agents and clinical courses are similar.

Frozen sections of sloughed epidermis can be used for rapid differentiation of TEN from SSSS while the practitioner awaits the definitive results of a skin biopsy.

Intensive supportive measures are required to avoid fluid and electrolyte losses and secondary bacterial infection. Respiratory distress syndrome has been reported in severe cases.

Morbidity and mortality are comparable to those in patients with Stevens-Johnson syndrome. In uncomplicated cases re-epithelialization of the skin occurs within several weeks and full recovery in 4–6 weeks. Scarring may develop in areas of secondary infection. Careful ongoing ophthalmologic evaluation is necessary to reduce the complications of severe conjunctival and corneal involvement.

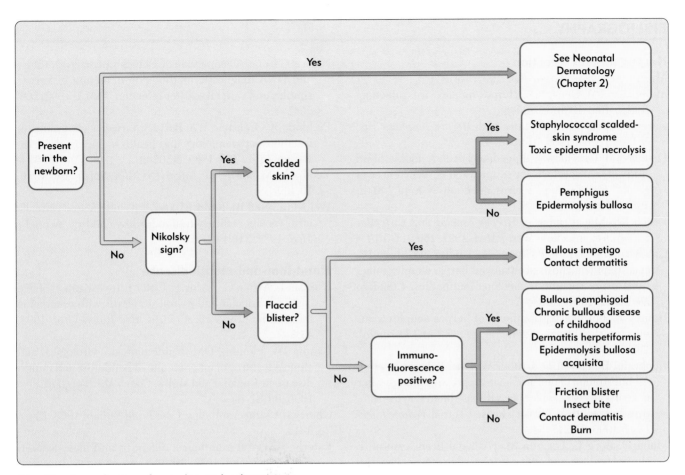

Algorithm for evaluation of vesiculopustular dermatoses.

BIBLIOGRAPHY

Herpes simplex infection

Abadi J. Acyclovir. *Pediatr Rev.* 1997; 18:70–1

Annunziato PW, Gershon A. Herpes simplex virus infection. *Pediatr Rev.* 1996, **17**:425–3.

Corey L, Spear PG. Infections with *Herpes simplex virus*. *N Engl J Med.* 1986, **314**:686–91.

Douglas JM. Critchlow C, Benedetti J et al. A double-blind study of oral acyclovir for suppression of recurrences of genital *Herpes simplex virus* infection. *N Engl J Med.* 1984, 310:1551–6.

Erlich KS. Management of *Herpes simplex* and *varicella-zoster virus* infection. *West J Med.* 1997, 166:211–15.

Goodyear HM, Wilson P, Cropper L, Laidler PW, Sharp IR, *et al*. Rapid diagnosis of cutaneous herpes simplex infections using specific monoclonal antibodies. *Clin Exp Dermatol.* 1994, 19:294–7.

Hamny R, Berman B. Treatment of herpes simplex virus infections with topical antiviral agents. *Eur J Dermatol.* 1998, 8:310–9.

Kimberlin D, Powell D, Gruber W, Diaz P, Arvin A, *et al*. Administration of oral acyclovir suppressive therapy after neonatal *Herpes simplex virus* disease limited to the skin, eyes and mouth: results of a Phase I/II trial. *Pediatr Infect Dis J.* 1996, 15:247–54.

Malm G, Berg U, Fosgren M. Neonatal herpes simplex: clinical findings and outcome in relation ot type of maternal infection. *Acta Paediatr.* 1995, **84**:256–60.

Malouf DJ, Oates RK. Herpes simplex virus infections in the neonate. *J Paediatr Child Health.* 1995, **316**:332–5.

Whitley RJ, Kimberlin DW. Treatment of viral infections in pregnancy and the neonatal period. *Clin Perinatal.* 1997, **24**:267–83.

Varicella-zoster infection

Alkalay A, Pomerance JJ, Rimoin DL. Fetal varicella syndrome. *J Pediatr.* 1987, **111**:320–3.

Baba K, Yabuuchi H, Takahashi M, Ogra P. Immunologic and epidemiologic aspects of varicella infection acquired during infancy and early childhood. *J Pediatr.* 1982, **100**:881–8.

Christian CW, Singer ML, Crawford JE, Dubin D. Perianal herpes zoster presenting as suspected child abuse. *Pediatrics.* 1997, 99:608–10.

Committee on Infectious Disease. The use of acyclovir in otherwise healthy children with varicella. *Pediatrics.* 1993, 91:674–6.

Dunkle LM, Arvin AM, Whitley RJ, *et al*. A controlled trial of acyclovir for chickenpox in normal children. *N Engl J Med.* 1991, 325:1539–44.

Krause PR, Klinman DM. Efficacy, immunogenicity, safety and use of attenuated chickenpox vaccine. *J Pediatr.* 1995, **127**:518–25.

Nahass GT, *et al*. Comparison of Tzanck smear, viral culture and DNA diagnostic methods on detection of herpes simplex and varicella-zoster infection. *JAMA.* 1992, **268**: 2541–4.

Preblud SR, Orenstein WA, Bart KJ. Varicella: clinical manifestations, epidemiology and health impact in children. *Pediatr Infect Dis.* 1984, 3:505–9.

Takahashi M. Varicella. *Infect Dis Clin North Am.* 1996, **10**:469–88.

Weibel Re, Neff BJ, Kuter BJ, *et al*. Live attenuated varicella virus vaccine: efficacy trial in healthy children. *N Engl J Med.* 1984, **310**:1409–15.

Hand-foot-and-mouth disease

B'arlean L, Avram G, Pavlov E, Cotor F. Investigation of five cases of vesicular enteroviral stomatitis with exanthema induced by *Coxsackie A5* virus. *Rev Roum Virol.* 1994, **45**:3–9.

Bendig JW, Fleming DM. Epidemiologic, virological and clinical features of an epidemic of hand, foot and mouth disease in England and Wales. *Comm Dis Rep CDR Rev.* 1996, 6:R81–6.

Cherry JD. Viral exanthems. *Curr Probl Pediatr.* 1983, **13**(6): 3–44.

Esterly NB. Viral exanthems: diagnosis and management. *Semin Dermatol.* 1984, 3:140–5.

Shelley WB, Hashim M, Shelley ED. Acyclovir in the treatment of hand, foot and mouth disease. *Cutis.* 1996, **57**:232–4.

Bacterial infections

See Chapter 2.

Pemphigus

Anhalt GJ, Labib RS, Vorhees JJ, Beals TF, Diaz LA. Induction of pemphigus in neonatal mice by passive transfer of IgG from patients with the disease. *N Engl J Med.* 1982, **306**:1189–96.

Grunwald MH, Zaninu E, Avinoach I, *et al*. Pemphigus neonatorum. *Pediatr Dermatol.* 1993, **10**:169–70.

Huilgol SC, Black MM. Management of immunobullous disorders. II. Pemphigus. *Clin Exp Dermatol.* 1995, **20**: 283–93.

Kanwar AJ, Dhar S, Kaur S. Further experience with pemphigus in children. *Pediatr Dermatol.* 1994, **11**:107–11.

Lyde CB, Cox SE, Cruz PD Jr. Pemphigus erythematous in a five year old child. *J Am Acad Dermatol.* 1994, **31**(5 Pt 2):906–909.

Smitt JH. Pemphigus vulgaris in childhood: clinical features, treatment and prognosis. *Pediatr Dermatol.* 1985, **2**: 185–90.

Bullous pemphigoid and chronic bullous dermatosis of childhood

Baldari U, Raccagni AA, Celli B, Righini MG. Chronic bullous disease of children following Epstein–Barr virus seroconversion, a case report. *Clin Exp Dermatol.* 1996, **21**:123–6.

Gereige RS, Washington KR. Pathologic case of the month. Linear IgA dermatosis of childhood (benign chronic bullous dermatosis of childhood). *Arch Pediatr Adolesc Med.* 1997, **15**:320–1.

Rye B, Webb JM. Autoimmune bullous disease. *Am Fam Physician.* 1997, **55**:2709–18.

Sweren RJ, Burnett JW. Benign chronic bullous dermatosis of childhood: a review. *Cutis.* 1982, **29**:350–7.

Wojnarowska F, Marsden RA, Bhogal B, Black MM. Chronic bullous dermatosis of childhood, childhood cicatricial pemphigoid and linear IgA disease of adults. *J Am Acad Dermatol.* 1988, **19**:792–805.

Zone JJ, Taylor TB, Kadunce DP, *et al.* IgA antibodies in chronic bullous disease of childhood react with 97 kDa basement membrane zone protein. *J Invest Dermatol.* 1996, **106**:1277–80.

Epidermolysis bullosa acquisita

Borok M, Heng MCY, Ahmed AR. Epidermolysis bullosa acquisita in an 8-year-old girl. *Pediatr Dermatol.* 1986, **3**:315–22.

Kawachi Y, Ikegami M, Tanaka T, Otsuka F. Autoantibodies to bullous pemphigoid and epidermolysis bullosa acquisita antigen in an infant. *Br J Dermatol.* 1996, **135**: 443–7.

Erythema multiforme and Stevens–Johnson syndrome

Kakourou T, Klontza D, Soteropoulou F, Kattamis C. Corticosteroid treatment of erythema multiforme major (Stevens–Johnson syndrome) in children. *Eur J Pediatr.* 1997, **156**: 90–3.

Noskin GA, Patterson R. Outpatient management of Stevens–Johnson syndrome: a report of four cases and management strategy. *Allergy Asthma Proc.* 1997, **18**:29–32.

Tay YK, Huff JC, Weston WL. *Mycoplasma pneumoniae* infection is associated with Stevens–Johnson syndrome, not erythema multiforme (von Hebra). *J Am Acad Dermatol.* 1996, **35**:757–60.

Toxic epidermal necrolysis

Amon RB, Dimond RL. Toxic epidermal necrolysis: rapid differentiation between staphylococcal and drug-induced disease. *Arch Dermatol.* 1975, **111**:1433–7.

Hawk RJ, Storer JS, Danon RS. Toxic epidermal necrolysis in a 6-week-old infant. *Pediatr Dermatol.* 1985, **2**:197–200.

Jones WG, Halebian P, Madden M, Finkelstein J, Goodwin CW. Drug-induced toxic epidermal necrolysis in children. *J Pediatr Surg.* 1989, **24**:167–70.

Revuz JE, Roujeau JC. Advances in toxic epidermal necrolysis. *Semin Cutan Med Surg.* 1996, **15**:258–66.

Schwartz RA. Toxic epidermal necrolysis. *Cutis.* 1997, **59**:123–8.

Weighton W. Toxic epidermal necrolysis. *Aust J Dermatol.* 1996, **37**:167–75.

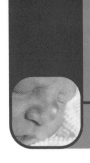

Chapter Five

Nodules and Tumors

INTRODUCTION

Nodules and tumors in the skin often raise fears of skin cancer. Fortunately, primary skin cancer is extremely rare in childhood, and most infiltrated plaques and tumors are benign (Fig 5.1). Hemangiomas, congenital nevi, and tumors of the newborn are reviewed in Chapter 2. The focus in this chapter is disorders of childhood and adolescence.

Several clinical clues, including the depth and color of lesions, aid in developing a differential diagnosis. Superficial growths are readily moved back and forth over the underlying dermis, whereas the overlying epidermis and superficial dermis may slide over deep-seated tumors. Some dermal and subcutaneous lesions characteristically produce tethering of the overlying skin. Epidermal tumors include warts, molluscum, and seborrheic keratoses. Milia, neurofibromas, granuloma annulare, mastocytomas, scars, keloids, xanthomas, xanthogranulomas, nevocellular nevi, and adnexal tumors involve the superficial and mid dermis. Leukemia, lymphoma, melanoma, lipomas, and metastatic solid tumors involve the dermis and/or fat and may extend deep into subcutaneous structures.

Color may suggest the specific cell types that comprise various cutaneous nodules and tumors. For instance, yellow tumors might include large quantities of fat in a lipoma or lipid-laden histiocytes in xanthomas or xanthogranulomas. Nevocellular nevi, epidermal nevi, mastocytomas, and seborrheic keratosis contain varying amounts of the brown pigment melanin in nevus cells or keratinocytes. Vascular tumors are usually red or blue, and primary or metastatic nodules may appear in various shades of red, purple, and blue, depending on their depth and degree of vascularity.

Finally, the diagnosis of certain genodermatoses associated with cutaneous and/or internal malignancies allows the clinician to develop strategies for close monitoring. Early recognition of malignancy in this setting may be lifesaving (Fig 5.2).

SUPERFICIAL NODULES AND TUMORS

Warts

Warts are benign epidermal tumors produced by human papillomavirus (HPV) infection of the skin and mucous membranes. In children they are seen most commonly on the fingers, hands, and feet. However, they can infect any area on the skin or mucous membranes (Figs 5.3–5.7). The incubation period for warts varies from 1 to 3 months and possibly up to several years, and the majority of lesions disappear within 3–5 years. Local trauma promotes inoculation of the virus. Thus, periungual warts are common in children who bite their nails or pick at hangnails.

Investigators have identified over 60 HPV types capable of producing warts, and many of these organisms produce characteristic lesions in specific locations. For instance, the discrete, round, skin-colored papillomatous papules typical of verruca vulgaris (common warts) are produced by HPV-2 and HPV-4 (Figs 5.3 and 5.5). The subtle, minimally hyperpigmented flat warts (verruca plana), which are caused by HPV-3, are frequently spread by deliberate or accidental scratching, shaving, or picking and may become widespread on the face, arms, and legs (Fig 5.6).

Plantar warts are most commonly caused by HPV-1 (Fig 5.4). Although not proved, the transmission of these warts probably occurs by contact with contaminated, desquamated skin in showers, pool decks, and bathrooms. Although often subtle on the surface, their large size may be hidden by a collarette of skin of normal appearance, and they often cause pain when the patient walks. While plantar warts may be confused with corns, calluses, or scars, they can be

Histologic diagnosis of 775 superficial lumps excised in children	
Type	**Number**
Epidermal inclusion cysts	459 (59%)
Congenital malformations (pilomatrixoma, lymphangioma, brachial cleft cyst)	117 (15%)
Benign neoplasms (neural tumors, lipoma, adnexal tumors)	56 (7%)
Benign lesions of undetermined origin (xanthomas, xanthogranulomas, fibromatosis, fibroma)	50 (6%)
Self-limited processes (granuloma annulare, urticaria pigmentosa, insect bite reaction)	47 (6%)
Malignant tumors	11 (1.4%)
Miscellaneous	35 (4%)

Fig 5.1 Histologic diagnosis of 775 superficial lumps excised in children. (Modified from Knight PJ, Reiner CB, *Pediatrics* 1983, **72**:147.)

Cancer-associated genodermatoses			
Disease	Associated cancer	Clinical manifestations	Inheritance
Basal cell nevus syndrome	Many basal cell carcinomas (mean age of onset 15 years) on sun-exposed and non-sun-exposed areas; meduloblastoma; astrocytoma	Many basal cell nevi, palmar and plantar pits, jaw cysts, calcification of the falx cerebri, ovarian fibromas, fused ribs	Autosomal dominant; gene locus 9q31
Hidrotic ectodermal dysplasia	Squamous cell carcinoma of palms, soles, nail bed	Normal sweating, total alopecia, severe nail dystrophy, palmar and plantar hyperkeratosis	Autosomal dominant
Basex syndrome	Basal cell carcinomas of the face (second to third decade)	Follicular atrophoderma, localized anhidrosis and/or generalized hypohidrosis	Autosomal dominant
Dysplastic nevus syndrome (familial, atypical, multiple-mole syndrome)	Cutaneous and intraocular melanoma, lymphoreticular malignancy, sarcomas	Multiple, large reddish-brown moles with irregular borders and nonuniform colors, usually on trunk and arms; familial occurrence of melanoma	Autosomal dominant
Multiple hamartoma syndrome (Cowden disease)	Carcinoma of the breast, colon, thyroid	Coexistence of multiple, ectodermal, mesodermal, and endodermal nevoid neoplasms; punctate keratoderma of the palms; multiple angiomas, lipomas	Autosomal dominant
Neurofibromatosis (von Recklinghausen disease)	Malignant degeneration of neurofibromas in 3—15% of cases; optic and acoustic neuromas, meningiomas, gliomas, pheochromocytoma, nonlymphocytic leukemia	Caf -au-lait spots, multiple skeletal anomalies, fibromatous skin tumors	Autosomal dominant; gene locus 17q11.2; spontaneous mutations in 50% of cases
Multiple mucosal neuroma syndrome (multiple endocrine neoplasia Type IIB)	Pheochromocytoma, medullary thyroid carcinoma	Pedunculated nodules on eyelid margins, lip; tongue with true neuromas	Autosomal dominant; gene locus 10q11.2; sporadic mutation in 50%
Intestinal polyposis II (Peutz—Jeghers syndrome)	Adenocarcinoma of the colon, duodenum; granulosa cell ovarian tumors	Pigmented macules on oral mucosa, lips, conjunctivae, digits; intestinal polyps	Autosomal dominant; spontaneous mutation in 40%
Intestinal polyposis III (Gardner syndrome)	Malignant degeneration of colon, adenomatous polyps; sarcomas, thyroid carcinoma	Polyps of the colon, small intestine; globoid osteoma of mandible with overlying fibromas; epidermoid cysts; desmoids	Autosomal dominant; gene locus 5q21—q22
Tuberous sclerosis	Rhabdomyoma of myocardium, gliomas, mixed tumor of kidney	Triad of angiofibromas, epilepsy, mental retardation; ash-leaf macules; shagreen patches; subungual fibromas; intracranial calcification in 50%	Spontaneous mutation in 75%; autosomal dominant in 25%; heterogeneous loci, 9q34, 16p13
Epidermolysis bullosa dystrophica dominant	Squamous cell carcinoma in chronic lesions	Lifelong history of bullae; phenotype not as severe as in recessive forms	Autosomal recessive, chromosome 3p21 (collagen type VII gene)
Epidermolysis bullosa dystrophica recessive	Basal, squamous cell carcinoma in skin, mucous membranes (especially esophagus)	Bullae develop at sites of trauma; present at birth or early infancy; may involve mucous membranes, esophagus, conjunctivae, cornea	Autosomal recessive, chromosome 3p (collagen type VII gene)
Albinism	Increased incidence of cutaneous malignancies	Lack of skin pigment, incomplete hypopigmentation of ocular fundi, horizontal congenital nystagmus, myopia	Tyrosinase positive: autosomal recessive, gene locus 15q11.2—q12 Tyrosinase negative: autosomal recessive, gene locus 11q14—q21

Fig 5.2 Cancer-associated genodermatoses.

Cancer-associated genodermatoses (continued)			
Disease	Associated cancer	Clinical manifestations	Inheritance
Bloom syndrome	High incidence of leukemia, lymphoma; squamous cell cancers of esophagus; adenocarcinoma of colon, often by 20 years of age	Small stature; cutaneous photosensitivity presenting as telangiectatic, facial (malar) erythema	Autosomal recessive; gene locus 15q26.1
Chédiak–Higashi syndrome	Malignant lymphoma	Decreased pigmentation of hair, eyes; photophobia; nystagmus; abnormal susceptibility to infection	Autosomal recessive
Rothmund–Thomson syndrome (poikiloderma congenitale)	Cutaneous malignancies	Poikiloderma, short stature, cataracts, photosensitivity, nail defects, alopecia, bony defects	Autosomal recessive; gene locus on chromosome 8
Xeroderma pigmentosum	Basal and squamous cell carcinoma of skin, malignant melanoma	Marked photosensitivity, early freckling, telangiectasia, keratoses, papillomas, photophobia, keratitis, corneal opacities	Autosomal recessive; gene loci – complementation group A–Chr. 9, group B–Chr. 2, group D–Chr. 19, group F–Chr. 15
Wiskott–Aldrich syndrome	Lymphoreticular malignances, malignant lymphoma, myelogenous leukemia, astrocytoma	Eczema, thrombocytopenia, bleeding problems (i.e. melena, purpura, epistaxis), increased susceptibility to skin infections, otitis, pneumonia, meningitis	X-linked recessive; gene locus Xp11.3–11.2
Dyskeratosis congenita	Squamous cell carcinoma of oral cavity, esophagus, nasopharynx, skin, anus	Reticulated hypo- and hyperpigmentation of skin, nail dystrophy, leukoplakia of oral mucosa, thrombocytopenia, testicular atrophy	X-linked recessive (most common); gene locus Xq26

Fig 5.2 Cancer-associated genodermatoses *continued*.

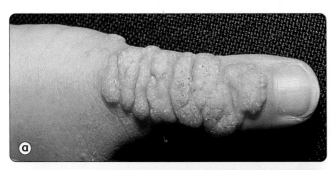
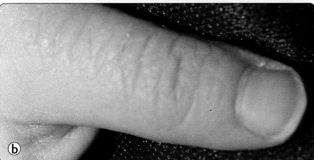

Fig 5.3 Warts. **(a)** Multiple common warts grew to confluence on the thumb of a 4-year-old boy. **(b)** Shortly before surgery was scheduled, the warts began to regress without treatment.

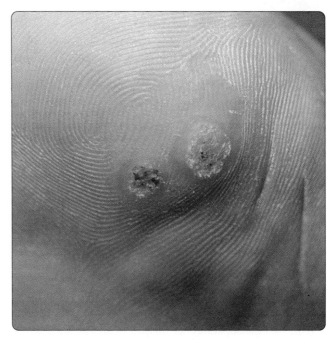

Fig 5.4 Plantar warts. Two painful papules are seen over the ball of the foot. Note how they interrupt the normal skin lines.

differentiated by their disruption of the normal dermatoglyphics. Characteristic black dots in the warts are thrombosed capillaries.

Warts can also be found on the trunk, oral mucosa, and conjunctivae. Condyloma acuminatum and flat warts in the anogenital area are usually caused by HPV-6 and HPV-11 (see Fig 5.7). Although sexual abuse must be considered in any child with anogenital warts, most are transmitted in a nonvenereal fashion.

Although warts are self-limited in most children, persistent, widespread lesions suggest the possibility of congenital or acquired immunodeficiency (Fig 5.8). In fact, warts may become a serious management problem in oncology and transplant patients who are chronically immunosuppressed.

Topical irritants, including salicylic acid and lactic acid in occlusive vehicles such as collodion or under tape occlusion, are safe, effective, and relatively painless preparations with which to treat warts that are not in sensitive areas such as the eyelids and perineum.

Recalcitrant lesions may respond to destructive measures, which include liquid nitrogen, electrocautery, and carbon

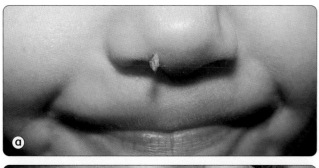

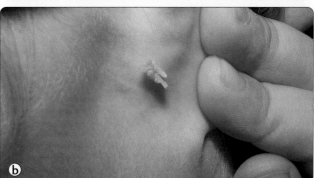

Fig 5.5 Verruca vulgaris. Filiform warts developed on (a) the nose and (b) ear of these children of school age.

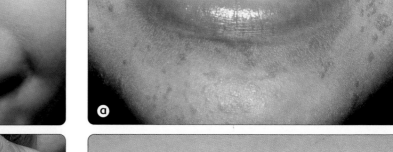

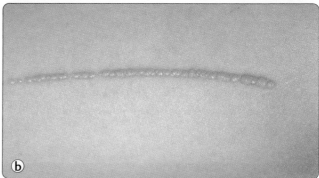

Fig 5.6 Verruca plana. (a) The tiny, light brown warts on the chin of a 12-year-old girl were spread by scratching. These asymptomatic warts were initially diagnosed as acne. (b) Flat warts were inoculated in a line on the flank of a 5-year-old girl.

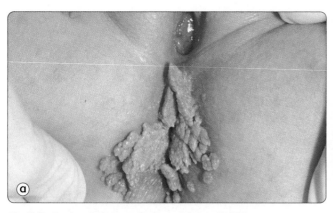

Fig 5.7 Anogenital warts and condyloma. (a) The warts developed at 8 months of age in this infant whose mother had extensive vaginal and cervical papillomavirus infection at delivery. These lesions resolved after treatment with podophyllotoxin. (b) Large condyloma enveloped the glans penis of this adolescent boy.

dioxide laser surgery. However, patients and parents must be cautioned about the risk of recurrence and scarring (Figs 5.9 and 5.10). Immunotherapy with topical contact sensitizers, such as dinitrochlorobenzene, diphencyclopropenone, and rhus extract is still considered experimental, and parents are counseled accordingly. Remember, most warts resolve without treatment in 3–5 years.

Large warts in the diaper area may cause itching, burning, bleeding, and secondary bacterial infection. Although not approved for use in children, judicious home application of topical podophyllotoxin is safe and effective in

symptomatic cases. Imiquimod, a new topical agent approved for treatment of genital warts in adults, may also gain acceptance in pediatric therapy. Scissors excision with electrocautery and carbon dioxide laser ablation may be effective in recalcitrant cases. However, painful destructive measures can only be performed with deep sedation or general anesthetic.

Several innocent epidermal growths are often confused with warts. Dermatosis papulosa nigra (DPN) describes a variant of seborrheic keratosis which appears in about a third of black individuals (Fig 5.11). Although seborrheic

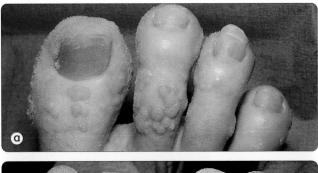
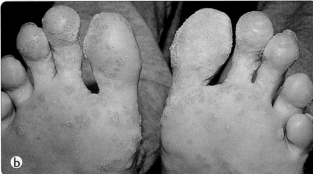

Fig 5.8 Extensive, recalcitrant warts spread over **(a)** the top and **(b)** bottom of the feet of a teenager with severe combined immunodeficiency.

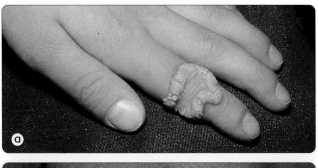
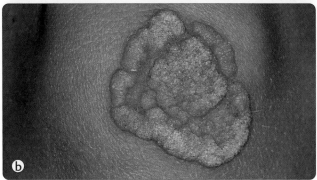

Fig 5.9 Recurrence of warts. **(a)** A 10-year-old boy developed a recurrent ring wart after liquid nitrogen treatment of a large common wart on the index finger. **(b)** A 10-year-old girl had a similar complication after treatment of a wart on her knee.

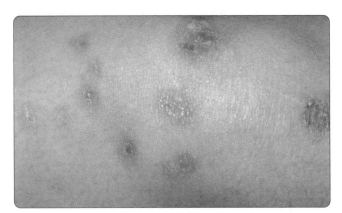

Fig 5.10 A 10-year-old boy developed multiple scars after liquid nitrogen therapy of warts on his knee.

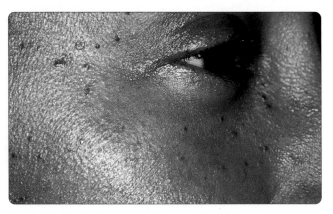

Fig 5.11 Small, brown papules typical of dermatosis papulosa nigra slowly increased in number and size on the face of this black adolescent. Her parents had similar lesions, which began to appear in late childhood.

keratoses usually do not erupt until middle age, small, brown, warty DPN typically begins to develop during adolescence in a symmetric, malar distribution on the face. The neck and upper trunk may also be involved. Although DPN is of no medical consequence, irritated or unsightly lesions may be snipped, frozen, or cauterized. Patients must be warned about the risk of postinflammatory pigmentary changes after treatment. Another type of innocent epidermal lesion, pearly penile papule, is often diagnosed as warts. Uniform, 1–3 mm diameter papules ring the corona at the base of the glans penis. Pearly penile papules are asymptomatic and probably represent a normal variant. No treatment is required.

Molluscum contagiosum

Molluscum contagiosum, caused by a large poxvirus, is characterized by sharply circumscribed single or multiple, superficial, pearly, dome-shaped papules (Fig 5.12a–d). They usually start as grouped, pinpoint papules and increase in size to 3–5 mm in diameter. Many lesions have umbilicated centers, which are best seen with a hand lens. Molluscum is endemic in young children, in whom involvement of the trunk, axillae, face, and diaper area is common. Lesions are spread by scratching and frequently appear in a linear arrangement (Fig 5.12c). In teenagers and adults, molluscum occurs frequently in the genital area as a sexually transmitted disease.

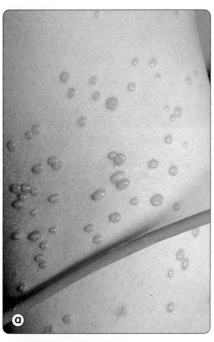

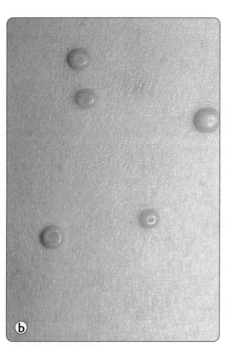

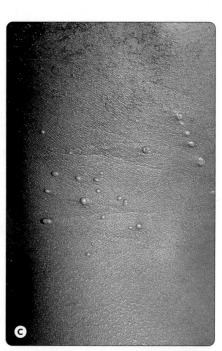

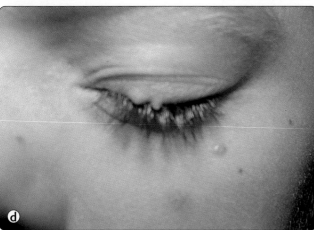

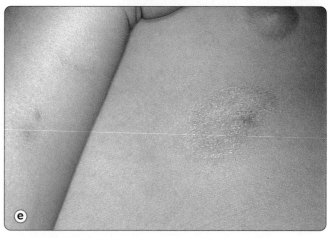

Fig 5.12 Molluscum contagiosum. **(a)** Multiple, pearly papules dot the arm of this 8-year-old girl with widespread molluscum. **(b)** A close-up view demonstrates the central umbilication present on mature molluscum lesions. **(c)** Note the linear spread of papules on the neck of this child, which followed scratching. **(d)** Molluscum on the eyelid margin and conjunctivae are particularly irritating and difficult to treat. **(e)** Red, scaly, dermatitic patches encircled this toddler's molluscum shortly before their resolution.

A white, cheesy core can be expressed from the center of the papule for microscopic examination, which reveals the typical molluscum bodies. Destruction of lesions by curetting their cores or by application of a blistering agent (cantharidin) and plastic tape, peeled off in 1–3 days, is curative of individual lesions. However, recurrences and the development of new papules are common, and most cases undergo spontaneous remission. Consequently, treatment is directed against symptomatic lesions only. Bacterial superinfection may be treated with appropriate topical or oral antibiotics. The development of scaly, red rings around old papules may herald the onset of a delayed hypersensitivity reaction and resolution of the infection (Fig 5.12e). As in children with warts, patients with widespread, recalcitrant molluscum are screened for congenital and acquired immunodeficiency.

Basal cell carcinoma

Basal cell carcinoma (BCC) presents as a nonhealing, pearly, reddish-gray to brown papule or plaque with a central dell or crust and peripheral telangiectasias (Fig 5.13). Although BCC occurs primarily in middle age and the elderly, the tumor is being recognized with increasing frequency in adolescents and young adults, particularly in fair-skinned individuals in sunny climates. The risk of developing BCC has been clearly linked to ultraviolet light exposure, and most lesions appear on sun-exposed sites, such as the face, ears, neck, and upper trunk. An indolent, superficial malignancy, BCC responds readily to electrodesiccation and curettage or simple excision. However, neglected lesions may become locally destructive and invade deep soft tissues, bone, and dura. Protection from excessive sun exposure, aggressive use of sunscreens, and careful skin surveillance should reduce the risk from BCC.

When BCC is diagnosed in sun-protected areas or in children, the practitioner must search for predisposing factors, such as radiation or arsenic exposure, a pre-existing nevus sebaceus or scar, or a hereditary condition such as basal cell nevus syndrome. In this autosomal-dominant disorder, numerous basal cell nevi are noted on the trunk, scalp, face, and extremities during the first decade (Fig 5.14). In time, many of these lesions begin to enlarge and develop into progressive BCCs. Other stigmata include palmar and plantar pits, jaw cysts, calcification of the falx cerebri, ovarian fibromas, and fused ribs. Early diagnosis and removal of enlarging BCCs reduces the need for more extensive and disfiguring surgery.

In children, BCC may be confused with warts, molluscum contagiosum, seborrheic keratoses, pigmented nevi, and other epidermal and superficial dermal growths. It should be considered in any slowly progressive, crusted, or ulcerated plaque, particularly if risk factors are present.

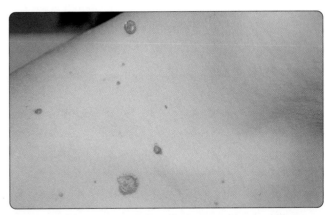

Fig 5.14 Basal cell nevus syndrome. Numerous 1–3 mm diameter papules composed of proliferating basaloid cells and two larger nodules, which demonstrated changes typical of basal cell carcinoma, are on the shoulder and neck of a 15-year-old girl with basal cell nevus syndrome. In addition to the widespread cutaneous tumors, she had subtle palmar and plantar pits and a history of jaw cysts. Her father, uncle, and grandmother had similar cutaneous lesions.

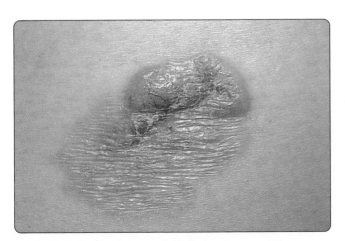

Fig 5.13 A slowly enlarging, reddish-tan plaque on the upper chest of an 18-year-old boy developed a nodular component with overlying telangiectasias. A skin biopsy demonstrated basaloid budding typical of basal cell carcinoma. The child had red hair, blue eyes, light complection, and a history of frequent sunburns since early childhood.

DERMAL NODULES AND TUMORS

Granuloma annulare

When fully evolved, granuloma annulare is an annular eruption histologically characterized by dermal infiltration of lymphocytes and histiocytes around altered collagen (Fig 5.15a–d). The lesion begins as a papule or nodule which gradually expands peripherally to form a ring 1–4 cm in diameter. Multiple rings may overlap to form large, annular plaques. In some cases the rings are broken up into segments. The overlying epidermis is usually intact and has the same color as adjacent skin. However, it may be slightly red or hyperpigmented. Most lesions are asymptomatic, although a few are reported to be mildly pruritic. Granuloma annulare most commonly erupts on the extensor surfaces of the lower legs, feet, fingers, and hands, but other areas may be involved.

Over months to years, old plaques and papules regress while new lesions appear. Eventually, granuloma annulare resolves without treatment. The origin is unclear, but some lesions may be associated with insect-bite reactions or other antecedent trauma. In adults, granuloma annulare, especially multiple eruptive lesions, have appeared in association with diabetes mellitus (Fig 5.15e). This is not the case in children.

Granuloma annulare is most commonly confused with tinea corporis or ringworm. However, the thickened, indurated character of the ring and lack of epidermal changes, such as scale, vesicles, or pustules, enable clinical distinction. A deep dermal or subcutaneous variant of granuloma annulare may be mistaken for rheumatoid nodules seen in rheumatic fever and other connective tissue disorders (Fig 5.16). These lesions are referred to as subcutaneous granuloma annulare and pseudorheumatoid nodules. Practitioners should avoid the latter term, because the subcutaneous variant is not associated with local symptoms or systemic disease. Subcutaneous nodules occur most commonly on the extremities and scalp, where they are often fixed to the underlying periosteum. The diagnosis is often suggested by the presence of typical annular dermal plaques. When necessary, skin biopsies reveal changes similar to the more superficial lesions.

Adnexal tumors

Neoplasms may arise from any structure in the skin. Although many tumors of the adnexal structures can only be differentiated by specific histopathology, some demonstrate distinctive clinical patterns.

Epidermal inclusion cysts

Epidermal inclusion cysts (EICs) are slow growing dermal or subcutaneous tumors that usually reach a size of 1–3 cm diameter and occur most commonly on the face, scalp, neck, and trunk. They also occasionally develop on the palms and soles. These cysts account for a majority of cutaneous nodules found in children and may be present at birth or appear anytime in childhood. Although they are usually associated with hair

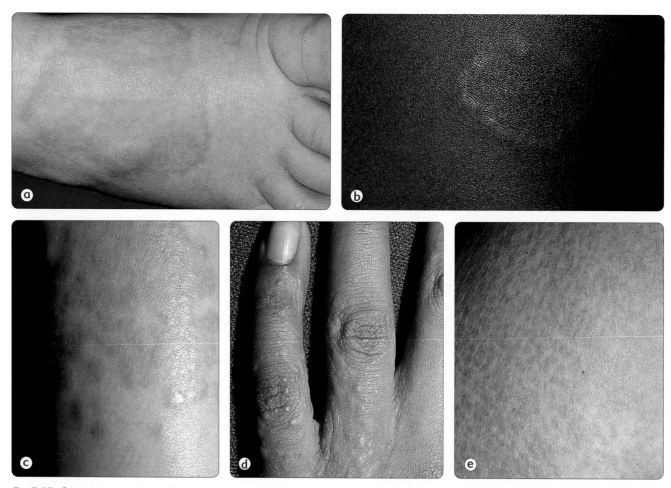

Fig 5.15 Granuloma annulare. Characteristic, doughnut-shaped, dermal plaques (a) on the foot of a white boy and (b) the thigh of a black girl. In both children the epidermal markings are preserved. (c) A large, confluent plaque is developing from merging papules on the arm of a 9-year-old boy. (d) Multiple, asymptomatic 2–4 mm diameter papules erupted on the hand of a teenager. (e) Disseminated granuloma annulare developed in a 20-year-old individual with insulin-dependent diabetes mellitus.

follicles, EICs may arise from the epithelium of any adnexal structure. Primary lesions probably represent a keratinizing type of benign tumor. Other cysts occur as a response to trauma or inflammation such as in nodulocystic acne (see Fig 8.21). Histologically, EICs consist of epidermal lined sacs, which arise most commonly from the infundibular portion of the hair follicle. Rupture of the cyst and spillage of the epithelial debris contained within results in acute and chronic dermal inflammation. These lesions may become red and painful. Noninflamed cysts can be readily excised. However, inflamed lesions may be settled down first with intralesional injections of corticosteroids and oral antibiotics before surgery is attempted.

Most EICs are solitary. When multiple lesions are present, the preceding injury or inflammatory process is usually apparent. In other cases, the development of multiple cysts suggests the diagnosis of Gardner syndrome or intestinal polyposis Type III. In this autosomal-dominant syndrome, increasing numbers of cysts, especially on the face and scalp, are associated with large-bowel polyposis and a 50% risk of malignant degeneration, osteomatosis that involves the bones of the head, and desmoid tumors, particularly of the abdominal wall. Members of affected families may now be screened for the genetic marker.

Milia represent miniature EICs that range from 1 to 3 mm in diameter. Although they occur commonly in the newborn (see Fig. 2.17), they may be acquired after acute and chronic cutaneous injury, such as abrasions, surgery, and recurrent blistering in epidermolysis bullosa (see Fig 2.53). Although milia often resolve without treatment, some remain indefinitely. Curettage or gentle puncture and expression with a comedone extractor is usually curative.

A number of other cystic tumors in the skin, including trichilemmal cysts, pilomatrixomas, vellus hair cysts, steatocystoma, and dermoid cysts, may be confused clinically with EICs.

Trichilemmal cysts

Trichilemmal cysts are clinically indistinguishable from EICs. However, they are less common than EICs, occur almost exclusively on the scalp, and appear as multiple lesions in a majority of patients. Trichilemmal cysts tend to be inherited in an autosomal-dominant pattern. Histologically, these lesions can be differentiated from epidermal cysts by the absence of a granular layer and the presence of a palisading arrangement of the peripheral cells in the cyst wall. The cyst cavity contains homogeneous, keratinous material, unlike the laminated, horny material seen in EICs.

Pilomatrixoma

Pilomatrixoma, or calcifying epithelioma of Malherbe, presents as a sharply demarcated, firm, deep-seated nodule covered by normal or tethered overlying skin (Fig 5.17). Superficial tumors develop a bluish-gray hue, and

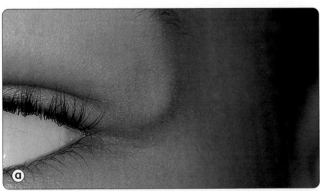

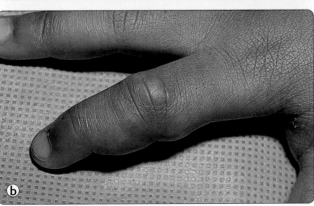

Fig 5.16 Subcutaneous granuloma annulare. Asymptomatic subcutaneous nodules persisted for over a year **(a)** on the upper eyelid of a 7-year-old boy and **(b)** on several fingers of a 10-year-old girl.

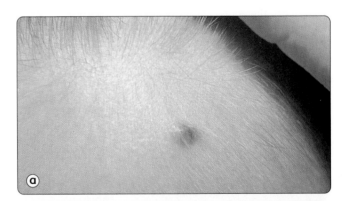

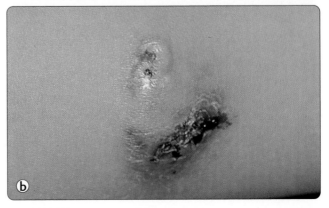

Fig 5.17 Pilomatrixoma. **(a)** A pilomatrixoma was removed from the forehead of a 7-year-old boy. Note the characteristic bluish-gray dermal papule. **(b)** This rock-hard nodule on the upper arm of a 5-year-old girl developed a central ulceration.

occasionally protuberant, red nodules are present. Lesions range in size from under 1 cm to over 3 cm diameter. Although pilomatrixomas may arise at any age, 40% appear before 10 years of age, and over 50% by adolescence. These tumors often come to the attention of anxious patients or parents when rapid enlargement follows hematoma formation after trauma.

Pilomatrixomas occur most commonly on the face, scalp, and upper trunk. They are usually solitary, but multiple lesions develop occasionally. Although most pilomatrixomas do not appear to be inherited, there are several reports of familial cases.

Histologically, this well-demarcated, encapsulated tumor demonstrates a distinctive pattern with islands of basophilic and shadow epithelial cells. Eosinophilic foci of keratinization and basophilic deposits of calcification are scattered throughout.

Although pilomatrixomas are usually asymptomatic, rapid enlargement or gradual progression to a large size may prompt surgical removal. They can usually be excised easily with local anesthetic.

Vellus hair cysts

Vellus hair cysts erupt as multiple, 1–2 mm diameter, follicular papules on the chest, abdomen, and arm flexures of children and young adults (Fig 5.18). Some of the papules have an umbilicated center, suggestive of molluscum contagiosum, and impacted, lightly pigmented vellus hairs may poke out of the center. These asymptomatic lesions resolve over months to years without treatment. Familial cases with autosomal-dominant inheritance have been described.

Steatocystoma

Steatocystoma may appear sporadically as a solitary tumor or in an autosomal-dominant pattern with numerous, nontender, 1–3 cm diameter, firm, rounded, cystic nodules

tethered to the overlying skin (Fig 5.19). Cysts usually begin to develop on the chest, arms, and face in childhood or adolescence. When ruptured, cysts exude an oily or milky fluid, and in some cases small hairs. The walls of the cyst characteristically contain flattened, sebaceous gland lobules or abortive hair follicles. Electron microscopy findings suggest that steatocystoma arises either from sebaceous ductal epithelium or from the hair outer-root sheath. A few bothersome cysts may be removed by simple excision. In some patients with hundreds of lesions, 13-*cis*-retinoid acid (isotretinoin) has been shown to shrink existing tumors and shut off the development of new ones.

Dermoid cysts

Dermoid cysts are congenital, subcutaneous cysts 1–4 cm in diameter, and are found most commonly around the eyes and on the head and neck (see Fig 2.21). On the head, most dermoids are nonmobile, because they are often fixed to the periosteum. Dermoid cysts grow slowly and may cause thinning of the underlying bone. Unlike epidermal cysts, the epithelial lining of dermoid cysts contains multiple adnexal structures, which include hair follicles, eccrine glands, sebaceous glands, and apocrine glands.

Multiple facial papules and nodules

Multiple facial papules and nodules suggest the diagnosis of syringomas, angiofibromas (see Fig 5.26), or trichoepitheliomas. Differentiation is made on the basis of clinical and histologic findings.

Syringomas

Syringomas appear as multiple, 1–2 mm diameter, skin-colored to yellow–brown papules on the lower eyelids and cheeks (Fig 5.20). Occasionally, they occur as isolated lesions or in a widely disseminated, eruptive form with hundreds of papules on the face, axillae, chest, abdomen, and genitals. Although they

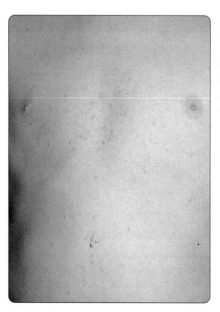

Fig 5.18 Multiple, asymptomatic, 1–3 mm diameter vellus hair cysts erupted on the chest of this 9-year-old boy.

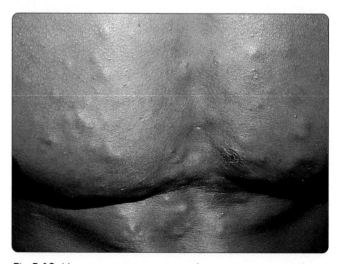

Fig 5.19 Numerous steatocystomas began to appear on the chest, neck, and face of this adolescent when he was 8 years old. His father and brother had similar nodulocystic lesions.

develop most commonly in adolescent girls and young women, they may appear at any age in males and females. They also develop more commonly in children with Down syndrome.

Histologic findings demonstrate characteristic, multiple, small ducts lined by two rows of flattened epithelial cells in the superficial dermis. The lumina of the ducts contain amorphous debris, and some ducts possess comma-like tails which give the appearance of tadpoles.

Although occasionally disfiguring, lesions are usually asymptomatic. Syringomas may be effectively removed by a number of methods, including carbon dioxide laser, electrocautery, cryosurgery, and surgical excision.

Trichoepitheliomas

Trichoepitheliomas occur most commonly as solitary, skin-colored tumors less than 2 cm in diameter on the face of children or young adults. Multiple lesions are inherited as an autosomal-dominant trait (Fig 5.21). In this setting, trichoepitheliomas appear first in childhood, and increase slowly in number and size. Numerous papules and nodules between 2 and 8 mm in diameter occur on the cheeks, nasolabial folds, nose, and upper lip. Histopathology shows a typical dermal tumor that consists of horn cysts of varying sizes and formations, resembling BCCs. Histologic differentiation from basal cell tumors is occasionally difficult.

Unfortunately, tumors may increase indefinitely and cause severe disfigurement. Surgical excision, electrocautery, and laser ablation have been used to deal with the most problematic lesions.

Xanthomas

Xanthomas are yellow dermal tumors that consist of lipid-laden histiocytes. They are usually associated with an abnormality of lipid metabolism, and their presence may provide a clue to an underlying systemic disease.

Poorly soluble lipids are transported in serum by lipoproteins. Abnormalities in lipid transport and metabolism may result in elevations of serum triglycerides and/or

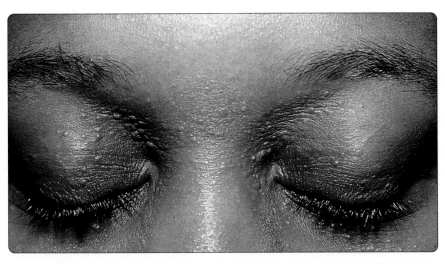

Fig 5.20 Syringomas dot the eyelids of this adolescent. The papules responded quickly to gentle vaporization with carbon dioxide laser.

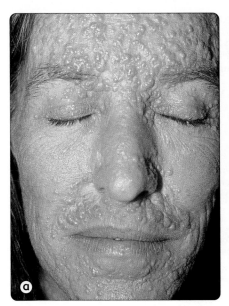
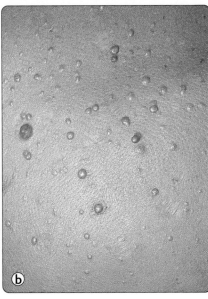

Fig 5.21 Trichoepitheliomas slowly increased in size and number on **(a)** the face and the **(b)** back of this 17-year-old boy. Note the involvement of the nasolabial folds and the upper lip. At least five individuals in three generations of his family were affected.

cholesterol. The deposition of these lipids in skin and soft tissue results in the development of xanthomas.

Although conditions such as fulminant hepatic necrosis from serum hepatitis and poorly controlled diabetes mellitus may trigger hyperlipidemia, a number of primary inherited dyslipoproteinemias have been defined (Fig 5.22).

The recognition of a number of clinical variants may help to define a particular systemic disorder (Fig 5.23a,b). Planar xanthomas present as soft, slightly infiltrated, yellow plaques at any site, but with a predilection for previously injured skin such as old lacerations and acne scars. Xanthelasma, an example of planar lesions on the eyelids, is associated with hypercholesteremia in about half of the cases. Diffuse

lesions may involve the extremities, trunk, face, and neck. In childhood, planar xanthomas occur in diabetes mellitus, liver disease, and histiocytosis syndromes.

Tuberous xanthomas arise as reddish-yellow nodules on the extensor surfaces of the extremities and buttocks. Although they may coalesce to cover a large area, tuberous lesions do not become adherent to the underlying soft-tissue structures, as do tendinous xanthomas. They may occur with elevations of cholesterol or triglycerides.

Tendinous xanthomas present as smooth, asymptomatic nodules on ligaments, tendons, and other deep, soft-tissue structures. They are usually several centimeters in size and occur most commonly on the ankles, knees, and elbows.

Hyperlipidemias and electrophoretic patterns								
Type (prevalence)	Pattern	Chol	TG	Inheritance	Possible mechanism	Clinical presentation	Age of detection	Secondary diseases
I (rarest)	Chyl	+	+++	AR	LDL defect or deficiency (fat induced)	Eruptive xanthomas (66%), abdominal pain, hepatosplenomegaly, lipemia retinalis, creamy plasma, pancreatitis	Early childhood	Pancreatitis, diabetes
IIa (common)	LDL	+++	+ or NI	AD	LDL receptors nonfunctional	Tendinous xanthomas (40–50%), xanthelasmas (23%), corneal arcus (10–15%), tuberous, xanthomas, atherosclerosis	Early childhood in homozygote	Hypothyroidism, nephrotic syndrome
IIb (common)	LDL, VLDL	+++	+ or NI	AD	VLDL overproduction	Same, abnormal GTT		Hepatic disease
III (relatively uncommon)	IDL	++ (variable)	+ (variable)	AR	Homozygous apolipoprotein E2, decreased remnant clearance, overproduction of VLDL	Xanthomas (75–80%; tuberous, palmar, tendinous, eruptive), abnormal GTT, hyperuricemia, atherosclerosis, obesity	Adult	Hepatic disease, dysglobulinemia, uncontrolled diabetes
IV (most common)	VLDL	+	++	AD	Carbohydrate induced	Atherosclerosis, abnormal GTT, eruptive or tuberous xanthomas	Adult	Hypothroidism, diabetes, pancreatitis, glycogen storage disease, nephrotic syndrome, multiple myeloma
V (uncommon)	Chyl, VLDL	+	++	AR	Overproduction of VLDL, defect in catabolism of VLDL	Abdominal pain, obesity, xanthomas (eruptive), hepatosplenomegaly	Early adult	Diabetes, insulin dependent; pancreatitis; alcoholism

Abbreviations: Chol, cholesterol; TG, triglycerides; Chyl, chylomicrons; LDL, low density lipoproteins; VLDL, very low density lipoproteins; IDL, intermediate density lipoproteins; AR, autosomal recessive; AD, autosomal dominant; GTT, glucose tolerance test; NI, normal

Fig 5.22 Hyperlipidemias and electrophoretic patterns.

Eruptive xanthomas develop suddenly as 1–4 mm diameter, yellowish–red papules over the extensor surfaces of the extremities, buttocks, and bony prominences (Fig 5.23c). Their appearance is usually associated with marked elevation in triglycerides, especially in poorly controlled diabetics or in patients with Types I, III, IV, and V hyperlipidemias.

Xanthomas must be differentiated from xanthogranulomas, which are not usually associated with systemic disease or elevated serum lipids (see Fig. 2.82). Xanthogranulomas rarely appear in large numbers; they are single in about 50% of the cases, and fewer than five nodules are present in most of the rest.

Fibrous tumors
Keloids

A number of benign dermal tumors result from the proliferation of fibroblasts in the dermis. During the healing process that follows an injury to the skin, loss of normal structures and the laying down of collagen by fibroblasts may result in the formation of a scar. In certain predisposed individuals the collagen may become particularly thick, which results in a hypertrophic scar. Over the ensuing 6–9 months many of these scars flatten. However, some may persist or develop into keloids that continue to thicken and extend beyond the margins of the initial injury (Fig 5.24). These rubbery nodules or plaques can be pruritic or tender, especially during the active growing

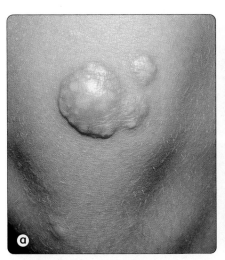
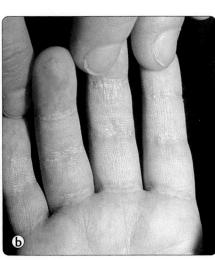
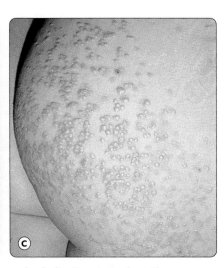

Fig 5.23 Xanthomas erupted in two children **(a, b)** with congenital biliary atresia and chronic liver failure. **(b)** Note the involvement of the hand and finger creases. The infiltrated nodules and plaques resolved after liver transplantation. **(c)** Widespread xanthomas erupted in this 19-year-old woman with primary biliary cirrhosis.

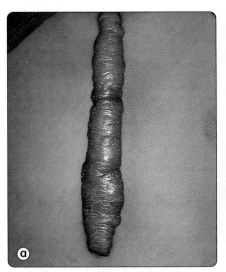
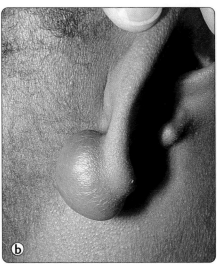
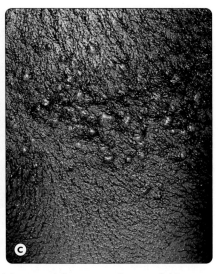

Fig 5.24 Keloids result from an abnormal reparative reaction to skin injury. They are characterized by proliferation of fibroblasts and production of collagen beyond the margins of the original wound. **(a)** A 5-year-old boy developed a progressive keloid in a thoracotomy scar. **(b)** A large nodule grew on the ear of this adolescent after ear piercing. **(c)** Acne keloidalis nuchae erupted on the back of the scalp of this 11-year-old boy. The appearance of multiple small keloids was preceded by pseudofolliculitis.

phase. Keloids may arise sporadically or occur in a familial form. They are most common in blacks, and have a predilection for the ear lobes, upper trunk, and shoulders. Fortunately, they are not seen on the mid-face. If treated early, hypertrophic scars and keloids may regress with intralesional corticosteroid injections alone or in combination with surgery. However, recurrences are common.

Dermatofibromas

Dermatofibromas present as firm, indolent, 0.3–1.0 cm diameter, reddish-brown dermal nodules (Fig 5.25). Although dermatofibromas are most common in adults, about 20% occur before 20 years of age, and they account for 2% of all cutaneous nodules found in children. Tumors may arise as single or multiple lesions (usually fewer than five) on any site, including the palms and soles. However, they appear most commonly on the arms and legs. Although the cause is unknown, many lesions are thought to follow minor trauma, such as insect bites or folliculitis.

On examination, dermatofibromas often demonstrate dimpling with lateral pressure because of attachment of the dermal nodule to an overlying, thickened, and hyperpigmented epidermis. Dermatofibromas may come to the attention of the patient after sudden enlargement following trauma and resultant hemorrhage. Histology, which reveals proliferating fibroblasts and histiocytes, permits easy differentiation from melanocytic tumors such as nevi and melanomas.

Angiofibromas

Although angiofibromas may develop as solitary papules in healthy individuals, their presence alerts the clinician to the diagnosis of tuberous sclerosis (Figs 5.26 and 5.27). In children with tuberous sclerosis, these dermal tumors gradually increase in size and number during childhood, involve the

scalp, cheeks, and nasolabial folds, and spare the upper lip. Subtle angiofibromas may be mistaken for flat warts, comedones, or seborrheic keratoses. Histopathology demonstrates a fibrous tumor with an increase in numbers of fibroblasts and

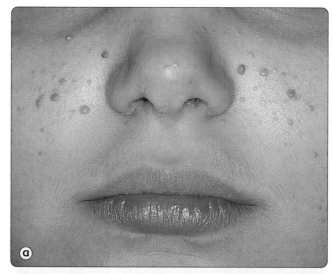

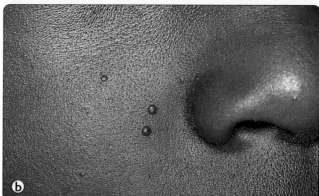

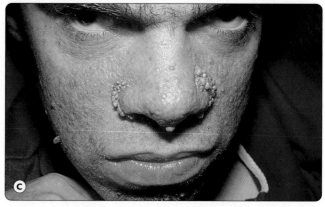

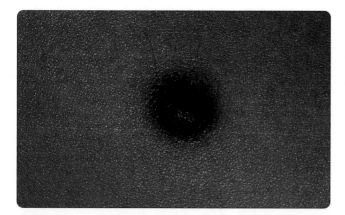

Fig 5.25 Dermatofibroma. An indolent, 5 mm diameter, firm, brown nodule appeared 2 years previously on the leg of this 17-year-old girl. The overlying epidermis was thickened and hyperpigmented.

Fig 5.26 Angiofibromas. **(a)** Small, reddish-brown facial papules were initially dismissed as acne. **(b)** Subtle, brown papules were diagnosed as moles. Both children were of normal intelligence and had no history of seizures. Skin biopsies demonstrated findings typical of angiofibromas. **(c)** This profoundly retarded boy with tuberous sclerosis developed progressive angiofibromas over much of his face. Note the involvement of the nasolabial folds and sparing of the upper lip.

amount of collagen, and capillary dilatation. The presence of acne-like papules beginning well before puberty suggests the diagnosis, even in otherwise healthy children of normal intelligence.

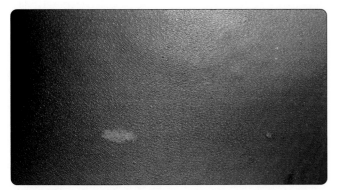

Fig 5.27 A teenager with tuberous sclerosis demonstrated hypopigmented macules and a shagreen patch (connective tissue nevus) on his back, in addition to facial angiofibromas.

Pyogenic granuloma

Pyogenic granuloma, also known as lobular capillary hemangioma, is a common, acquired, benign vascular tumor that resembles a small capillary hemangioma (Fig 5.28). Although it is usually thought to represent an overgrowth of granulation tissue following trauma or reaction to a foreign body, such as a thorn or splinter, the majority of pyogenic granulomas probably arise *de novo*. Lesions are usually solitary, bright red, soft papules, which are often pedunculated and range in size from 2 mm to 2 cm diameter. Two-thirds arise on the head and neck, followed in frequency by the trunk, upper extremities, and lower extremities. Although they are seen most commonly in children and young adults, they may appear at any age.

The term pyogenic granuloma is misleading, because the tumor is neither an infectious pyoderma nor a granuloma. Skin biopsy demonstrates proliferating capillaries in a loose, edematous, fibrous matrix. The surface may become friable and secondarily infected. Minimal trauma results in profuse bleeding, which prompts a visit to the practitioner. Treatment consists of surgical excision, laser

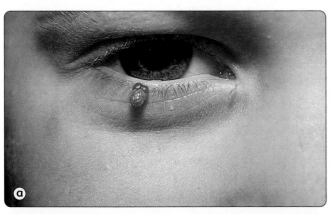

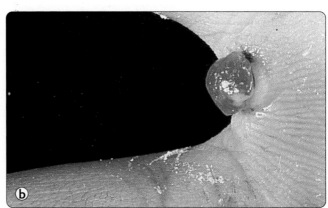

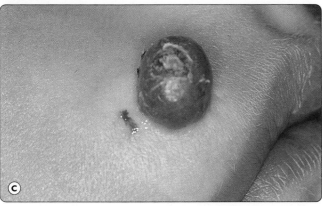

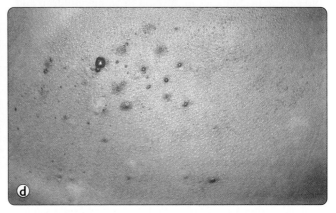

Fig 5.28 Pyogenic granuloma. **(a)** A hemorrhagic papule developed on the lower eyelid of this 8-year-old boy. **(b)** Another rapidly growing, friable lesion is present between the fingers of a 5-year-old boy. **(c)** This 8 mm diameter nodule with a central crust bled profusely several times before surgical removal. **(d)** Multiple satellite lesions erupted on the back of a 10-year-old boy several months after the appearance of a single pyogenic granuloma.

ablation, or shave excision with electrodesiccation of the base. Care must be taken to destroy residual vessels or the lesion will recur. Occasionally, surgical removal of pyogenic granulomas is followed by the eruption of multiple satellite lesions. These may regress spontaneously, but further surgery may be required. Laser surgery may be particularly useful in the management of recurrent or multiple lesions.

Neural Tumors
Neurofibromas
Neurofibromas are the most common tumors of neural origin for which a patient might seek dermatologic consultation (Fig 5.29). These soft, compressible, skin-colored, 0.5–3 cm diameter tumors arise in the dermis and occasionally in the subcutaneous fat. Neurofibromas occur sporadically as solitary lesions or progressively in large numbers in patients with neurofibromatosis (see Fig 6.1).

Neuromas
Neuromas arise in three settings. Traumatic neuromas are solitary, painful nodules that develop in scars after surgery or trauma. Pain resolves quickly after surgical excision. Traumatic neuromas also include amputation neuromas and congenital, rudimentary, supernumerary digits, which occur most commonly on the ulnar side of the base of the fifth finger (see Fig 2.22). Idiopathic neuromas are rare lesions that develop in early childhood through adult life as solitary or multiple 0.2–1 cm diameter dermal nodules on the skin and oral mucosa (Fig 5.30). They are not associated with multiple endocrine neoplasia. Finally, multiple, mucosal neuromas are part of an autosomal-dominant syndrome (multiple endocrine neoplasia Type IIB) in which numerous small tumors begin to appear on the lips, oral mucosa, and face in early childhood. Recognition of this syndrome is important because of the associations with medullary thyroid carcinoma, which can develop in young children and adults, and pheochromocytoma in adolescents and adults.

In multiple mucosal neuroma syndrome, facial lesions may be confused with angiofibromas, trichoepitheliomas, multiple trichilemmomas in Cowden disease, and extensive papillomavirus infection. However, the large numbers of nerve bundles seen on skin biopsy are distinctive. Nodules on the trunk and extremities cannot be differentiated from other dermal tumors without a biopsy.

Lymphocytoma cutis
Lymphocytoma cutis presents as asymptomatic nodules and plaques most commonly on the face, but any site may be involved. Although multiple lesions may erupt, solitary nodules ranging from less than 1 cm to several centimeters in diameter are the rule (Fig 5.31). Most tumors develop in adolescents and young adults.

The differentiation from a non-Hodgkin lymphoma, which also presents as a single nodule, may be impossible. Histologic findings demonstrate a mixed dermal infiltrate of large and small lymphocytes separated from the epidermis

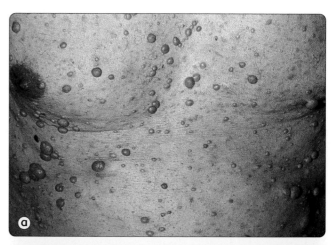

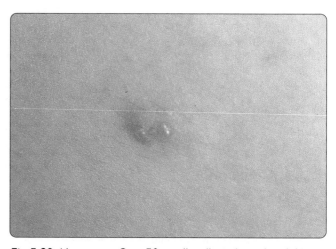

Fig 5.29 Neurofibromas. **(a)** Widespread, compressible tumors developed over much of the body surface of this young man with neurofibromatosis Type I. The neurofibromas began to appear when he was 10 years old. His 4-year-old son had multiple café-au-lait spots, but no cutaneous tumors. **(b)** A giant, plexiform neurofibroma slowly grew to involve most of this teenager's back. Note the multiple, overlying, cutaneous neurofibromas and café-au-lait spots.

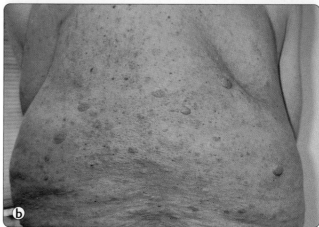

Fig 5.30 Neuromas. Over 50 small, yellow, dermal nodules erupted on the face, neck, trunk, and extremities of a 3-year-old girl. She has no signs of multiple endocrine neoplasia, and the family history is negative.

by a small band of normal collagen. The infiltrate may become organized into structures that resemble lymph follicles. The frequent presence of an admixture of plasma cells and/or eosinophils speaks against malignancy. Unfortunately, the histology is not specific, and the usual innocent nature of the eruption in children is defined by the clinical course. Nodules heal without treatment over months to years. Some patients may benefit from intralesional corticosteroids.

Clinically, lymphocytoma cutis is indistinguishable from cutaneous nodules found in lymphoma and leukemia, and all children deserve a careful history and complete physical examination to exclude signs and symptoms of systemic disease (Figs 5.32 and 5.33). Other infiltrative processes, such as histiocytosis X, follicular mucinosis (Fig 5.34), and mastocytomas, as well as insect-bite reactions, sarcoidosis, deep fungal infections (Fig 5.35), mycobacterial infections (Fig 5.36), and dermatofibromas may resemble lymphocytoma cutis. The clinical course, histologic findings, and culture results help to define these entities. Rarely, other malignancies, such as leukemia, rhabdomyosarcoma, neuroblastoma, and renal carcinoma, present initially with cutaneous nodules. Their rapid growth and histologic pattern differentiate these malignancies from benign lymphocytoma cutis.

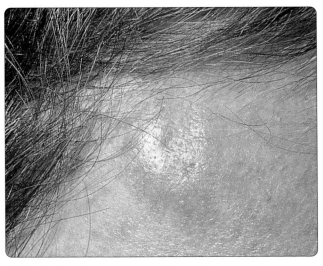

Fig 5.31 Lymphocytoma cutis. A 1 cm diameter, painless nodule persisted for over a year on the forehead of a teenage boy. A skin biopsy from the center of the lesion demonstrated a lymphocytic infiltrate in the dermis that formed lymphoid, follicle-like structures. Intralesional corticosteroids resulted in some improvement.

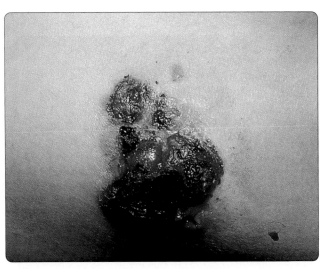

Fig 5.32 Lymphoma. An indolent nodule on the thigh of a 7-year-old boy was initially diagnosed as a persistent insect-bite reaction. During the following year several new nodules appeared on his legs and buttocks and regressed without treatment. Biopsy of the initial lesion shown here, which persisted throughout the period, demonstrated a lymphoma positive to Ki-1 marker.

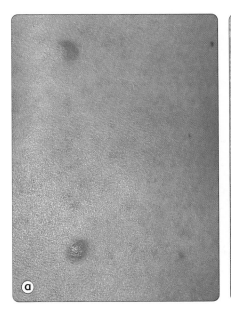

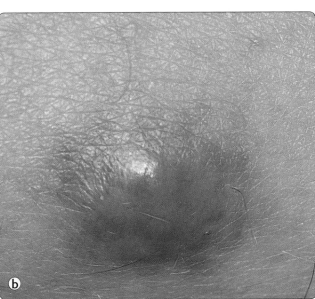

Fig 5.33 Leukemia cutis. An adolescent with myelogenous leukemia developed **(a)** small, cutaneous nodules on his scalp and **(b)** several larger tumors on his trunk and extremities, associated with a recurrence of disease in his bone marrow.

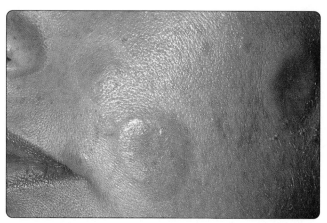

Fig 5.34 Follicular (alopecia) mucinosis. Multiple nodules and indurated plaques appeared on the face and neck of an 18-year-old girl. Histopathology of a skin biopsy showed intracellular edema, formation of cystic spaces, and accumulation of mucin in the external root sheaths of involved hair follicles and sebaceous glands. Several plaques were treated successfully with intralesional injections of corticosteroids. The remainder resolved over several years without treatment.

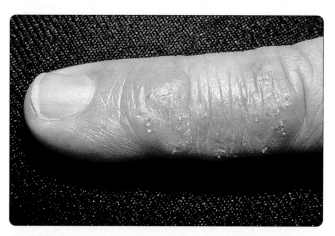

Fig 5.35 Sporotrichosis. A teenage boy developed a slowly expanding, painless, violaceous, indurated plaque on his left fifth finger. Sporotrichosis was diagnosed on a skin biopsy and confirmed by fungal culture. The lesion healed in 3 months with oral administration of a saturated solution of potassium iodide.

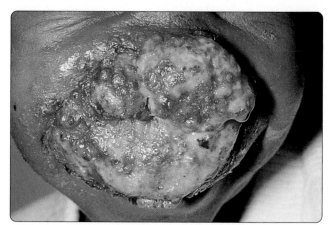

Fig 5.36 Cutaneous tuberculosis. This infection began as a small nodule on the nose and grew into a large, infiltrative tumor that involved the center of her face. The diagnosis was confirmed by skin biopsy and mycobacterial culture. She responded to antibiotics with almost complete clearing of the tumor in 4 months.

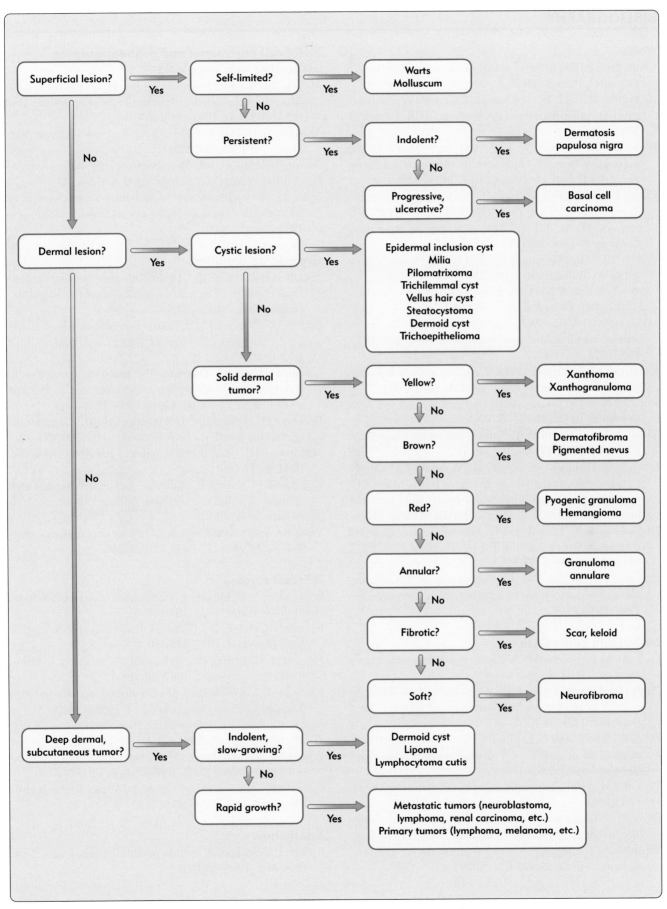

Algorithm for evaluation of nodules and tumors.

BIBLIOGRAPHY

Warts

Androphy EJ. Human papillomavirus: current concepts. *Arch Dermatol.* 1989, **135**:683–5.

Barnett N, Mark H, Winkelstein JA. Extensive verrucosis in primary immunodeficiency diseases. *Arch Dermatol.* 1983, **119**:5–7.

Borovoy MA, Borovoy M, Elson LM, Sage M. Flashlamp pulsed dye laser (585 nm). Treatment of resistant verrucae. *J Am Pediatr Med Assoc.* 1996, **86**:547–50.

Cohen BA, Honig PG, Androphy E. Anogenital warts in children. *Arch Dermatol.* 1990, **126**:1575–80.

Cohen BA. Warts and children: can they be separated? *Contemp Pediatr.* 1997, **14**:128–49.

Frasier LD. Human papillomavirus infection in children (Review). *Pediatr Ann.* 1994, **23**:354–7.

Glass AT, Solomon BA. Cimetidine for recalcitrant warts in adults. *Arch Dermatol.* 1996, **132**:680–2.

Ingelfinger JR, Grupe WE, Topor M, *et al.* Warts in a pediatric renal transplant population. *Dermatologica.* 1977, **155**:7–12.

Kimble-Haas S. Primary care treatment approach to non genital verruca. *Nurse Pract.* 1996, **21**:29–33, 36.

Lutzner MA. The human papillomaviruses. A review. *Arch Dermatol.* 1983, **119**:631–5.

Messing AM, Epstein WL. Natural history of warts. *Arch Dermatol.* 1963, **87**:306–10.

Obalek S, Jablonska S, Favre M, Walczak L, Orth G. Condylomata acuminata in children: frequent association with human papillomavirus responsible for cutaneous warts. *J Am Acad Dermatol.* 1990, **23**:205–13.

Ordoukhanian E, Lane A. Warts and molluscum: beware of treatments worse than the disease. *Postgrad Med.* 1997, **101**:223–6, 229–32, 35.

Rampen FH, Steijlen PM. Diphencyprone in the management of refractory warts: an open study. *Dermatology.* 1996, **193**:236–8.

Molluscum contagiosum

Gottieb SL, Myskowski. Molluscum contagiosum. *Int J Dermatol.* 1994, **33**:453–61.

Pauly CR, Artis WM, Jones HE. Atopic dermatitis, impaired cellular immunity, and molluscum contagiosum. *Arch Dermatol.* 1978, **114**:391–3.

Pierard-Franchimont C, Legrain A, Pierard GE. Growth and regression of molluscum contagiosum. *J Am Acad Dermatol.* 1983, **9**:669–72.

Prasad SM. Molluscum contagiosum. *Pediatr Rev.* 1996, **17**:118–9.

Steffen C, Markman JA. Spontaneous disappearance of molluscum contagiosum. *Arch Dermatol.* 1980, **116**:923–4.

Weston WL, Lane AT. Should molluscum be treated? *Pediatrics.* 1980, **65**:865–6.

Basal cell carcinoma and genodermatoses associated with neoplasia

Mallory SB. Genodermatoses with malignant potential. In: Alper JC (ed). *Genetic disorders of the skin.* Mosby Year Book, St Louis, 1991, pp. 256–61.

Milstone E, Helwig E. Basal cell carcinoma in children. *Arch Dermatol.* 1978, **108**:523.

Sasson M, Mallory SB. Malignant primary skin tumors in children. *Curr Opin Pediatr.* 1996, **8**:372–7.

Spitz JL. *Genodermatoses, a full-color clinical guide to genetic skin disorders.* Williams and Wilkins, Baltimore, 1995.

Granuloma annulare

Argent JD, Fairhurst JJ, Claude NM. Subcutaneous granuloma annulare: four cases and review of the literature. *Pediatr Radiol.* 1994, **24**:527–9.

Barron DF, Cootauco MH, Cohen BA. Granuloma annulare, a clinical review. *Lippincott's Primary Care Practice.* 1997, **1**:33–9.

Calista D, Landi G. Disseminated granuloma annulare in acquired immunodeficiency syndrome: case report and review of the literature. *Cutis.* 1995, **55**:158–60.

Dicken CH, Carrington SG, Winkelmann RK. Generalized granuloma annulare. *Arch Dermatol.* 1969, **99**:556–63.

Mulhbauer JE. Granuloma annulare. *J Am Acad Dermatol.* 1980, **3**:217–30.

Rapelanoro-Rabenja F, Maleville J, Taieb A. Granulome annulaire localisé chez l'enfant: évolution de 30 cas. *Arch Pediatr.* 1995, **2**:1145–8.

Wells RS, Smith MA. The natural history of granuloma annulare. *Br J Dermatol.* 1963, **75**:199–206.

Adnexal tumors

Brownstein MH, Helwig EB. Subcutaneous dermoid cysts. *Arch Dermatol.* 1973, **107**:237–9.

Esterly NB, Fretxin DF, Pinkus H. Eruptive vellus hair cysts. *Arch Dermatol.* 1977, **113**:500–3.

Friedman SJ, Butler DF. Syringoma presenting as milia. *J Am Acad Dermatol.* 1987, **16**:310–14.

Kligman AM, Kirschbaum JD. Steatocystoma multiplex: a dermoid tumor. *J Invest Dermatol.* 1964, **42**:383–7.

Knight PJ, Reiner CB. Superficial lumps in children. What, when, and why. *Pediatrics.* 1983, **72**:147–53.

Pariser RJ. Multiple hereditary trichoepitheliomas and basal cell carcinomas. *J Cutan Pathol.* 1986, **13**:111–17.

Pollard ZF, Robinson HD, Calhoun J. Dermoid cysts in children. *Pediatrics.* 1976, **57**:379–82.

Xanthomas

Parker F. Xanthomas and hyperlipidemias. *J Am Acad Dermatol.* 1985, **13**:1–30.

Fibrous tumors

Murray JC, Pollack SV, Pinnell SR. Keloids: a review. *J Am Acad Dermatol*. 1981, **4**:461–70.

Niemi KM. The rare benign fibrocystic tumors of the skin. *Acta Derm Venereol (Stockh)*. 1970, **50**(Suppl.):43–66.

Pyogenic granuloma

Amerigo J, Gonzales-Camara R, Galera H, *et al*. Recurrent pyogenic granuloma with multiple satellites. *Dermatologica*. 1983, **166**:117–21.

Patrice SJ, Wiss K, Mulliken JB. Pyogenic granuloma (lobular capillary hemangioma): a clinicopathologic study of 178 cases. *Pediatr Dermatol*. 1991, **8**:267–76.

Neural tumors

Holm TW, Prawer SE, Sahl WJ Jr, *et al*. Multiple cutaneous neuromas. *Arch Dermatol*. 1973, **107**:608–10.

Khairi MRA, Dexter RN, Burzynski NJ, *et al*. Mucosal neuroma, pheochromocytoma and medullary thyroid carcinoma: multiple endocrine neoplasia type 3 (review). *Medicine (Baltimore)*. 1975, **54**:89–112.

Lymphocytoma cutis

Burg G, Kerl H, Schmoekel C. Differentiation between malignant B-cell lymphomas and pseudolymphomas of the skin. *J Dermatol Surg Oncol*. 1984, **10**:271–5.

VanHale HM, Winkelmann RK. Nodular lymphoid disease of the head and neck: lymphocytoma cutis, benign lymphocytic infiltrate of Jessner, and their distinction from malignant lymphoma. *J Am Acad Dermatol*. 1985, **12**:455–61.

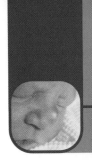

Chapter Six

Disorders of Pigmentation

INTRODUCTION

Although most disorders of pigmentation in infancy and childhood are of cosmetic importance only, some lesions provide clues to the diagnosis of multisystem disease. Disorders of pigmentation may be differentiated clinically by the presence of increased or decreased pigmentation in a localized or diffuse distribution.

HYPERPIGMENTATION

Localized areas of hyperpigmentation are frequently developmental or hereditary in origin, and appear early in childhood. However, pigmented lesions may also be acquired later in childhood following inflammatory rashes in the skin or environmental exposure to actinic, traumatic, chemical, or thermal injury. Epidermal melanosis occurs when increased numbers of epidermal melanocytes are present in the basal cell layer or increased quantities of melanin are present in epidermal keratinocytes. Dermal melanosis results from increased melanin in dermal melanocytes or melanophages. Although epidermal melanosis may result in the development of dark-brown or black macules and papules, most lesions appear tan or light-brown in color. Dermal melanosis tends to produce slate-gray, dark-brown, and bluish-green lesions.

Epidermal melanosis
Café-au-lait spots
Café-au-lait spots are discrete, tan macules that appear at birth or during childhood in 10–20% of normal individuals. Lesions vary from the size of freckles to 20 cm or more in diameter and may involve any site on the skin surface (Fig 6.1).

Although most affected children are normal, café-au-lait spots, particularly six or more lesions over 0.5 cm in diameter if less than 15 years old, and over 1.5 cm in diameter for older individuals, provide a marker for classic neurofibromatosis (von Recklinghausen disease or National Institutes of Health classification NF-1). Conversely, 90% of individuals with neurofibromatosis have at least one lesion. Although café-au-lait spots are often present at birth, they usually increase in size and number throughout childhood, particularly during the first few years of life in children with neurofibromatosis. Other stigmata, including neurofibromas and Lisch nodules, may not appear until later childhood or adolescence (Fig 6.1b,c). Axillary freckling is also a characteristic sign of neurofibromatosis.

Histologic findings include increased numbers of melanocytes and increased melanin in melanocytes and keratinocytes. Giant pigment granules have been identified in the café-au-lait spots of neurofibromatosis, but they may also be seen in sporadic café-au-lait spots, nevi, freckles, and lentigines.

Café-au-lait spots are not specific for neurofibromatosis and have also been associated with tuberous sclerosis, Albright syndrome, LEOPARD syndrome, epidermal nevus syndrome, Bloom syndrome, ataxia–telangiectasia, and Silver–Russell syndrome (Fig 6.2).

Freckles (ephelides)
Freckles or ephelides are 2–3 mm in diameter, reddish-tan and brown macules that appear on sun-exposed surfaces, particularly the face, neck, upper chest, and forearms (Fig 6.3). They typically arise in early childhood on lightly pigmented individuals. Lesions tend to fade in the winter and increase in number and pigmentation during the spring and summer months. Photoprotection with clothing, sunblocks, and sunscreens may decrease the summer exacerbation of freckles, which are generally of cosmetic importance only. The development of progressive, widespread freckling in sun-exposed sites may suggest an underlying disorder of photosensitivity (see pages 174–176, Chapter 7).

Histologically, freckles demonstrate hyperpigmentation of the basal cell layer of the epidermis. The number of melanocytes may actually be decreased, but those that are present are larger and show more numerous and prominent dendritic processes.

Freckles must be differentiated from lentigines, which are more uniform and darker in color, fewer in number, and do not demonstrate seasonal variation. Lentigines vary from 2 to 5 mm in diameter and may involve any site on the skin or mucous membranes.

Lentigo simplex
Lentigo simplex arises most commonly during childhood and does not show a predilection for sun-exposed surfaces. The lentigines are scattered, 2–5 mm in diameter, uniformly pigmented macules that range from brown to black in color and may be indistinguishable clinically from junctional pigmented nevi.

Microscopically, lentigo simplex shows elongation of the rete ridges, an increase in concentration of melanocytes in the basal layer, an increase in melanin in both melanocytes and basal keratinocytes, and melanophages in the upper dermis.

Several special variants of lentigo simplex are recognized, which include lentiginosis profusa, LEOPARD syndrome (multiple lentigines syndrome), and speckled lentiginous nevus.

Lentiginosis profusa

Lentiginosis profusa is characterized by the presence of diffuse, multiple, small, darkly pigmented macules from birth or infancy. They are not usually familial, and children are otherwise healthy and develop normally. This entity must be differentiated from LEOPARD syndrome, in which diffuse lentigines are associated with multisystem disease.

LEOPARD syndrome

In LEOPARD syndrome, the lentigines are tan or brown in color, begin to appear in early infancy, and increase in number throughout childhood (Fig 6.4). Axillary freckling and café-au-lait spots appear frequently. Other anomalies, which are suggested by the LEOPARD mnemonic and variably occur, include electrocardiographic conduction abnormalities (E), ocular

hypertelorism (O), pulmonic stenosis (P), abnormal genitalia (A), growth retardation (R), and neural deafness (D). This disorder is inherited as an autosomal-dominant trait. In both lentiginosis profusa and LEOPARD syndrome the mucous membranes are spared. In a related disorder, LAMB syndrome, multiple lentigines are associated with atrial myxoma (A), cutaneous papular myxomas (M), and blue nevi (B).

Speckled lentiginous nevus

Speckled lentiginous nevus, or nevus spilus, presents at birth as a discrete tan or brown macule, which becomes dotted with darker, pigmented macules during childhood (Fig 6.5). The light-brown patch demonstrates histologic changes typical of lentigo simplex, while the dark, pigmented macules show nests of nevus cells at the dermal–epidermal junction.

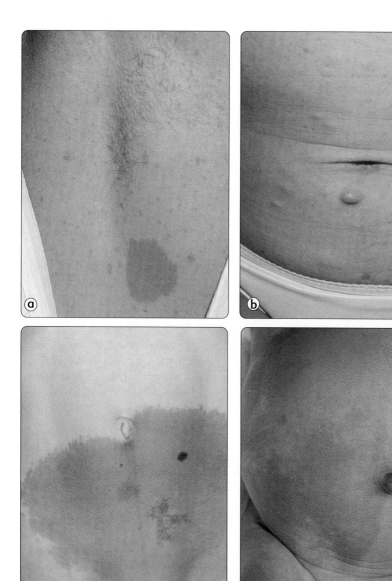
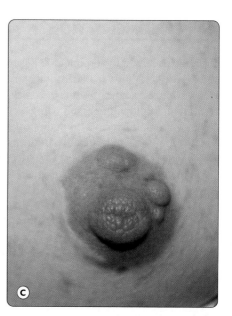

Fig 6.1 Café-au-lait spots. **(a–c)** This 16-year-old girl with neurofibromatosis had multiple café-au-lait spots since early childhood. **(a)** Her axilla demonstrates a 4 cm in diameter café-au-lait spot and diffuse freckling. **(b)** At puberty she began to develop widespread neurofibromas. Note the variable size of the dermal tumors on her abdomen. **(c)** Cutaneous neurofibromas also erupted on her nipples. Note the extensive freckling on her breasts. **(d)** In the center of a large café-au-lait spot, which was present at birth, this 6-year-old girl developed a spongy tumor. Skin biopsy of the mass demonstrated a neurofibroma. Note the dark-brown, pigmented nevus within the café-au-lait spot. **(e)** A large, unilateral café-au-lait spot was noted at birth on this infant's abdomen. She subsequently developed other findings typical of Albright syndrome.

Café-au-lait spots		
Disorder	**Other skin findings**	**Systemic involvement**
Neurofibromatosis	Axillary freckling, Lisch nodules (iris), neurofibromas	Skeletal abnormalities, neurologic involvement
Albright syndrome	Few large café-au-lait spots	Precocious puberty in girls, polyostotic fibrous dysplasia
Watson syndrome	Axillary freckling	Pulmonary stenosis, mental retardation
Silver–Russell dwarfism	Hypohidrosis in infancy	Small stature, skeletal asymmetry, clinodactyly of fifth finger
Ataxia–telangiectasia	Telangiectasia in bulbar conjunctivae and on face, sclerodermatous changes	Growth retardation, ataxia mental retardation, lymphopenia, IgA, IgE, lymphoid tissue, respiratory infections
Tuberous sclerosis	Hypopigmented macules, shagreen patch, adenoma sebaceum, subungual fibromas	Central nervous system, kidneys, heart, lungs
Turner syndrome	Loose skin especially around neck, lymphedema in infancy, hemangiomas	Small stature, gonadal dysgenesis, skeletal anomalies, renal anomalies, cardiac defects
Bloom syndrome	Telangiectatic erythema of cheeks, photosensitivity, ichthyosis	Short stature, malar hypoplasia, risk of malignancy
Multiple lentigines (LEOPARD syndrome)	Lentigines, axillary freckling	Electrocardiogram abnormalities, ocular hypertelorism, pulmonic stenosis, genital abnormalities, growth retardation, sensorineural deafness
Westerhof syndrome	Hypopigmented macules	Growth and mental retardation

Fig 6.2 Café-au-lait spots.

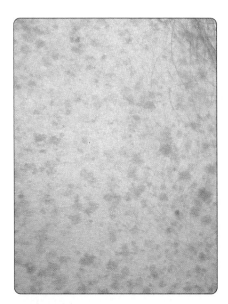

Fig 6.3 Ephelides. Freckles cover sun-exposed areas of this red-haired, blue-eyed girl. The pigmented macules darken and increase in number during the summer.

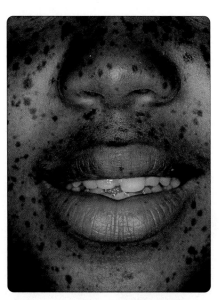

Fig 6.4 Lentigo. Multiple lentigines persisted all year round on the face, upper trunk, and extremities of this 13-year-old boy with LEOPARD syndrome. The lips and mucous membranes were spared, but he did have axillary freckling. His sister, father, and grandfather had similar cutaneous findings.

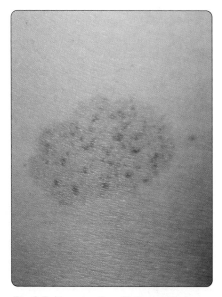

Fig 6.5 Nevus spilus. This speckled nevus remained unchanged since it was noted shortly after birth.

The risk of malignant change is unknown, but may be increased, as in small congenital pigmented nevi.

Peutz–Jeghers syndrome

Peutz–Jeghers syndrome is differentiated by the presence of diffuse, small, slate-gray to black macules on the skin and mucous membranes at birth or during early childhood. Lesions increase in number throughout childhood. The face is most commonly involved, in particular the vermilion border of the lips and buccal mucosa, but macules may appear on the hands, arms, trunk, and perianal and genital skin (Fig 6.6). Axillary freckling may also occur in this autosomal-dominant disorder. Cutaneous lesions occasionally occur alone. However, they are characteristically associated with intestinal polyposis, which is usually restricted to the small bowel. Although the risk of malignant change in the gastrointestinal tract is low, polyps may act as the lead point for intussusception and result in bleeding or obstruction.

Although the lesions in Peutz–Jeghers syndrome are clinically indistinguishable from lentigines, the histology reveals only increased pigmentation in the basal cell layer. Some investigators have found increased numbers of melanocytes, which suggests that this disorder may represent a distinct form of epidermal melanosis.

Cutaneous macules may become disfiguring and respond well to destructive measures, such as gentle liquid nitrogen freezing or carbon dioxide laser ablation. The new pigmented-lesion lasers (Q-switched ruby, neodymium: yttrium–aluminum–garnet, and alexandrite lasers) also provide a safe, effective, relatively painless therapeutic alternative.

Solar lentigines

Solar lentigines usually do not become apparent until the fourth and fifth decades of life. However, these irregularly shaped, darkly pigmented macules, which range from a few millimeters to a few centimeters in diameter on sun-exposed skin may begin to appear in later childhood or adolescence, particularly in lightly pigmented individuals who spend long hours outdoors. Although the risk of malignant degeneration is minimal, they provide a marker of significant sun exposure. Children and parents should be counseled regarding the cumulative risk of actinic damage and use of protective clothing and sunscreens.

Becker nevus

Becker nevus (hairy epidermal nevus) typically develops as a unilateral patch of hyperpigmentation on the trunk of an older child or adolescent (Fig 6.7). This common lesion is usually followed by the appearance of hypertrichosis within 2 years. Although it occurs most frequently in boys on the shoulder, chest, or back, girls occasionally develop lesions, and any skin site may be involved. Pigmentation is usually uniform and well demarcated, but reticulated patches may be present. The coarse, long hairs may extend beyond the area of hyperpigmentation.

Histologically, the epidermis demonstrates acanthosis and rete ridge elongation in association with increased pigment in the basal cell layer and melanophages in the upper dermis. Smooth muscle bundles may be increased in some cases, reminiscent of the changes seen in congenital smooth muscle hamartomas.

As in other epidermal melanoses, gentle destructive measures and the new pigmented-lesion lasers may result in improvement of hyperpigmentation. Use of photoprotection decreases darkening from sun exposure during the summer months. Bleaching agents that contain hydroquinone (e.g. Solaquin Forte®, Melanex®) may also be effective.

However, patients should be made aware that inadvertent contact of the drug with normal contiguous skin may result in hypopigmentation. The pigmented-lesion lasers are also effective for eradicating the pigment in Becker nevus and café-au-lait spots, but pigment can recur within 1–2 years. Shaving, depilatories, and electrolysis may be helpful for nevi with prominent hair.

Acanthosis nigricans

Acanthosis nigricans is marked by distinctive, velvety, warty hyperpigmentation in intertriginous areas. Four types are recognized. The inherited type usually erupts during infancy or childhood, but occasionally at puberty (Fig 6.8a). Lesions

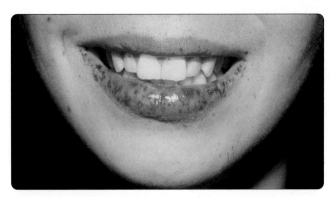

Fig 6.6 Peutz–Jeghers syndrome. This smiling, 12-year-old girl developed progressive lentigines on her face, particularly her lips, in early childhood. She also has involvement of the extremities, trunk, and mucous membranes.

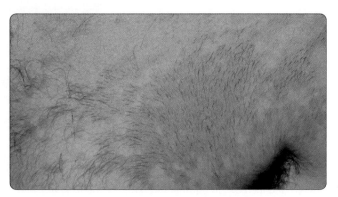

Fig 6.7 Becker nevus. Progressive, mottled hyperpigmentation began at 13 years of age and was followed by the development of dark, coarse hair on the upper chest of this 17-year-old boy.

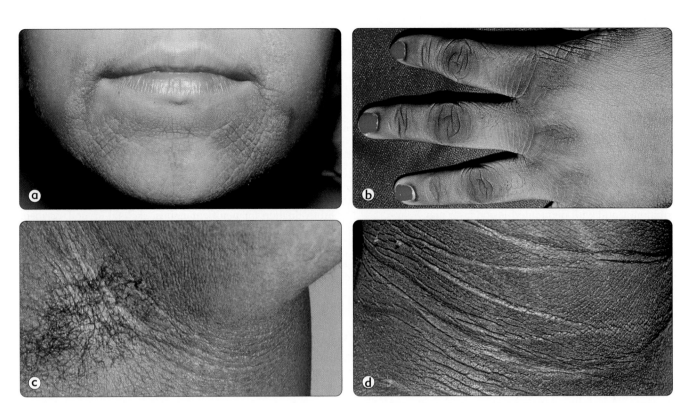

Fig 6.8 Acanthosis nigricans. **(a)** Progressive, leathery thickening of the skin and hyperpigmentation developed on the face, neck, chest, back, and flexures of this healthy 9-year-old boy with familial acanthosis nigricans. Note the symmetric patches on his chin and cheeks. **(b–d)** Symmetric, velvety patches appeared over the bony prominences and flexures of this obese, black adolescent with benign acanthosis nigricans. Lesions were most prominent over **(b)** the knuckles, **(c)** axilla, and **(d)** neck.

tend to intensify in adolescence and may fade somewhat during adulthood. No association has been found with underlying medical disorders, and the inheritance is autosomal dominant. The endocrine type is usually associated with a pituitary tumor or polycystic ovary syndrome and insulin resistance. Obesity is a variable feature. Malignant acanthosis nigricans can usually be differentiated from the other types by its extensive and more florid lesions, progressiveness, and onset in middle age. The malignant type is only rarely seen in childhood. Associated tumors include gastric carcinoma, lymphoma, Hodgkin disease, and osteogenic sarcoma. Idiopathic acanthosis nigricans is the most common type (Fig 6.8b–d). There is no associated endocrine disorder, malignancy, or genetic predisposition. Idiopathic lesions occur most commonly in healthy, obese adolescents. Pigmentation may decrease after puberty, particularly in patients who experience a weight reduction.

Although brown-to-black pigmentation and thickening of the skin is most intense in skin creases of the neck, axilla, and groin, skin over bony prominences, including the knuckles, elbows, knees, and ankles, may be affected. In cases of malignant acanthosis nigricans, mucous membranes are occasionally involved.

Histopathology demonstrates hyperkeratosis, minimal acanthosis, and marked papillomatosis. Although there may be a slight increase in melanin in the basal cell layer, hyperpigmentation probably results from compact hyperkeratosis.

Melasma

Melasma occurs primarily in pubertal girls and women, but also occasionally in adolescent boys (Fig 6.9). Although this symmetric, patchy, facial melanosis may be idiopathic, it is often associated with pregnancy or the ingestion of oral contraceptives. Lesions tend to increase after sun exposure.

Histologically, epidermal and dermal types of melanization are recognized, but many patients demonstrate pigment in both sites. Increased numbers of epidermal melanocytes

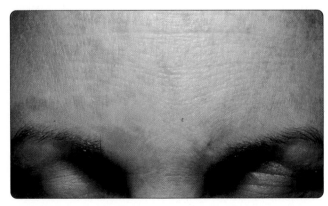

Fig 6.9 Melasma. Diffuse, mottled, tan pigmentation developed on the forehead and cheeks of this young woman shortly after she began taking oral birth-control pills.

occur and increased pigment is found in epidermal keratinocytes and dermal melanophages.

Clinically, melasma must be differentiated from postinflammatory hyperpigmentation and phytophotocontact
(berloque) dermatitis. Berloque dermatitis frequently
appears after inadvertent application of a photosensitizer
such as musk ambrette, a common component of perfumes,
and sun exposure.

Pigmentation often wanes after pregnancy or the discontinuation of oral contraceptives. However, treatment with
potent topical sunscreens and bleaching agents (hydroquinone), and with pigmented-lesion laser may help.

Dermal melanosis
Mongolian spots
Mongolian spots are poorly circumscribed, slate-gray to
blue–green congenital macules (Fig 6.10a,b). Lesions range
from a few millimeters to over 20 cm in diameter and are
found on the trunk and proximal extremities of 80–90% of
black infants, 75% of Asians, and 10% of white infants. Nearly
75% of lesions appear on the lumbosacral region. Mongolian
spots do not require therapy and usually fade or are camouflaged by normal pigment by the age of 3–5 years. When
lesions are clinically confused with a pigmented nevus, skin
biopsy reveals characteristic melanocytes in the dermis in a
mongolian spot.

Special variants of the mongolian spot, the nevus of Ota
and nevus of Ito tend to persist into adult life.

Nevus of Ota
Nevus of Ota (nevus fuscoceruleus ophthalmomaxillaris) represents a unilateral, patchy, dermal melanosis of the skin of
the face in the distribution of the trigeminal nerve (Fig 6.10c).
Although most cases are sporadic, rare family clusters have
been reported. Lesions tend to be slate-gray to brown in
color with a 'powder-blast burn' appearance. The forehead,
temple, periorbital area, cheek, and nose are commonly
involved. Rarely, pigmentation is bilateral and large areas of
the face and oral mucous membranes are affected. Melanin
pigment involves the eye in about half the cases. About 50%
of lesions are present at birth, and the remainder appear
during puberty. Although lesions are most common on Asians
and blacks, all races are affected, and the majority of patients
are female.

Nevus of Ito
Nevus of Ito (nevus fuscoceruleus acromiodeltoideus) is a
similar pathologic process to nevus of Ota in which unilateral
pigmentation is located over the supraclavicular, deltoid, and
scapular regions. Although it usually occurs as an isolated
lesion, nevus of Ota may also be present.

Nevus of Ito and nevus of Ota are benign dermal
melanoses. However, there are rare reports of malignant
degeneration. Extensive lesions are amenable to corrective,
cosmetic camouflage. The Q-switched ruby laser results in
safe, effective destruction of the abnormal pigment with little
risk of recurrence.

Incontinentia pigmenti
Incontinentia pigmenti is an inherited, multisystem disorder
that is defined by its splashy, reticulated hyperpigmentation
(see Fig 2.63). An inflammatory phase in the newborn
precedes the pigmentary change in over 90% of affected
children. Another disorder in children, which should be
differentiated from incontinentia pigmenti, presents with
localized or diffuse whorled pigmentation without antecedent
inflammation (Fig 6.11). These children demonstrate variable
genetic mosaicism in the skin and occasionally multiple organ
system malformations. Consequently, they also require a careful evaluation for neurocutaneous, skeletal, dental, cardiac,
and other anomalies. Inheritance also varies from the typical
X-linked dominant pattern of incontinentia pigmenti.

Postinflammatory hyperpigmentation
The most common cause of increased pigmentation is postinflammatory hyperpigmentation. This alteration in normal
pigmentation follows many inflammatory processes in the
skin, such as a diaper dermatitis, insect bites, drug reactions,
and traumatic injury. Lesions are usually localized and typically follow the distribution of the resolving disorder (Fig
6.12). Although epidermal melanocytes appear normal, aberrant delivery of melanin to the surrounding keratinocytes
results in deposition of pigment in the dermal melanophages.
Areas of hyperpigmentation are more marked in darkly
pigmented children. No therapy is necessary, and lesions
usually fade over several months.

Fixed drug eruption
A special subset of drug reactions known as a fixed drug eruption
produces peculiar, persistent hyperpigmentation, particularly on
the face, genitals, and scattered on the trunk and extremities (see
Fig 7.3). After exposure to certain medications, such as tetracycline, ibuprofen and other nonsteroidal anti-inflammatory drugs,
phenobarbital, and phenolphthalein, patients develop acutely
inflamed, dusky-red, edematous, round to oval, 1–3 cm diameter plaques, which may become frankly bullous in the center.
These target lesions are clinically and histologically indistinguishable from target lesions found in erythema multiforme
minor. When the drug is discontinued the reaction subsides to
leave residual postinflammatory pigmentation. On re-exposure to
the inciting agent, new lesions may appear, but the old lesions
recur in the same 'fixed' spots. The reactivity of the skin seems
to reside in the dermis, because normal epidermis grafted over
affected dermis becomes reactive, whereas involved epidermis
grafted onto normal dermis loses its sensitivity.

Acquired nevomelanocytic nevi
Acquired nevomelanocytic nevi, also referred to as pigmented nevi and pigmented moles, begin to develop in early
childhood as small, pigmented macules 1–2 mm in diameter.
In these early, flat nevi, nevus cells are located at the
dermal–epidermal junction and are called junctional nevi
(Fig 6.13a). They then enlarge slowly, and become papular.
In elevated lesions, the nevus cells have spread into the
dermis to become compound nevi (Fig 6.13b). Many nevi

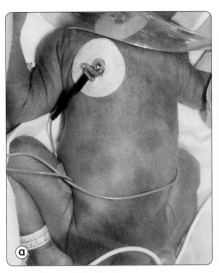

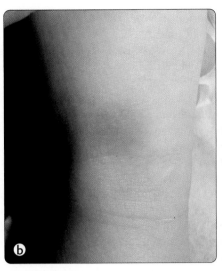

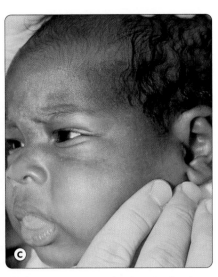

Fig 6.10 Mongolian spot. **(a)** Widespread and confluent mongolian spots were noted at birth on this premature black infant. The pigment was slate-gray in color. **(b)** Note the solitary, blue mongolian spot on the shin of a white newborn. **(c)** A nevus of Ota involved the forehead, cheek, and contiguous scalp of an otherwise healthy black infant. The lids and conjunctivae were spared.

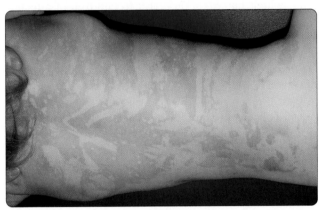

Fig 6.11 Nevoid hyperpigmentation. A 9-year-old girl with profound mental retardation and seizures was noted at birth to have swirling hyperpigmentation following the lines of Blaschko. No history of an antecedent inflammatory eruption was found. Genetic studies of fibroblasts from the hyperpigmented skin demonstrated a ring chromosome 22 anomaly, which was also evident in some peripheral lymphocytes.

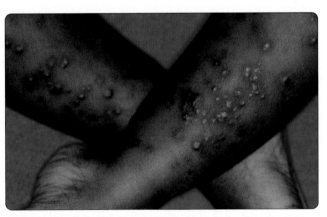

Fig 6.12 Postinflammatory hyperpigmentation. Marked hyperpigmentation developed in this 5-year-old boy from recurrent insect bites. Although the pigment faded somewhat, it was still noticeable 2 years later.

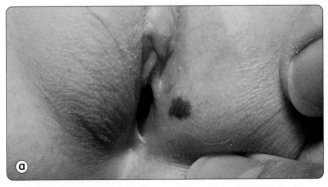

Fig 6.13 Acquired nevomelanocytic nevus. **(a)** This brown macule on the labia of a 3-year-old girl was flat on palpation. Darkening and increase in size of the macule prompted a biopsy, which revealed a benign junctional nevus. **(b)** A shave excision of this facial nodule showed a compound nevomelanocytic nevus.

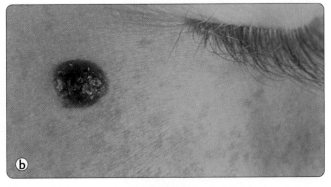

become fleshy or pedunculated over a period of years, particularly those on the upper trunk, head, and neck. Histopathology of these nevi demonstrates nevus cells restricted to the dermis, hence the so-called intradermal nevus.

During puberty, nevi show an increase in darkening, size, and number. However, most normal acquired nevomelanocytic nevi do not exceed 0.5 cm in diameter, and retain their regularity in color, contour, texture, and symmetry. The majority of nevi appear on sun-exposed areas, but lesions may involve the palms, soles, buttocks, genitals, scalp, mucous membranes, and eyes. Generally, nevi change slowly over months to years and warrant observation only.

Sudden enlargement of a nevus, with redness and tenderness, may occur because of an irritant reaction or folliculitis. Trauma from clothing or scratching may produce hemorrhage or crust formation that heals uneventfully. Another more gradual change that causes concern in patients and parents is the appearance of a hypopigmented ring and mild local pruritus around a benign nevus (Fig 6.14). This so-called halo nevus is caused by a cytotoxic T-lymphocyte reaction against both the nevus cells and contiguous melanocytes. As a result, the nevus tends first to lighten and then disappear completely, and the halo eventually repigments. Occasionally, halo nevi are associated with vitiligo or the loss of pigmentation in areas of normal skin that have no nevi.

As long as the clinical appearance of a nevus is innocent, excision is unnecessary. However, a number of changes in pigmented lesions may portend the development of melanoma, and include:
- change in size, shape, or contours with scalloped, irregular borders;
- change in the surface characteristics, such as the development of a small, dark, elevated papule or nodule within an otherwise flat plaque and flaking, scaling, ulceration, or bleeding;

- change in color, with the appearance of black, brown, or an admixture of red, white, or blue;
- burning, itching, or tenderness, which may be an indication of an immunologic reaction to malignancy.

Melanomas

Fortunately, melanomas are rare in children. However, the incidence is increasing, and curative treatment is contingent on early diagnosis and prompt excision. A keen awareness of diagnostic features is important.

Melanomas in children may occur *de novo* or within acquired or congenital nevi (Fig 6.15; see Fig 2.81). Family history of malignant melanoma and the presence of multiple, unusually large, and irregularly pigmented, bordered, and textured nevi carries a high lifetime risk of melanoma, which may approach 100%. Malignant melanoma in this hereditary setting is referred to as familial atypical mole syndrome (familial dysplastic nevus syndrome). During early childhood, children in such families may develop only innocent-looking nevi. However, the predisposition for the development of malignant melanoma is autosomal dominant, which imparts a 50% risk to children of affected parents. The presence of a large number of nevi, particularly on the scalp and sun-protected sites in prepubertal children, may be an early marker for atypical mole syndrome. Children in these high-risk families must be observed carefully for the development of dysplastic nevi, at least through their adolescent years. Changing nevi of unusual appearance must be biopsied to exclude malignant degeneration. As many as 5% of light-pigmented individuals with a negative family history of melanoma may also develop atypical moles. Although the risk of melanoma is probably lower than in people with a positive family history, patients with sporadic atypical mole syndrome should also be observed for malignant changes.

A rare cause of melanoma in the pediatric age group is transplacental spread of maternal melanoma. Neonates born

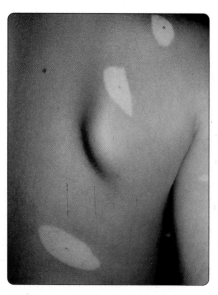

Fig 6.14 Halo nevus. Large, depigmented halos surround innocent-looking nevi on the back of a 9-year-old boy.

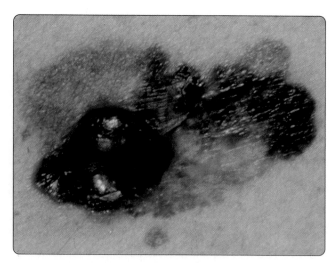

Fig 6.15 Melanoma. This lesion shows the irregularity of outline, color, and thickness typical of a melanoma.

to mothers with a history of melanoma must be examined and followed carefully. Conversely, mothers of infants born with melanoma must be examined thoroughly for signs of the malignancy.

Differential diagnosis of childhood melanoma includes congenital and acquired nevomelanocytic nevi, the blue nevus (a small, firm, blue papule that consists of deep nevus cells; Fig 6.16), traumatic hemorrhage (especially under the nails, on the heels, or in the mucous membranes), and a number of innocent vascular lesions such as pyogenic granuloma or hemangioma.

Spindle and epithelial cell nevus

Spindle and epithelial cell nevus, also known as Spitz nevus after the clinician who first described it in 1948, is an innocent nevomelanocytic nevus that may be clinically and histologically confused with malignant melanoma (Fig 6.17). Initially, Spitz nevus was also referred to as 'benign juvenile melanoma'. However, this term should be discarded, because 'melanoma' is misleading and these lesions have also been described in adults. Spitz nevi frequently appear as rapidly growing, dome-shaped, red papules or nodules on the face or extremities. Occasionally they contain large quantities of melanin and may appear brown or black. In most histopathologic specimens, malignant melanoma can be readily excluded. Consequently, simple excision is usually adequate.

Diffuse hyperpigmentation

Diffuse hyperpigmentation has rarely been reported as progressive familial hyperpigmentation. Affected infants are born with splotches of macular hyperpigmentation that slowly increase in size and number to involve much of the skin surface. This can usually be differentiated from the normal pigmentary darkening that occurs during the first year of life in many infants, particularly those of dark-skinned races.

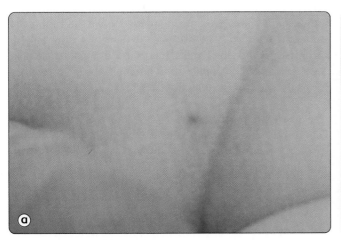

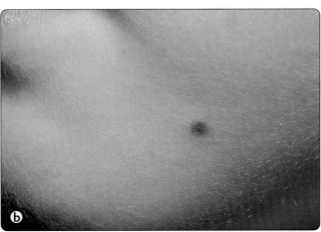

Fig 6.16 Blue nevus. The blue papules are made up of deep nevus cells. **(a)** The blue nevus on the infant's buttock was present at birth. **(b)** A 6-year-old boy developed a similar nevus on the lower cheek.

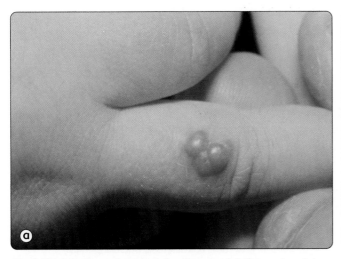

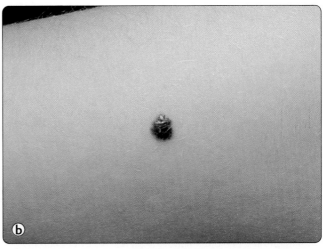

Fig 6.17 Spindle and epithelial cell nevus. **(a)** This red nodule stabilized at 1 cm in diameter a month after it first appeared. **(b)** Rapidly growing pigmented nevus on the arm of a 7-year-old boy showed histologic changes typical of a Spitz nevus.

Generalized bronze pigmentation may develop after photo-therapy for hyperbilirubinemia, particularly in infants with a high direct bilirubin component. Most cases have resolved uneventfully after discontinuation of phototherapy, but occasional hepatic abnormalities and deaths have been reported.

Generalized hyperpigmentation may also occur after exposure to certain drugs (e.g. heavy metals, phenothiazines, antimalarials) and in association with a number of systemic endocrine and inflammatory disorders. In adrenocortical insufficiency, Cushing syndrome, and acromegaly, melano-tropin-stimulating hormone or other hormones with similar properties of pigment-production stimulation trigger generalized hyperpigmentation. Pigmentation may be particularly marked in skin creases on the palms and soles, and on mucous membranes. Increased epidermal and dermal melanin also occurs in hemochromatosis, chronic renal and hepatic disease, and extensive cutaneous fibrosis associated with dermatomyositis and scleroderma.

HYPOPIGMENTATION AND DEPIGMENTATION

Partial or complete pigmentary loss may be congenital or acquired in a localized or diffuse pattern. Localized disorders of pigmentation include hypopigmented macules of the newborn, incontinentia pigmenti achromians, piebaldism, postinflammatory hypopigmentation, and vitiligo. Generalized pigmentary disturbances occur in albinism and progressive vitiligo.

Localized hypopigmentation
Hypopigmented macules
Localized hypopigmentation is characteristic of several nevoid phenomenon, which include hypopigmented macules, incontinentia pigmenti achromians, and piebaldism. Although 0.1% of normal newborns have hypopigmented macules (ash leaf macules), they may be a marker for tuberous sclerosis (Fig 6.18). These macules appear at birth as 2 mm to 3 cm diameter lesions on the trunk of 70–90% of individuals with tuberous sclerosis. Although macules are typically lancet shaped, small confetti spots and oval, round, or irregularly shaped patches may appear on any body site.

The identification of hypopigmented macules may be enhanced in lightly pigmented children by the use of Wood light. The visible purple light that passes through the Wood filter is absorbed by melanin. In a darkened room, subtle areas of depigmentation or hypopigmentation appear bright violet, whereas normally pigmented skin absorbs most of the light and appears dull purple or black.

Children with hypopigmented macules require close neurodevelopmental observation. Onset of other cutaneous findings (adenoma sebaceum, angiofibromas, or subungual fibromas) and systemic symptoms of tuberous sclerosis (seizures, intracranial tumors) may be delayed for years (see Fig 5.26). Tuberous sclerosis is transmitted as an autosomal-dominant trait, but 25–50% of children represent new mutations. A careful family history and cutaneous examination of other family members may demonstrate subtle findings of tuberous sclerosis. The presence of asymptomatic rhabdo-myomas, calcified intracranial tubers, renal angiolipomas, and cystic lesions in the kidneys and lungs also support the diagnosis in otherwise healthy individuals.

Nevus depigmentosus
The term nevus depigmentosus (achromic nevus) should probably be used to describe the majority of children with one or two hypopigmented macules and no other signs of neurocutaneous disease (Fig 6.19). However, nevus depigmentosus has rarely been reported in association with hemi-hypertrophy and mental retardation without findings of tuberous sclerosis. Hypopigmented macules on cosmetically important areas are readily camouflaged by rehabilitative cosmetics such as Dermablend® and Covermark®.

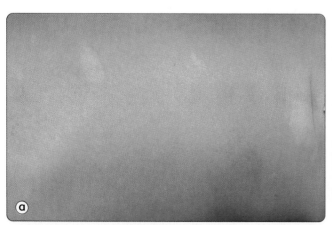

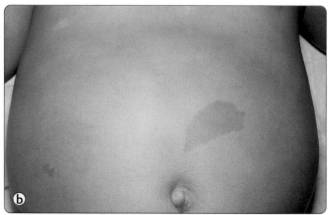

Fig 6.18 Ash leaf macules. **(a)** A 4-month-old boy was admitted to the pediatric neurology service for evaluation of seizures. Several hypopigmented macules were discovered on his back. A computed tomography scan of the head demonstrated tumors typical of tuberous sclerosis. **(b)** This 10-month-old boy with tuberous sclerosis had congenital, hypopigmented macules on the upper trunk and café-au-lait spots scattered on the abdomen.

Nevus anemicus

Nevus anemicus is often misdiagnosed as an ash leaf macule. This congenital patch, usually located on the trunk, appears pale compared with surrounding normal skin (Fig 6.20). However, Wood lamp examination demonstrates the presence of normal pigment. Rubbing the area results in erythema from vasodilatation in surrounding normal skin, while the lesion remains unchanged. A persistent increase in vascular tone, which results in maximal vasoconstriction in the nevus, seems to account for this phenomenon.

Incontinentia pigmenti achromians

Incontinentia pigmenti achromians (also known as hypomelanosis of Ito, after the physician who first described the disorder in 1952) is characterized by congenital, hypopigmentation with a marble-cake pattern. This dyspigmentation, which follows embryonic cleavage lines known as the lines of Blaschko, resembles the pattern of hyperpigmentation found in incontinentia pigmenti (Fig 6.21). Genetic mosaicism has been demonstrated in some patients when gene markers from hypopigmented skin are compared with those of normal skin and peripheral lymphocytes. Although many of the children with cutaneous lesions are otherwise healthy, some patients manifest associated neurologic, developmental, dental, skeletal, and ophthalmologic anomalies. Affected children require a careful medical, neurologic, and ocular examination, and close neurodevelopmental observation. Further studies are tailored to the clinical findings.

Piebaldism

Piebaldism (partial albinism) is a rare, autosomal-dominant disorder characterized by a white forelock and circumscribed congenital leukoderma (Fig 6.22). The typical lesions include a triangular patch of depigmentation and white hair on the frontal scalp, with the apex pointing toward the nasal bridge

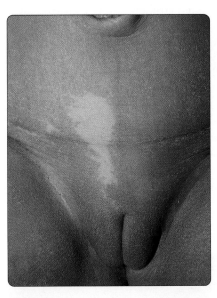

Fig 6.19 Nevus depigmentosus. At birth an otherwise healthy infant was noted to have a hypopigmented patch on the suprapubic area.

Fig 6.20 Nevus anemicus. This adolescent had a congenital pale patch on his back which was initially diagnosed as nevus depigmentosus. Note that the patch becomes better defined after scratching the surrounding skin. This patch tans normally in the summer and does not enhance with Wood light.

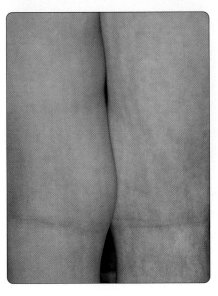

Fig 6.21 Incontinentia pigmenti achromians. Hypopigmented streaks covered the trunk and extremities of this 6-year-old girl. Some of the most prominent hypopigmentation was present on the back of her right leg.

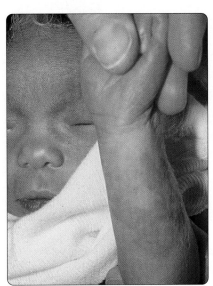

Fig 6.22 At birth a patch of mottled hypopigmentation was discovered on this infant's forearm. Also note the white forelock characteristic of Waardenburg syndrome.

and hypopigmented or depigmented macules on the face, neck, ventral trunk, and/or flanks. However, depigmented patches may involve any part of the skin surface. Within areas of decreased pigmentation, scattered patches of normal pigment or hyperpigmentation may occur. The lesions are stable throughout life, although some variability in pigmentation may occur with sun exposure. Special variants of piebaldism include Waardenburg syndrome (in which leukoderma is associated with lateral displacement of the inner canthi and inferior lacrimal ducts, a flattened nasal bridge, and sensorineural deafness) and Wolf syndrome, an autosomal-recessive disorder associated with multiple neurologic defects.

Postinflammatory hypopigmentation

Postinflammatory hypopigmentation may appear after any inflammatory skin condition. Patches are usually variable in size and irregularly shaped, although they may be remarkably symmetric in disorders such as seborrheic and atopic dermatitis (see Fig 3.27). Areas of pigmentary alteration are usually seen in association with the primary lesions of the underlying disorder. Concomitant hyperpigmentation is also a frequent finding.

Postinflammatory hypopigmentation may be differentiated from vitiligo, which demonstrates well-demarcated depigmentation, and nevus depigmentosus, which appears at birth. In tinea versicolor (see Fig 3.52), the lesions are usually uniform in size and shape, minimally scaly, and prominent in the seborrheic areas on the trunk.

Vitiligo

Vitiligo is an acquired disorder of pigmentation in which there is complete loss of pigment in involved areas. Lesions are macular and usually appear progressively in a characteristic distribution around the eyes, mouth, genitals, elbows, hands, and feet (Fig 6.23). Spontaneous but slow repigmentation, particularly after exposure to the summer sun, may occur from the edges of active lesions and hair follicles within, which results in a speckled appearance. Transient hyperpigmentation of the contiguous normal skin or hypopigmentation at the advancing edge may produce a trichrome, with depigmentation centrally and normal pigmentation around the area of hyper- or hypopigmentation. Histologically, melanocytes are absent in areas of vitiligo, and evidence suggests that these are destroyed by an autoimmune mechanism. Rarely, the pigment in the eye may become involved. Consequently, a thorough eye examination is carried out for all patients with vitiligo.

Early in the course of vitiligo, some children respond to twice daily applications of medium-potency topical corticosteroids. Topical therapy may stabilize lesions in the winter until sunlight is readily available in the spring and summer. Some adolescents are pleased with the temporary camouflage provided by rehabilitative cosmetics (e.g. Dermablend®, Covermark®) and topical dyes (e.g. Neo-Dyoderm®, Vita-Dye®). Most patients with progressive vitiligo that fails to respond to sunlight or topical corticosteroids will repigment at least partially with phototherapy. Light therapy may be administered with an oral or topical psoralens photosensitizer and sunlight (PUVA-sol) or artificial long-wavelength ultraviolet light (PUVA). Topical phototherapy is restricted to small areas of the skin and administered under close supervision because of the high risk of inducing an accidental burn. This risk is reduced with oral psoralens. However, systemic therapy is rarely associated with cataract formation and requires diligent use of protective goggles and regular

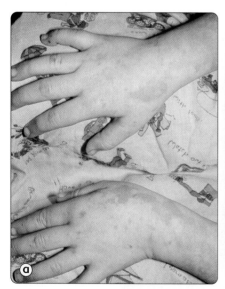 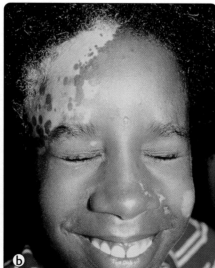 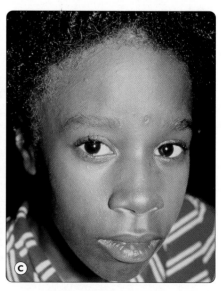

Fig 6.23 Vitiligo. **(a)** Extensive depigmented patches developed on the back of the hands of a 10-year-old girl. These patches were difficult to detect in the winter when her tan faded. **(b)** A progressive, disfiguring patch of vitiligo on the forehead of a 9-year-old girl was **(c)** well camouflaged with a corrective cosmetic.

ophthalmologic follow-up. Although some investigators recommend autoimmune screening (antithyroid, antiadrenal, antigastrin antibodies, etc.) in patients with vitiligo, the results of studies comparing children with vitiligo with age-matched controls have been equivocal.

Vitiligo can be readily differentiated from nevoid pigmentary disorders, which are stable and usually congenital. Vitiligo is rare in infancy, but appears before 20 years of age in about 50% of affected individuals. In postinflammatory hypopigmentation, careful observation reveals residual pigmentation. Tinea versicolor can also be excluded by the presence of pigment and fine scale, which reveals spores and pseudohyphae on potassium hydroxide preparation (see Fig 1.7).

Diffuse hypopigmentation
Albinism

Albinism is a heterogeneous group of inherited disorders manifested by generalized hypopigmentation or depigmentation of the skin, eyes, and hair (Fig 6.24). It occurs as an autosomal-recessive, oculocutaneous form and as an X-linked ocular variant (Fig 6.25).

In oculocutaneous albinism (OCA), both sexes and all races are equally involved. On the basis of clinical findings and biochemical markers, OCA may be divided into a number of variants. Tyrosinase-negative and tyrosinase-positive forms have been established based on the ability of plucked hairs incubated in tyrosine to produce pigment. Recently, the discovery of gene markers in some variants has allowed for specific DNA diagnosis in patients and carriers. In classic tyrosinase-negative OCA, children are born without any trace of pigment. Affected individuals have snow-white hair, pinkish-white skin, and blue eyes. Nystagmus is

common, as is moderate-to-severe strabismus and poor visual acuity. Although children with tyrosinase-positive OCA may be clinically indistinguishable from their tyrosinase-negative counterparts at birth, they usually develop variable amounts of pigment with increasing age. Eye color may vary from gray to light brown, and hair may change to blond or light brown. Most black patients acquire as much pigment as light-skinned whites.

In tyrosinase-negative albinism, the enzyme tyrosinase is either absent or nonfunctional. Tyrosinase-positive albinism results from a number of different defects in pigment synthesis and transport.

In both tyrosinase-positive and -negative variants of albinism, 'clear cells' are noted in the basal cell layer of the epidermis. However, epidermal melanocytes form pigment when incubated with dopa only in the tyrosinase-positive variants. Electron microscopy demonstrates the presence of small amounts of melanin and mature melanosomes in tyrosinase-positive cases, but no melanin and only early stages of melanosome development in tyrosinase-negative patients.

Patients with OCA require aggressive sun protection to prevent actinic damage and early development of basal cell and squamous cell skin cancers. Strabismus and macular degeneration may also be associated with a progressive decrease in visual acuity. Consequently, ongoing ophthalmology input is also important.

Although the skin and hair appear clinically normal in ocular albinism, characteristic macromelanosomes have been demonstrated by electron microscopy. This finding is a reliable marker and may be used to confirm the diagnosis and identify asymptomatic female carriers. When available, DNA analysis can also establish a specific diagnosis.

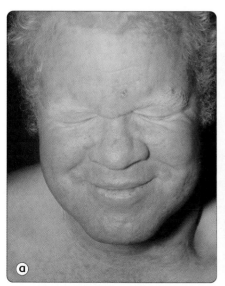 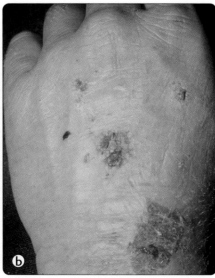 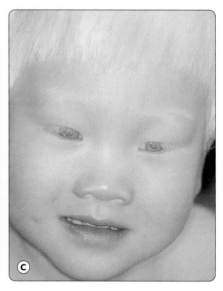

Fig 6.24 Albinism. **(a)** This 19-year-old black man with oculocutaneous albinism already has extensive actinic damage. He works outdoors by the waterfront and has not used sunscreens. **(b)** Numerous actinic keratoses were removed from his face, upper back, and hands. The crusted plaque on the middle of his hand was a squamous cell carcinoma. **(c)** This 18-month-old boy had no detectable pigment. He had white hair, pale skin, nystagmus, and poor visual acuity.

Oculocutaneous albinism					
Disorder	Incidence	Inheritance	Pathogenesis	Clinical findings	Comments
Tyrosinase-negative	1:28,000 African–Caribbeans 1:39,000 Caucasians Male = female	Autosomal recessive; gene locus 11q14–q21	No tyrosinase activity	White hair and skin; blue-to-gray irides; no retinal pigment; nystagmus; poor visual acuity	Hair-bulb test negative; DNA analysis available for prenatal diagnosis; no improvement with age
Tyrosinase-positive	1:15,000 African–Caribbeans 1:37,000 Caucasians Male = female	Autosomal recessive; gene locus 15q11.2–q12	Some due to mutations in p-locus on chromosome 15q	White-to-cream color skin, light hair at birth darkening with age; blue, tan, hazel irides; minimal retinal pigment; nystagmus; photophobia; poor-to-fair visual acuity	Hair-bulb test positive; DNA linkage analysis and mutation detection available for prenatal diagnosis; pigment may improve with age
Yellow mutant	Rare, initially described in Amish, now in numerous races	Autosomal recessive	Melanocytes produce pigment, but hair-bulb test negative Hairs produce pheomelanin when incubated with L-tyrosine and cysteine	White-to-light tan skin darkens somewhat with sun and age; white hair at birth turns yellow with age; blue eyes at birth may darken with age; some retinal pigment; poor visual acuity may improve with age	
Albinoidism	Unknown	Autosomal dominant		Marked pigment dilution of the skin may mimic tyrosinase-positive albinism, but only minimal involvement of the eyes; normal visual acuity	
Hermansky–Pudlak syndrome	Over 200 cases reported Male = female	Autosomal recessive	Tyrosinase-positive Bleeding secondary to platelet storage pool defect Lysosomal membrane defect results in accumulation of ceroid lipofuscin in macrophages in lung and gastrointestinal tract	Creamy white to almost normal skin varying with race; cream-to-red-brown hair; blue-to-brown irides; reduced retinal pigment; nystagmus; photophobia; poor visual acuity Increased bleeding with dental procedures, surgery, childbirth; epistaxis, menorrhagia, gingival bleeding Pulmonary fibrosis, granulomatous colitis, cardiomyopathy from ceroid deposition in viscera	
Chédiak–Higashi syndrome	Rare, fewer than 100 cases reported Male = female	Autosomal recessive, high consanguinity	Lysosomal storage disease involving neutrophils, melanocytes, neurons, platelets, lymphocytes	White skin; blond-to-silver hair; blue-to-brown eyes with variable retinal pigment; photophobia; strabismus Recurrent sinusitis, pneumonia Progressive neurologic dysfunction with ataxia, muscle weakness, sensory loss, seizures Pancytopenia resulting in bleeding diathesis, anemia, sepsis	Fetoscopy at 18–21 weeks reveals fetal blood cells with characteristic neutrophilic granules
Cross syndrome	Rare	Autosomal recessive		White skin; white-to-blond hair; blue-to-gray irides; poor visual acuity; microphthalmia; cataracts Spastic diplegia, mental retardation	
Griscelli syndrome	Rare	Autosomal recessive		Silver color hair; severe combined immunodeficiency	Microscopic examination of hairs shows clumping of pigment in hair shafts, normal melanosomes, but reduced melanocyte dendritic processes

Fig 6.25 Oculocutaneous albinism.

Oculocutaneous albinism (continued)					
Disorder	Incidence	Inheritance	Pathogenesis	Clinical findings	Comments
Prader–Willi syndrome	Unknown	Sporadic	Chromosomal and molecular changes of chromosome 15 at the q11–q13 region	Light skin compared with relatives; normal-to-light hair; blue-to-brown irides; variable retinal pigment, normal to slightly reduced visual acuity Neonatal hypotonic hyperphagia; obesity; developmental delay; mental retardation	Chronic scratching and picking may result in persistent cutaneous ulcers
Angelman syndrome	Unknown	Sporadic, autosomal recessive?	Chromosomal and molecular changes of the proximal region of chromosome 15 similar to those of Prader–Willi syndrome	Light skin compared with relatives; normal-to-light hair; blue-to-brown eyes; variable retinal pigment; normal to slightly reduced visual acuity Growth retardation, developmental delay, mental retardation Ataxia, jerky gait, seizures Dysmorphic facies (microcephaly, flat occiput, protuberant tongue)	

Fig 6.25 Oculocutaneous albinism (continued).

Other disorders associated with diffuse hypopigmentation

Diffuse hypopigmentation may suggest a number of other systemic disorders associated with defects in melanin synthesis in the skin, hair, and eyes. Children with inborn errors of amino acid metabolism (e.g. phenoketonuria, histidinemia, and homocystinuria) often demonstrate widespread pigment dilution. Hypopigmentation of skin and hair in Menke (kinky hair) syndrome results from a defect in copper metabolism that interferes with the normal activity of copper-dependent tyrosinase (see Fig 8.9). Hypohidrotic ectodermal dysplasia and deletion of the short arm of chromosome 18 are also associated with diffuse hypopigmentation and light hair color. Finally, children with malnutrition, particularly kwashiorkor, may develop hypopigmentation, which resolves when adequate calorie and protein intake resume.

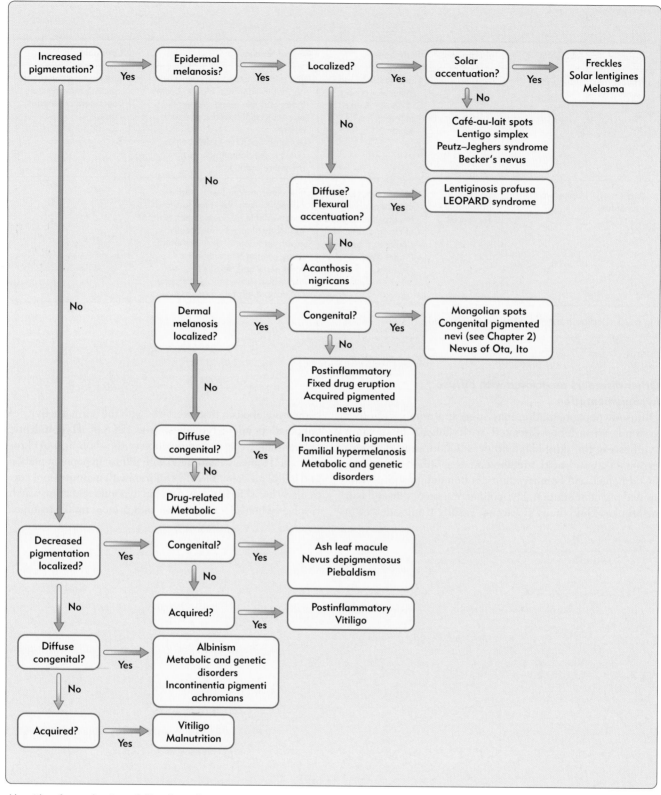

Algorithm for evaluation of disorders of pigmentation.

BIBLIOGRAPHY

Café-au-lait spot

Goldberg Y, Dibbern K, Klein J, Riccardi VM, Graham JM Jr. Neurofibromatosis type 1 – an update and review for the primary pediatrician. *Clin Pediatr (Philadelphia).* 1996, **35**:545–61.

Johnson BL, Charneco DR. Café-au-lait spots in neurofibromatosis and in normal individuals. *Arch Dermatol.* 1970, **102**:442–6.

Korf BR. Diagnostic outcome in children with cafe au lait spots. *Pediatr.* 1992, **90**:924–7.

Riccardi VM. Neurofibromatosis and Albright syndrome. In: Alper JA (ed). *Genetic disorders of the skin.* Mosby Year Book, St Louis, 1991, pp. 163–9.

Shen MH, Harper PS, Upadhyaya M. Molecular genetics of neurofibromatosis type 1 (NF1). *J Med Genet.* 1996, **33**:2–17.

Yamamoto T, Ozono K, Kaayama S, *et al.* Increased IL-6 production by cells isolated from the fibrous bone dysplasia tissue in patients with McCune–Albright syndrome. *J Clin Invest.* 1996, **98**:30–5.

Lentigo

Arnsmeier SL, Paller A. Pigmentary anomalies in the multiple lentigines syndrome: is it distinct from LEOPARD syndrome? *Pediatr Dermatol.* 1996, **13**:100–4.

Atherton DJA, Pitcher DW, Wells RS, *et al.* A syndrome of various cutaneous pigmented lesions, myxoid neurofibromata and atrial myxoma; the NAME syndrome. *Br J Dermatol.* 1980, **103**:421–9.

Cohen HJ, Minkin W, Frank SB. Nevus spilus. *Arch Dermatol.* 1970, **102**:433–7.

Coppin BD, Temple IK. Multiple lentigines syndrome (LEOPARD syndrome or progressive cardiomyopathic lentiginosa). *J Med Genet.* 1997, **34**:582–6.

Jozwiak S, Schwartz RA, Jannuger CK. LEOPARD syndrome (cardiocutaneous lentiginosa syndrome). *Cutis.* 1996, 57:208–14.

Kaufmann J, Eichman A, Neves C, *et al.* Lentiginosa profusa. *Dermatologica.* 1976, **153**:109–28.

Tovar JA, Eizaguirre I, Albert A, *et al.* Peutz–Jeghers in children: report of two cases and review of the literature. *J Pediatr Surg.* 1983, **18**:1–6.

Becker nevus

Becker SW. Concurrent melanosis and hypertrichosis in distribution of nevus unius lateris. *Arch Dermatol Syph.* 1949, **60**:155–60.

Happle R, Koopman RJ. Becker nevus syndrome. *Am J Med Genet.* 1997, **68**:357–61.

Kopera D, Hohenlentner U, Landthaler M. Quality-switched ruby laser treatment of solar lentigines and Becker's nevus: a histopathologic and immunohistochemical study. *Dermatology.* 1997, **194**:338–43.

Urbanek RW, Johnson WC. Smooth muscle hamartoma associated with Becker nevus. *Arch Dermatol.* 1978, **114**:98–9.

Acanthosis nigricans

Brockow K, Steinkraus V, Rinninger F, Abeck D, Ring J. Acanthosis nigricans: a marker for hyperinsulinemia. *Pediatr Dermatol.* 1995, **12**:323–6.

Panidis D, Skiadopoulos S, Rousso D, Ionnides D, Panidou E. Association of acanthosis nigricans with insulin resistance in patients with polycystic ovary syndrome. *Br J Dermatol.* 1995, **132**:936–41.

Stuart CA, Gilkison CR, Keenan BS, Nagamani M. Hyperinsulinemia and acanthosis nigricans in African Americans. *J Natl Med Assoc.* 1997, **89**:523–7.

Melasma

Grimes PE. Melasma. Etiologic and therapeutic considerations. *Arch Dermatol.* 1995, **131**:1453–7.

Sanchez NP, Pathak MA, Sato S, *et al.* Melasma: a clinical, light microscopic, ultrastructural, and immunofluorescence study. *J Am Acad Dermatol.* 1981, 4:698–710.

Mongolian spot

Cordova A. The mongolian spot. *Clin Pediatr.* 1981, **20**: 714–22.

Goldberg DJ. Laser treatment of pigmented lesions. *Dermatol Clin.* 1997, **15**:397–407.

Hidano A, Kajima H, Ikeda S, *et al.* Natural history of nevus of Ota. *Arch Dermatol.* 1967, **95**:187–95.

Kopf AW, Weidman AJ. Nevus of Ota. *Arch Dermatol.* 1962, **85**:195–208.

Mevorah B, Frenk E, Delacretaz J. Dermal melanocytosis. *Dermatologica.* 1977, **154**:107–14.

Smalek JE. Significance of mongolian spots. *J Pediatr.* 1980, **97**:504–5.

Stanford DG, Georgourajk E. Dermal melanocytosis: a clinical spectrum. *Aust J Dermatol.* 1996, **37**:19–25.

Fixed drug eruption

Cohen HA, Cohen Z, Frydman M. Fixed drug eruption of the scrotum due to hydroxyzine hydrochloride (Atarax). *Cutis.* 1996, **57**:431–2.

Korkij W, Soltani K. Fixed drug eruption. A brief review. *Arch Dermatol.* 1984, **120**:520–4.

Masu S, Seiji M. Pigmentary incontinence in fixed drug eruptions. *J Am Acad Dermatol.* 1983, **8**:525–32.

Sharma VK, Dhas S, Gill AN. Drug related involvement of specific sites in fixed eruption: a statistical evaluation. *J Dermatol.* 1996, **23**:530–4.

Pigmented nevi

Casso EM, Grin-Jorgensen CM, Grant-Kels JM. Spitz nevi. *J Am Acad Dermatol.* 1992, **27**:901–13.

English DR, Armstrong BK. Melanocytic nevi in children. I. Anatomic sites and demographic and host factors. *Am J Epidemiol.* 1994, **139**:390–401.

Gallagher RP, McLean DI. The epidemiology of acquired melanocytic nevi. A brief review. *Dermatol Clin.* 1995, **13**:595–603.

Hughes BR, Cunliffe WJ, Bailey CC. Excess benign melanocytic naevi after chemotherapy for malignancy in childhood. *BMJ.* 1989, **299**:88–91.

Luther H, Altmeyer P, Garber C, *et al.* Increase of melanocytic nevus counts in children during 5 years of follow-up and analysis of associated factors. *Arch Dermatol.* 1996, 132:1473–8.

Mehregan AH, Mehregan DA. Malignant melanoma in childhood. *Cancer.* 1993, **71**:4096–103.

National Institutes of Health Consensus Development Conference. Precursors to malignant melanoma. *J Am Acad Dermatol.* 1984, **10**:683–8.

Nicholls EM. Development and elimination of pigmented moles, and the anatomical distribution of primary malignant melanoma. *Cancer.* 1973, **32**:191–5.

Novakovic B, Clark WH Jr, Fears TR, Fraser MC, Tucker MA. Melanocytic nevi, dysplastic nevi, and malignant melanoma in children from melanoma-prone families. *J Am Acad Dermatol.* 1995, **33**:631–6.

Smith CH, McGregor JM, Barker JN, Morris RW, Rigder SP, McDondal DM. Excess melanocytic nevi in children with renal allografts. *J Am Acad Dermatol.* 1993, **28**:51–5.

Weedon D, Little JH. Spindle and epithelioid cell nevi in children and adults. A review of 211 cases of the Spitz nevus. *Cancer.* 1977, **40**:217–25.

Hypopigmented macules

Fitzpatrick TB, Szabo G, Hori Y, *et al.* White leaf-shaped macules. *Arch Dermatol.* 1968, **98**:1–6.

Fryer AE, Osborne JP. Tuberous sclerosis – a clinical appraisal. *Pediatr Rev Commun.* 1987, 1:239–55.

Norio R, Oksanen T, Rantanen J. Hypopigmented skin alterations resembling tuberous sclerosis in normal skin. *J Med Genet.* 1996, **33**:184–6.

Vanderhooft SL, Francis JS, Pagon RA, Smith LT, Sybert VP. Prevalence of hypopigmented macules in a healthy population. *J Pediatr.* 1996, **129**:355–61.

Nevus anemicus

Fleisher TL, Zeligman I. Nevus anemicus. *Arch Dermatol.* 1969, **100**:750–5.

Incontinentia pigmenti achromians

Delaporte E, Janin A, Blondel V, *et al.* Linear and whorled nevoid hypermelanosis versus incontinentia pigmenti: is pigment incontinence really a distinctive feature? *Dermatology.* 1996, **192**:70–2.

Happle R. Tentative assignment of hypomelanosis of Ito to 9q33-qter. *Hum Genet.* 1987, **75**:98–9.

Ishikawa T, Kanayama M, Sugiyama, *et al.* Hypomelanosis of Ito associated with benign tumors and chromosomal abnormalities: a neurocutaneous syndrome. *Brain Dev.* 1985, **7**:45–9.

Sybert VP. Hypomelanosis of Ito: a description, not a diagnosis. *J Invest Dermatol.* 1994, **103**(Suppl. 5):1415–38.

Vitiligo

Hatchome N, Aiba S, Kato T, *et al.* Possible functional impairment of Langerhans cells in vitiliginous skin. *Arch Dermatol.* 1987, **123**:51–4.

Majumder PP, Nordlund JJ, Nath SK. Pattern of familial aggregation of vitiligo. *Arch Dermatol.* 1993, **129**:994–8.

Nordlund JJ, Lerner AB. Editorial: Vitiligo. It is important. *Arch Dermatol.* 1982, **118**:5–8.

Norris DA, Kissinger RM, Naughton GM, *et al.* Evidence for immunologic mechanisms in human vitiligo: patient's sera induce damage to human melanocytes *in vitro*. *J Invest Dermatol.* 1988, **1982**:783–9.

Shullreuter KU, Lemke R, Brandt O, *et al.* Vitiligo and other diseases: coexistence or true association? Hamberg study of 321 patients. *Dermatology.* 1994, **188**:269–75.

Albinism

Boissay RE, Nordlund JJ. Molecular basis of congenital hypopigmentary disorders in humans: a review. *Pigment Cell Res.* 1997, **10**:12–24.

Hayashibe K, Mishima Y. Tyrosinase-positive melanocyte distribution and induction of pigmentation in human piebald skin. *Arch Dermatol.* 1988, **124**:381–6.

Orlow SJ. Albinism: an update. *Semin Cut Med Surg.* 1997, **16**:24–9.

Shimizu H. Prenatal diagnosis of inherited skin diseases. *Keio J Med.* 1996, **45**:28–36.

Spritz RA. Piebaldism, Waardenburg syndrome, and related disorders of melanocyte development. *Semin Cut Med Surg.* 1997, **16**:15–23.

Waardenburg PJ. A new syndrome combining developmental anomalies of the eyelids, eyebrows and nose root with pigmentary defects of the iris and head hair and with congenital deafness. *Am J Hum Genet.* 1951, **3**:195–253.

Witkop CJ Jr, Hill CW, Desnick SJ, *et al.* Ophthalmologic, biochemical, platelet and ultrastructural defects in the various types of oculocutaneous albinism. *J Invest Dermatol.* 1973, **60**:443–56.

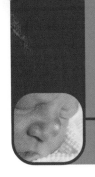
Reactive Erythema

INTRODUCTION

The term reactive erythema refers to a group of disorders characterized by erythematous patches, plaques, and nodules that vary in size, shape, and distribution. Unlike other specific dermatoses, they represent cutaneous reaction patterns triggered by a variety of endogenous and environmental agents. In children, the most common reactive erythemas include drug eruptions, urticaria, viral exanthems, erythema multiforme (EM), erythema nodosum, vasculitis, photosensitive eruptions, and collagen vascular disorders.

DRUG ERUPTIONS

Of all patients admitted to hospital, 2–3% experience an adverse drug reaction, and about half of these develop a rash. Drug-induced rashes are also a frequent diagnostic problem in the outpatient setting. Although the skin rash often occurs alone, it may be accompanied by fever, arthritis, and other systemic findings. Nearly 50% of the rashes are morbilliform, followed by urticaria in 25%, fixed drug reactions in 10%, EM in 5%, and exfoliative, lichenoid, and acneiform eruptions in less than 5% each. Early recognition of drug-related rashes and discontinuation of the inciting agent may prevent progressive, life-threatening complications.

Morbilliform drug eruptions

Morbilliform (measles-like, maculopapular, exanthematous) rashes account for the majority of drug-induced rashes.

Typically, after 5–10 days of drug therapy, red macules and papules erupt on the extremities and spread centrally to involve the trunk. Not infrequently, however, the trunk is the first area to be involved and the rash spreads centripetally (Fig 7.1). Lesions may become confluent, but the perioral and perinasal areas are often spared. Conjunctival and oral mucosal erythema may be prominent. Although the rash is often asymptomatic, pruritus may be severe. The skin may be the only organ system involved, but fever, arthralgias, and general malaise may follow. Occasionally, the rash resolves despite continuation of the medication.

However, lesions rarely progress to EM or toxic epidermal necrolysis (TEN) with widespread necrosis of the epidermis. Almost any drug can trigger a morbilliform rash. Common categories include antibiotics, anticonvulsants, and antihypertensives. Prompt diagnosis and discontinuation of the drug usually results in improvement in 1–2 days and resolution within 1 week. Occasionally, the rash does not appear until several days after the drug course has been completed.

Unfortunately, morbilliform rashes often appear in febrile children who are placed on antibiotics for treatment of presumed bacterial infections such as sinusitis and otitis media. The differentiation of a viral infection with associated exanthems from a drug rash is usually impossible, and many of these children are labeled antibiotic allergic. In some patients, recognition of specific viral exanthems and serologic confirmation supports an infectious etiology. Moreover, some drugs may interact with certain viruses to produce an exanthem such as the rash seen in up to 90% of children

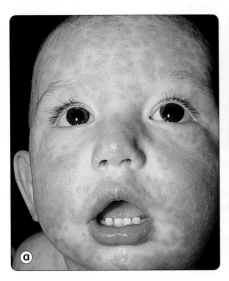
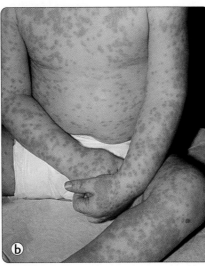

Fig 7.1 A morbilliform reaction to phenobarbital developed in a toddler after 2 weeks of treatment for febrile seizures. Lesions were most prominent on **(a)** the face, and **(b)** upper trunk and extremities. Note the perioral and perinasal sparing.

with mononucleosis who are accidentally treated with ampicillin (Fig 7.2). The differential diagnosis also includes graft versus host disease and Kawasaki syndrome, but the medical history and associated findings help to exclude these disorders.

Erythema multiforme

Both EM and TEN are distinctive, acute hypersensitivity syndromes that may be caused by a number of drugs, as well as by viruses, bacterial infections, foods, and immunizations. The former accounts for less than 5% of drug reactions. However, the clinician must recognize the reaction pattern early to avoid or effectively deal with potentially serious complications. Classic EM minor, EM major, or Stevens–Johnson syndrome, and TEN are described in Chapter 4.

Fixed drug eruption

Fixed drug eruption is a distinctive reaction pattern characterized by the sudden development of EM-like annular, erythematous, edematous plaques from 1 cm to over 5 cm in diameter that occur after exposure to a number of medications (Fig 7.3). Intense edema may result in bulla formation. When the drug is withdrawn, lesions flatten, erythema fades, and prominent postinflammatory hyperpigmentation persists for weeks to months. On re-exposure to the allergen, old lesions reappear and new plaques may develop and slowly progress.

Although the rash may develop on any site, lips and genitals are the most commonly involved. The most frequent triggering agents include trimethoprim–sulfamethoxazole, aspirin, tetracycline, phenolphthalein (present in laxatives), barbiturates, and nonsteroidal anti-inflammatory drugs.

Although the mechanism is not known, T-lymphocytes that reside in the dermis are thought to be responsible for the acute reaction as well as the cutaneous memory function of the fixed

drug eruption. Histologic findings are similar to those of EM, but pigment incontinence tends to be intense. This explains the impressive, discrete hyperpigmentation, which may be the only clinical finding between episodes. Once the diagnosis is considered, the allergen can be identified and avoided.

Urticaria

Urticaria, commonly known as hives, is characterized by the sudden appearance of transient, well-demarcated wheals that are usually intensely pruritic, especially when they arise as part of an acute, IgE-mediated hypersensitivity reaction (Fig 7.4). Individual lesions usually last several minutes to several hours, but they may rarely persist for up to 24 hours. Wheals may have a red center with an edematous white halo – or the reverse, an edematous white center with a red halo. Size can vary from a few millimeters to giant lesions over 20 cm in diameter. Central clearing with peripheral extension may lead to the formation of annular, polycyclic, and arcuate plaques that simulate EM and erythema marginatum. The reaction may involve the mucous membranes and can spread to the subcutaneous tissue to

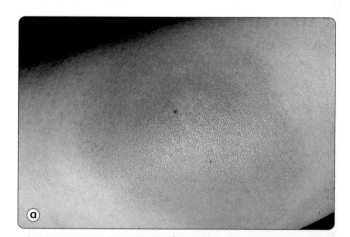

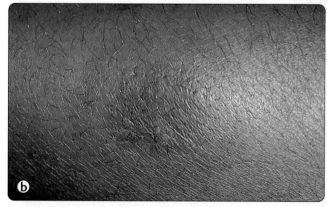

Fig 7.2 A teenager who was initially diagnosed with streptococcal pharyngitis was started on ampicillin. After 4 days, a morbilliform rash erupted on the trunk and spread to the face and extremities. A monospot test was positive in the office, and the antibiotic was discontinued.

Fig 7.3 Fixed drug eruption. **(a)** A red, edematous plaque recurred on the arm of a 16-year-old girl each month when she took a nonsteroidal anti-inflammatory agent for menstrual cramps. Some residual hyperpigmentation is present in the center of the plaque from prior flares. **(b)** This 10-year-old, darkly pigmented boy developed a recurrent target lesion in the same spot on his arm after exposure to a cold remedy. Note the dusky center with marked hyperpigmentation.

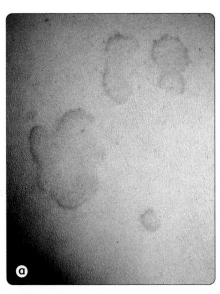
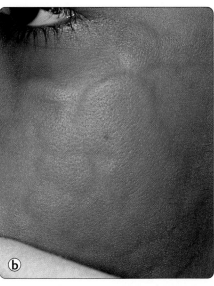
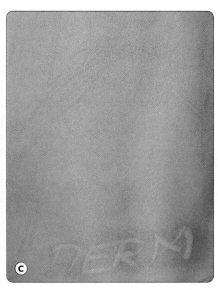

Fig 7.4 Urticaria. **(a)** Widespread urticaria developed during a course of amoxicillin for otitis media. Note the discrete annular plaques on the trunk of this 3-year-old infant. **(b)** Wheals have become confluent on the face of this boy. **(c)** Dermatographism, which is common in patients with urticaria, was produced by the examiner on the back of this child with chronic hives.

produce woody edema known as angioedema (Fig 7.5). Histopathology usually demonstrates a mild, lymphocytic, perivascular infiltrate with marked dermal edema.

Urticaria can be triggered by a variety of immunologic mechanisms, including IgE antibody response, complement activation, and abnormal response to vasoactive amines. Most cases of acute urticaria, which lasts less than 6 weeks, are caused by a hypersensitivity reaction to drugs, food, insect bites, contact antigens, inhaled substances, or acute infections. Physical agents, which include cold, heat, water, exercise, and mechanical pressure, may also trigger hives. Less than 5% of patients evolve into chronic urticaria, which lasts from 6 weeks to many years.

Specific drugs and foods known to cause hives should be avoided because of the risk of inducing anaphylaxis on subsequent exposure. Exhaustive laboratory studies in an otherwise healthy child are unlikely to be rewarding. Laboratory evaluation is guided by findings on history and physical examination. Patients with chronic disease require intermittent re-examination, particularly if other problems such as arthritis, diarrhea, or fever develop.

Extensive urticaria associated with pruritus may respond readily to H$_1$ antihistamines such as diphenhydramine, hydroxyzine, or chlorpheniramine. Dosages should be increased to twice the recommended level or until unacceptable adverse reactions are noted. Most children accommodate quickly to sedation associated with these medications. In resistant cases, the addition of an H$_2$ antihistamine, such as cimetidine or ranitidine, and/or β-adrenergic agonists, such as ephedrine and terbutaline, may be helpful. Several nonsedating antihistamines, which include astemizole, terfenadine, and cetirizine are particularly useful in some children with chronic urticaria. Epinephrine (adrenaline) may be lifesaving in urticaria and angioedema that

involve the airway. Systemic corticosteroids are reserved for patients with life-threatening disease.

Urticarial eruptions may appear early in the course of serum sickness reactions triggered by infectious agents or drugs. Asymptomatic or painful, red papules and expanding annular plaques with hemorrhagic borders are associated with fever, arthralgias, periarticular swelling, and occasionally arthritis. Skin lesions differ from classic urticaria by the lack of pruritus and persistence beyond 24 hours. Serum sickness reactions have been reported recently with cefaclor, but may also occur with a number of other antibiotics (Fig 7.6). Skin biopsies

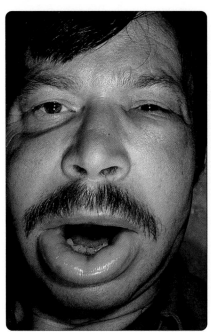

Fig 7.5 This young man developed recurrent episodes of idiopathic angioedema. Fortunately, although his face and lips were frequently involved, he did not experience layrngeal edema or dyspnea.

usually demonstrate a lymphohistiocytic, dermal, inflammatory infiltrate, but occasionally vasculitis may be present.

Erythema marginatum, one of the major criteria for rheumatic fever and which occurs in 20% of patients, may be confused with hives. This eruption is characterized by transient, asymptomatic, red papules that enlarge over several hours to form annular, scalloped, and serpiginous expanding plaques with narrow borders and central clearing (Fig 7.7). Successive crops appear on the trunk and extremities as old plaques fade. New lesions typically flare with evening fever spikes, and involvement is restricted predominantly to the trunk and proximal extremities. The absence of pruritus helps to distinguish erythema marginatum from hives, and skin biopsies show predominantly a perivascular neutrophilic infiltrate. The diagnosis of rheumatic fever is dependent on the recognition of other well-defined criteria.

Urticaria must also be distinguished from the figurate erythemas and other reactive erythemas discussed later in this chapter.

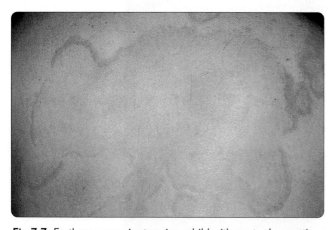

Fig 7.6 A 10-month-old girl developed urticaria on the lower trunk and thighs while being treated with cefaclor for an ear infection. Although the drug was stopped, the annular plaques progressed and became purpuric centrally. The rash was accompanied by arthralgias, joint swelling, and fever consistent with a serum sickness picture.

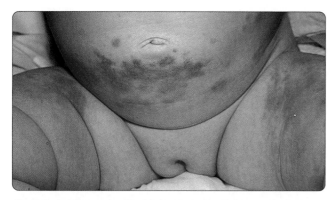

Fig 7.7 Erythema marginatum in a child with acute rheumatic fever. Note the scalloped margins and distribution on the trunk.

Exfoliative, lichenoid, and acneiform drug reactions

Drugs can also trigger reactions that mimic other cutaneous conditions. In an exfoliative erythroderma, widespread inflammation in the skin is associated with generalized erythema and scale. The entire surface is involved, including the scalp, palms, and soles. Although this reaction pattern usually evolves from a primary cutaneous disorder, such as atopic dermatitis, seborrheic dermatitis, psoriasis, or T-cell lymphoma, a number of medications, which include allopurinol, barbiturates, captopril, carbamazepine, cimetidine, diltiazem, griseofulvin, gold, thiazide diuretics, isoniazid, hydantoins, D-penicillamine, quinidine, and sulfonamides, have been implicated in some patients. A history of drug exposure, preceding rashes, and associated findings provides clues to the cause of the erythroderma. Histopathology usually reveals a chronic dermatitis. However, the presence of eosinophils may suggest a hypersensitivity reaction, while other distinct findings indicate an underlying skin disorder.

In lichenoid drug reactions, clinical findings are usually indistinguishable from those of lichen planus. However, the dermal infiltrate may contain eosinophils, which is unusual for classic lichen planus. Withdrawal of medications may result in improvement of the eruption over weeks to months. Drugs that have been reported to cause lichenoid reactions include thiazide diuretics, streptomycin, isoniazid, methyldopa, β-blockers, naproxen, and captopril.

Acneiform drug reactions may be differentiated from typical acne vulgaris by the presence of uniform, inflammatory papules and pustules (rather than mixed comedones and inflammatory lesions in acne vulgaris), involvement of the usual acne areas (face, shoulders, upper trunk), as well as the lower trunk, arms, and legs, acute onset with introduction of the inciting drug, and resistance to standard therapy. Medications may also exacerbate pre-existing acne. Commonly identified drugs include corticosteroids, corticotropin, isoniazid, lithium, iodides, cyclosporine, and anticonvulsants. Although the eruption may improve with systemic and topical acne preparations, severe or recalcitrant cases may require a decrease or discontinuation of the medication if possible.

VIRAL EXANTHEMS

A number of viral infections have cutaneous manifestations that provide a clue to the diagnosis. In some, the skin rash is the major finding. Early recognition of distinct exanthems also helps to differentiate viral infections from drug reactions, bacterial and rickettsial rashes, and other reactive erythemas.

In the early twentieth century, clinicians commonly referred to childhood exanthems by number. Scarlet fever and measles were known as first and second disease, but the two rashes were frequently confused. Rubella was established as an entity distinct from measles and known as third disease. In 1900 Duke described fourth disease, which probably does not represent a distinct condition but a combination of rubella and scarlet fever. Fifth disease is recognized today as erythema infectiosum, and roseola finishes off the numbered exanthems as sixth disease. Many other viruses produce distinct reaction patterns in the skin. Infections from herpes- and poxviruses are readily diagnosed by their characteristic vesiculobullous eruptions, while infections from picornaviruses (which include the enteroviruses) are well recognized for their maculopapular exanthems.

Viruses trigger exanthems by a number of mechanisms. Direct infection of the skin occurs in varicella, enteroviruses, and herpertic infections. Other rashes, such as measles and rubella, probably result from a combination of viral spread to the skin and host immunologic response. Some host–viral interactions are activated by exposure to certain drugs, exemplified by the generalized maculopapular eruption that occurs in over 95% of individuals with Epstein–Barr virus infection who receive ampicillin.

Measles and rubella

In the prevaccine era, measles and rubella were common and their exanthems became a paradigm for other 'morbilliform' rashes. Although the usual late winter to early spring epidemics have been interrupted by widespread vaccina-tion in industrialized nations, failure to immunize significant numbers of children during the past decade has resulted in intermittent outbreaks in the US.

Measles

Measles (rubeola, red measles, 10-day measles) is a highly contagious, potentially severe illness with a prodrome characterized by fever, malaise, dry cough, coryza, conjunctivitis, and severe photophobia (Fig 7.8a). Several days into the course, diagnostic Koplik spots appear on the buccal and labial mucosae (Fig 7.8b). Lesions consist of 1–3 mm diameter, bluish-white papules surrounded by red halos, which increase in number and fade over 2–3 days. Unfortunately, this characteristic enanthema is often transient and goes unnoticed.

On the third or fourth day of illness, the exanthem first appears on the face as a blanching, red, maculopapular eruption, which spreads cephalocaudally over 3 days, and ultimately involves the palms and soles (Fig 7.9). Once generalized, lesions become confluent on the face, trunk, and extremities in succession. Older lesions commonly develop a rusty hue from capillary leak and hemosiderin deposition. The rash begins to

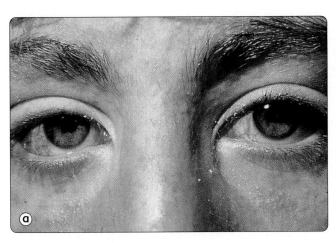
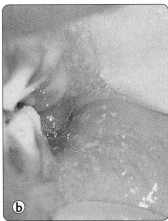

Fig 7.8 Rubeola/measles. (a) During and after the prodromal period, the conjunctivae are injected and produce a clear discharge. This is associated with marked photophobia. (b) Koplik spots, bluish-white dots surrounded by red halos, appear on the buccal and labial mucosae a day or two before the exanthem and begin to fade with the onset of the rash.

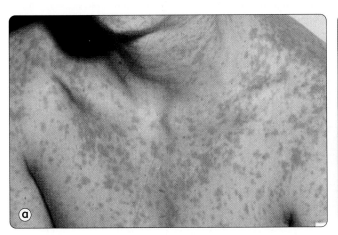
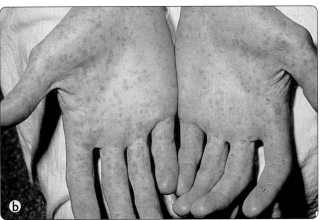

Fig 7.9 The measles exanthem. (a) A blotchy, erythematous, blanching eruption appears at the hairline and spreads cephalocaudally over 3 days. (b) Ultimately, the exanthem involves the palms and soles. With evolution, lesions become confluent on the face, neck, and upper trunk.

fade after 3 days and clearance is complete 3 days later, a total duration of 10 days for the illness. Widespread desquamation may appear 1–2 weeks after resolution of the rash.

Patients are contagious 4 days before the exanthem until 4 days after it appears. During the illness fever may be persistent and severe. Generalized adenopathy is common. Morbidity and mortality is highest in patients compromised by hereditary or acquired immunodeficiency and in developing countries in which malnutrition is rampant. Potential complications that result from primary viral infection or secondary bacterial infection include otitis media, pneumonitis, meningitis, acute encephalitis, and obstructive laryngotracheitis. Atypical measles is an unusual syndrome that occurs in individuals who received killed measles vaccine, when it was available between 1963 and 1967, and are subsequently exposed to the measles virus. Unlike typical measles, the exanthem begins and remains primarily on the extremities and often develops a petechial component. Koplik spots are absent, fevers are high, and pneumonitis is usually severe. This disorder probably represents a hypersensitivity reaction to the virus and is most frequently confused with Rocky Mountain spotted fever and collagen vascular disease.

Rubella

Rubella (German measles) is known as 3-day measles, because the pink maculopapular exanthem, which mimics a mild case of measles, usually evolves over 1–3 days. In fact, nearly 25% of patients may have only mild upper respiratory symptoms with little or no rash.

Rubella is typically associated with several days of low-grade fever, adenopathy, headache, sore throat, and coryza. In young children, fever may last for less than 24 hours. Forschheimer spots consist of transient, small, red papules on the soft palate and are seen in some patients at the beginning of the rash. This enanthema helps to differentiate this otherwise nonspecific eruption from other viral exanthems.

As with measles, peak incidence occurs in the late winter and early spring. Serologic testing may be useful to make a specific diagnosis, particularly if the patient is pregnant. Although complications are rare in children, the fetus is particularly vulnerable to intrauterine infection with

complications that include spontaneous abortion, diffuse cataracts, microphthalmia, glaucoma, and congenital heart disease. Up to 25% of infected newborns develop severe, disseminated disease with jaundice, pneumonitis, meningoencephalitis, bony abnormalities, thrombocytopenia, blueberry muffin lesions, and a morbilliform exanthem. Babies with congenital infection may shed virus in urine, stools, and respiratory secretions for up to 1 year and should be isolated from other infants and pregnant women.

Erythema infectiosum (Fifth disease)

In 1983, erythema infectiosum (or fifth disease) was linked to human parvovirus B19. Since then, investigators have defined the clinical features and epidemiology of infection in normal and compromised patients.

In its most commonly recognized clinical presentation, viral infection presents in children of school age with asymptomatic, slapped cheek erythema on the face and a lacy or reticulated, blanching erythema on the trunk and extremities (Fig 7.10). Although the exanthem usually fades over 2–3 weeks, lesions may recur for up to 3 months, especially when cutaneous blood flow is increased as after fever or vigorous physical activity.

The prevalence of B19 antibody is about 5–10% in children under 5 years of age and rises to over 50% in adults. Human volunteer studies suggest that the virus is spread in respiratory secretions. After an incubation period of 5–7 days, infectivity peaks during the viremia, which lasts 5–7 days. The end of viremia is marked by a rise in IgM and then IgG antibody, and followed 2–5 days later by the appearance of the rash. Consequently, the risk of infection is low when the exanthem is diagnosed, and children can remain in school.

Associated symptoms, which include fever and arthralgias, are usually mild or absent in young children. However, arthralgias or frank arthritis may be severe in adolescents and adults. At least a quarter of patients with serologic evidence of disease do not develop the exanthem, and the arthropathy may develop before, after, or without the rash.

Early in the infection most patients experience a transient reticulocytopenia for 7–10 days and a clinically insignificant drop in hemoglobin level. This phenomenon, however, may trigger an aplastic crisis in patients with severe hemoglobino-

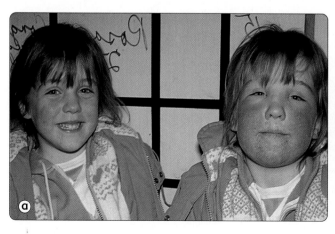

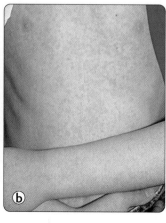

Fig 7.10 Fifth disease. **(a)** These sisters demonstrate the slapped cheek erythema typical of erythema infectiosum. Despite the edema in one girl, both were completely asymptomatic. **(b)** A diffuse, morbilliform eruption was present in an otherwise healthy 9-year-old boy. The reticulated erythema on his arms flared intermittently for 6 weeks.

pathies. The virus has also been implicated as a cause of hydrops fetalis in pregnant women with no other evidence of clinical disease. However, recent reports suggest that parvovirus can rarely cause fetal malformations. In hereditary or acquired immunodeficiency syndromes, B19 may produce persistent infection and chronic, life-threatening anemia.

The reticulated exanthem of erythema infectiosum may be confused with livedo reticularis, a persistent, lacy, blanching, violaceous erythema that occurs in primary and secondary forms (Fig 7.11). In the idiopathic variant, lesions are symmetric and widespread with poorly defined borders. Unlike cutis marmorata in neonates, the pattern does not resolve with warming. This occurs most commonly in young women who are otherwise healthy. The secondary variant is more common in men and has been reported in association with periarteritis nodosa, hepatitis, syphilis, and a number of other infections, connective tissue diseases, and malignancy.

Exanthema subitum (Roseola)

Roseola, or exanthema subitum (the 'surprise' rash), has been recognized by pediatricians for over a century. The classic clinical course occurs in children between 6 months and 3 years old. After a 3–5 day illness marked by high-spiking fevers, which occasionally trigger febrile seizures, a sudden end to the fever is followed by the appearance of a widely disseminated,

pink, papular rash (Fig 7.12). As in fifth disease, the end of viremia is marked by the development of the rash and a rise in antibody to the causative agent: human herpesvirus (HHV) 6. Consequently, the risk of infection is greatest during the febrile period and minimal after the appearance of the rash.

Serologic studies show an almost universal exposure of the population to HHV6. Although only a third of infants develop clinical disease, prevalence of antibody increases from less then 10% in children under 6 months of age to 75–90% in adults. Consequently, a large number of children develop asymptomatic infection. Conversely, seroprevalence studies of febrile infants demonstrate that viral infection may commonly produce a febrile illness without a rash. A similar febrile disorder has been associated with HHV7 in some children.

Also, HHV6 has been linked to a mononucleosis-like illness in young adults, and its role as an immunomodulator is being investigated in the immunodeficient host.

Papular acrodermatitis

In 1956, Gianotti and Crosti described a distinctive exanthem associated with anicteric hepatitis, lymphadenopathy, and hepatitis B surface antigenemia, subtype *ayw*. The skin rash consists of flat-topped, 3–10 mm diameter, skin-colored to red, edematous papules that involve the arms, legs, buttocks, and face (Fig 7.13). Lesions on the calves and extensor

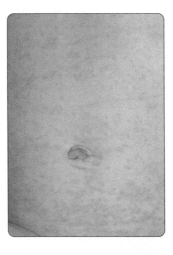

Fig 7.12
Roseola/exanthema subitum. A generalized, pink, maculopapular rash suddenly appeared on this infant after 3 days of high fever.

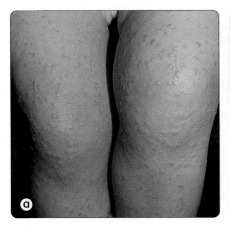

Fig 7.11 Widespread livedo reticularis was particularly prominent on the proximal extremities of this adolescent with secondary syphilis.

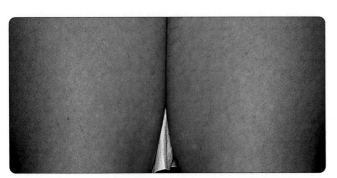

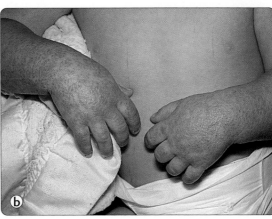

Fig 7.13 Papular acrodermatitis. (a) A symmetric, acrally distributed, red, papular rash developed in this toddler with low-grade fever and loose stools. Note the discrete, edematous papules on the knees and calves. (b) In some areas on his hands and forearms the lesions were confluent.

surfaces of the arms may become so edematous as to appear vesicular, and occasionally frank vesicles are present.

During the past 15 years it has become apparent that most cases in the US are caused by various viruses, including enteroviruses, respiratory viruses, and Epstein–Barr virus. As most children are asymptomatic, no treatment is necessary. However, parents are counseled that the eruption may persist for up to several months.

Papular acrodermatitis can be differentiated from lichen planus, which is usually extremely pruritic. A negative history of recent drug exposure excludes a lichenoid drug eruption. Other viral eruptions also may be confused with papular acrodermatitis. Unfortunately, the histopathology is not specific and shows focal spongiosis and exocytosis in the epidermis overlying a perivascular, lymphocytic, dermal infiltrate.

Other viral exanthems

Exanthems associated with the enteroviruses are quite variable and usually follow a shorter incubation period than the classic viral exanthems. Although they occur all year round, the incidence peaks in the late summer and early fall. Morbilliform, vesicular, petechial, and urticarial eruptions are variably present, usually in association with fever (Fig 7.14). Other symptoms may include meningitis, conjunctivitis, cough, coryza, pharyngitis, and pneumonia. Hand-foot-and-mouth disease is a distinctive entity associated with papulovesicular lesions on the palms, soles, palate, and (not infrequently) the trunk, particularly the buttocks. Cocksackieviruses A5, A10, and A16 and enterovirus 71 have been identified in patients with this syndrome. Papulovesicular rashes may be differentiated from varicella-zoster and herpes simplex infections by obtaining a Tzanck smear. The clinical course and, if necessary, cultures and serologic studies help to make a specific diagnosis. Although meningococcal infections tend to peak during the winter and spring, occasionally

cases occur during the summer and fall enteroviral season. Consequently, the child with a petechial exanthem and presumed enteroviral meningitis must be evaluated carefully to exclude a bacterial infection.

Infection with cytomegalovirus, Epstein–Barr virus, and respiratory viruses may be associated with macular, morbilliform, or urticarial exanthems, which are difficult to differentiate from drug rashes. Children who require medications and develop intercurrent viral infections may remain on their medications while under close observation. These minor viral exanthems usually fade in several days, while drug reactions tend to persist or intensify. However, drugs must be discontinued in any patients who develop urticaria, angioedema, EM, or other signs of progressive allergic reactions.

SCARLATINIFORM RASHES

The rash of scarlet fever provides a model for a number of important disorders that must be differentiated by other signs and symptoms. Bacterial toxins, viral infections, drugs, and Kawasaki syndrome have all been associated with scarlatiniform eruptions.

Scarlet fever

Scarlet fever is characterized by a fine, red, papular, sandpaper-like rash that begins on the face and neck and generalizes to the trunk and extremities within 1–2 days (Fig 7.15). The skin is warm and flushed, and some patients complain of mild pruritus. Circumoral pallor is typical, but not diagnostic. The rash ranges from a subtle pink to fiery red color and usually follows the onset of streptococcal pharyngitis by 24–48 hours. Pastia lines are the accentuation of the rash from linear petechiae, which occurs in the flexural creases of the arms, legs, and trunk (Fig 7.15a). Other associated symptoms include nausea, vomiting, fever, headache, general malaise, and abdominal pain. The palms, soles, and conjunctivae are usually spared. In classic cases, the pharynx is beefy red with palatal petechiae, purulent tonsilitis, and tender, cervical adenopathy. Early in the course the lingual papillae poke through a white membrane (white strawberry tongue; Fig 7.16). Shedding of the membrane by days 4–5 results in a bright red, strawberry tongue. In many patients, the throat infection is mild or completely asymptomatic. Scarlet fever may also be associated with streptococcal impetigo.

The rash is triggered by one of three antigenically distinct erythrotoxins, which are produced by most strains of Group A β-hemolytic streptococci. Development of antibodies against the streptococcal organism and erythrotoxin is protective and results in resolution of the symptoms and rash within 4–5 days. This is followed 1–2 weeks later by generalized desquamation, which is particularly marked on the finger tips and toes (Fig. 7.15b). While both oral and cutaneous infections with nephritogenic streptococci can trigger glomerulonephritis, only pharyngeal infections have been associated with subsequent development of rheumatic fever. Treatment of patients with amoxicillin or penicillin (erythromycin in penicillin-allergic patients) may shorten the

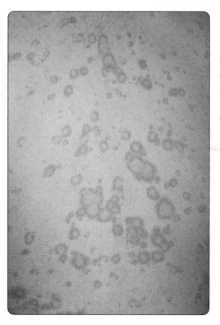

Fig 7.14 An urticarial viral exanthem spread from the trunk to the face and extremities in this infant. Lesions faded over several days.

course of fever and other symptoms. If antibiotics are initiated within 10 days of the onset of pharyngitis, the risk of rheumatic fever may be reduced from 3% to less than 1%. Unfortunately, early treatment of nephritogenic strains has not been shown to decrease the incidence of poststreptococcal renal disease. Moreover, asymptomatic pharyngeal infection may escape detection until after the development of late complications.

Several other toxin-mediated syndromes may be confused with scarlet fever. Children with staphylococcal scarlet fever develop a rash which may be indistinguishable from streptococcal disease. Nikolsky sign may be present, but pharyngeal signs are usually absent. Cultures from the typical purulent conjunctivitis or the oral or nasal pharynx invariably demonstrate *Staphylococcus aureus*. Unlike streptococcal scarlet fever, desquamation begins early in the course (by day 2) and is complete within a week. The clinical signs and course probably vary with the source of the infection, amount of staphylococcal exotoxin present, and host response. A similar eruption may accompany toxic shock syndrome. However,

the eruption is usually accompanied by hyperemia of the conjunctivae, oral and vaginal mucosa, a strawberry tongue, and severe multisystem disease. The early findings in both staphylococcal scalded-skin syndrome and TEN may mimic scarlet fever. However, the presence of Nikolsky sign and progression to widespread sloughing of skin quickly differentiate these disorders. Scarlatiniform viral exanthems may occur with a number of different organisms. The course may be similar to that of scarlet fever and can only be differentiated by serologic studies and the absence of streptococci in throat or skin cultures.

Kawasaki syndrome

Although the exact etiology of Kawasaki syndrome is unknown, the epidemiology, clinical findings, and course suggest an as yet unidentified infectious agent. Over 75% of patients are under 4 years old and 50% less than 2 years of age. Cases occur all year round, with slight peaks in the late spring and late fall. Epidemics have also been reported. Although all races may be affected, the increased incidence

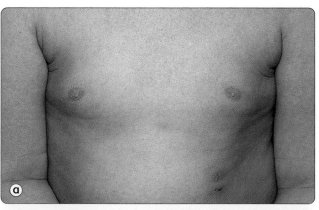

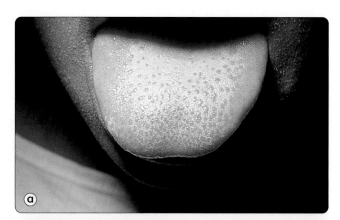

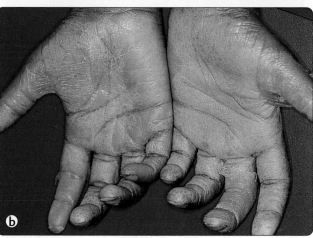

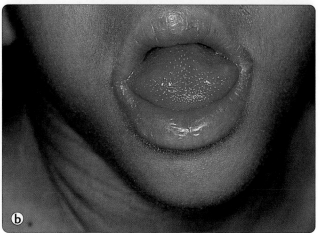

Fig 7.15 Scarlet fever. (a) A generalized, bright red, sand-paper-like papular rash developed in a 7-year-old boy with a streptococcal pharyngitis. Note the accentuation of the rash at the neck and axillary and antecubital creases.
(b) Widespread desquamation appeared in this 8-year-old girl 10 days after the onset of symptoms and rash, and was most prominent on the hands and feet.

Fig 7.16 Scarlet fever. (a) A white strawberry tongue is usually followed by (b) a red strawberry tongue as the erythrotoxin-mediated enanthema evolves.

among Japanese and intermediate risk of Japanese–Americans supports a genetic predisposition.

Kawasaki syndrome is defined clinically by the presence of five out of six major criteria, which are fever, usually unresponsive to antipyretics for at least 5 days, conjunctivitis, pharyngitis, erythema and edema of the hands and feet, rash, and adenopathy (Fig 7.17). The acute phase, which lasts 10–14 days, begins with an abrupt onset of high fever and extreme irritability. A rash usually appears shortly after the fever and may take the form of a scarlatiniform, morbilliform, or urticarial exanthem. It is commonly accentuated in intertriginous areas, where maceration and scaling may be prominent, particularly on the perineum and inguinal creases (Fig 7.17d). Facial swelling and pallor are commonly present. Other findings during the acute phase include nonpurulent, conjunctival injection, erythema, edema, and cracking of the lips, palatal erythema and a strawberry tongue, painful erythema and edema of the hands and feet, and painful, unilateral, cervical adenopathy. Arthritis, diarrhea, abdominal pain, aseptic meningitis, hepatitis, urethritis, otitis, and hydrops of the gallbladder may also be present.

The subacute phase begins 10–14 days after the onset of symptoms, as the fever and rash improve. It is during this period that carditis associated with coronary angiitis becomes apparent. Although up to 20% of children may have findings on echocardiography, only about 1% develop serious heart disease. By 3 weeks most patients experience a thrombocytosis of over 1 million platelets/cm^3, which may further increase coronary morbidity. Widespread desquamation occurs 1–2 weeks after resolution of the rash, particularly over the fingers and toes where the skin is shed in large sheets. Although no specific laboratory tests are available for Kawasaki syndrome, leukocytosis is common and acute-phase reactants, which include C-reactive protein and erythrocyte sedimentation rate, are markedly elevated.

The convalescent phase begins in the fourth or fifth week and ends when the sedimentation rate returns to normal. Children require cardiac re-evaluation at least through this stage and for a year or more if aneurysms are detected.

The differential diagnosis includes viral exanthems, toxin-mediated bacterial disorders, connective tissue disease, and a number of other reactive erythemas.

Acral erythema and edema, one of the classic findings during the acute phase of Kawasaki syndrome, is also typical of papular acrodermatitis and other viral exanthems, Rocky Mountain spotted fever, erythromelalgia, pernio, and acrodynia (pink disease). Papular acrodermatitis is easily differentiated from Kawasaki syndrome by the lack of fever and other systemic symptoms. The specific criteria and course of Kawasaki syndrome usually help to differentiate it from other viral infections that produce urticarial lesions and edema of the extremities. The findings in rickettsial diseases are also distinctive.

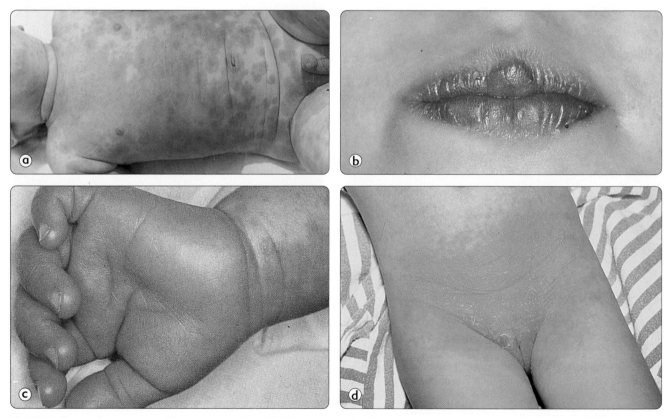

Fig 7.17 Kawasaki syndrome. Characteristic clinical findings demonstrated include **(a)** a generalized, morbilliform, erythema multiforme-like rash, **(b)** erythema and fissuring of the lips, **(c)** palmar and plantar erythema with edema of the hands and feet, and **(d)** erythema and scaling in the groin creases.

ACRAL ERYTHEMA

Erythromelalgia

Erythromelalgia is an unusual entity characterized by paroxysms of painful erythema of the hands and feet, which last for minutes to hours (Fig 7.18). Patients often complain of warmth of the distal extremities followed by marked erythema and pain, which is initially improved by elevation and then only by increasing periods of emersion in cold water. Although the primary variant is usually familial, secondary erythromelalgia may be triggered by polycythemia vera, lymphoproliferative disorders, hypertension, and disorders associated with hyperviscosity. When the underlying condition is treated, symptoms improve. Unfortunately, primary disease is often recalcitrant and cold-water exposure results in an 'immersion foot', with progressive vascular injury, recurrent ulcerations, and secondary bacterial infection.

Pernio

Pernio results from cold exposure, usually just above freezing, and recurrent trauma. It is commonly reported in temperate climates, where women and children are most commonly affected. Typical lesions consist of painful nodules and plaques that overlie bony prominences on the hands and feet (Fig 7.19). Histopathology demonstrates intense edema of the papillary dermis and endothelial swelling associated with a mononuclear, perivascular infiltrate. Inflammation may extend to vessels in the deep dermis and fat. Equestrians, scuba divers, and individuals who participate in fall and winter sports are particularly prone to develop lesions.

Acrodynia

Acrodynia, or pink disease, occurs in infants and toddlers as a result of chronic exposure to mercury. Painful, persistent erythema and swelling of the hands and feet is accompanied by other signs of sympathetic stimulation, which include tachycardia, hyperhidrosis, restlessness, and irritability. Treatment is directed toward removing the source of mercury exposure and chelation therapy.

PURPURAS

Bleeding into the skin may be an innocent finding in minor trauma or the first sign of a life-threatening disease. Early diagnosis and treatment, when necessary, requires that the practitioner recognize and carefully evaluate any patient with purpura.

Cutaneous hemorrhage can be differentiated from hyperemia that results from increased blood flow through dilated vessels by failure of the hemorrhagic area to blanch when pressure is applied across the surface (diascopy). Diascopy can be demonstrated by pressing the skin apart between the thumb and index finger or by applying a glass or plastic slide. Pinpoint areas of hemorrhage are called petechiae; large, confluent patches are referred to as ecchymoses. Purpura results from extravascular, intravascular, and vascular phenomena.

Extravascular purpura

Trauma is the most common cause of extravascular purpura in children. Nonblanching, purple patches caused by accidental trauma vary from a few millimeters to many centimeters in diameter and are usually located over bony prominences, such as the knees, elbows, the extensor surfaces of the lower legs, the forehead, nose, and chin. Petechiae are only occasionally present in otherwise healthy children, although they may occur on the face and chest after vigorous coughing or vomiting.

The presence of purpura on protected or nonexposed sites, such as the buttocks, spine, genitals, upper thighs, and upper arms, suggests the possibility of deliberately induced trauma. In some cases the shape of the bruise gives a clue as to the weapon used to inflict the injury.

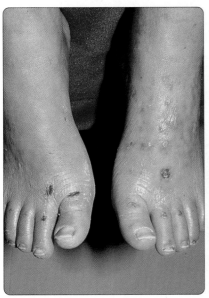

Fig 7.18 Erythromelalgia. Necrotic blisters and ulcerations recurred chronically in this 11-year-old girl who received relief from throbbing, debilitating foot pain by dunking her feet in near-freezing water for up to 12 hours a day. Her brother also had erythromelalgia, but his symptoms were mild and usually resolved with leg elevation alone.

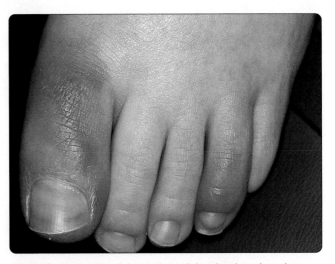

Fig 7.19 Pernio. Painful, purple nodules developed on the sides of the feet and toes in this 13-year-old boy after walking with wet boots in a cold stream.

Scars, sun damage, nutritional deficiency, inherited disorders of collagen and elastic tissue, and other factors that decrease the tensile strength of the skin may increase the risk of bruising caused by extravascular phenomena, even after minor trauma (Fig 7.20).

Intravascular purpura

Intravascular purpura results from any disorder that interferes with normal coagulation. Petechiae and ecchymoses are present on the skin, mucosal bleeding may be seen, and in severe cases bleeding may occur in the kidneys, gastrointestinal tract, and central nervous system. Among the causes are autoimmune thrombocytopenic purpura (ATP), acute leukemia, aplastic anemia, sepsis, and clotting factor deficiencies.

Autoimmune thrombocytopenic purpura

In children, ATP is the most common cause of intravascular purpura. Patients typically present in the late winter and early spring, a few weeks to several months after a viral illness, with purpura of all sizes and no history of trauma. When injuries occur, ecchymoses may be impressive. Bleeding of the gums occurs regularly with brushing, and occult blood may be detected in the urine and stool. Fortunately, severe bleeding is unusual and most cases are self-limited, with improvement in platelet counts from less than 10,000/mm^3 to over 100,000/mm^3 within 1–2 months. The presence of ATP is associated with the development of an immunoglobulin G (IgG) that binds to platelets and results in increased destruction by the reticuloendothelial system. Antiplatelet antibodies have also been reported in patients with lupus erythematosus, leukemia, lymphoma, and drug reactions. Moderate-to-severe cases usually respond to treatment with intravenous immunoglobulin. Resistant patients may require systemic corticosteroids and/or splenectomy.

Patients with ATP may be clinically indistinguishable from those with leukemia and aplastic anemia (Fig 7.21). Associated symptoms, which include fatigue, general malaise, fever, weight loss, and bone pain, suggest the diagnosis of leukemia. In leukemia, blasts may be discovered in the peripheral smear as well as the bone marrow. In ATP, the bone marrow demonstrates increased numbers of megakaryocytes, whereas they are usually decreased in leukemia. In aplastic anemia, purpura may be the first sign of marrow failure. All blood elements are decreased in the peripheral blood as well as in the bone marrow. Severe bacterial infection is a common complication. Children with inherited clotting-factor disorders bruise easily and may develop hemarthroses and bleeding into viscera. Petechiae are not usually seen in these patients.

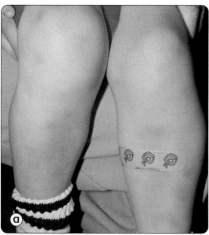
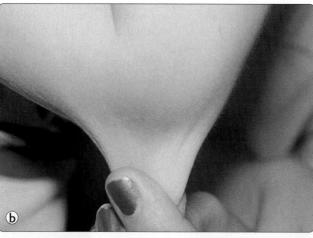
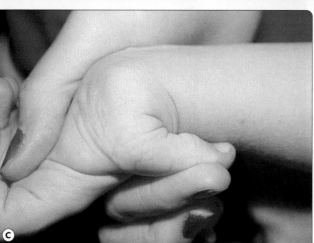
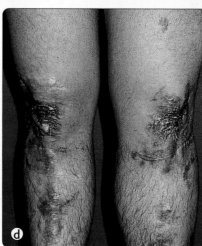

Fig 7.20
Ehlers–Danlos syndrome. This child demonstrates a number of classic features of the disorder, which include
(a) increased bruisability,
(b) hyperelastic skin, and
(c) hyperextensible joints. His father
(d) had multiple, wide, atrophic purple scars over the shins, which accumulated over the years from trauma.

Disseminated intravascular coagulation

Bacterial sepsis, disseminated viral infection, malignancy, and medications may rarely trigger disseminated intravascular coagulation, with widespread bleeding into the skin and viscera. Ecchymoses may progress rapidly to cover large areas of the body surface in minutes to hours (Fig 7.22). Unfortunately, necrosis may develop in the center of some areas of purpura. In survivors, healing occurs with scarring and occasionally loss of digits or limbs.

Patients are usually critically ill and death may ensue quickly unless supportive measures, including urgent volume expansion, vasopressors, and parenteral antibiotic therapy, are begun immediately. Some intensivists recommend treatment with heparin and fresh frozen plasma. Laboratory studies demonstrate thrombocytopenia, decreased fibrinogen, prolonged bleeding time, and elevations in fibrin split products. In children, meningococcemia, Rocky Mountain spotted fever, and streptococcal infections are the most common cause.

Vascular purpura

Vascular purpura develops when an inflammatory process involves the vessel wall (vasculitis). In leukocytoclastic vasculitis, the inflammation is predominantly neutrophilic. In lymphocytic vasculitis and late stages of leukocytoclastic vasculitis, vascular damage is caused by infiltrating mononuclear cells. Sweet syndrome shows primarily leukocytoclastic changes, whereas pyoderma gangrenosum shares features of leukocytoclastic and lymphocytic vasculitis.

Leukocytoclastic vasculitis

Leukocytic vasculitis results from immune complex deposition in dermal blood vessels and subsequent complement-activated leukocyte infiltration. Infections, medications, autoimmune disorders, and malignancy can trigger vasculitis.

Henoch–Schönlein purpura

Henoch–Schönlein purpura (HSP), also known as anaphylactoid purpura or allergic vasculitis, is the most common form of leukocytoclastic vasculitis to occur in children, with peak incidence found in children between 4 and 8 years old. However, HSP also has been reported in infants and adults.

Although the rash is characterized by palpable purpura, the typical 2–10 mm diameter, purpuric papules may be preceded by several days of urticaria. Lesions most commonly pepper the buttocks and the extensor surfaces of the arms and legs. However, any site may be involved including

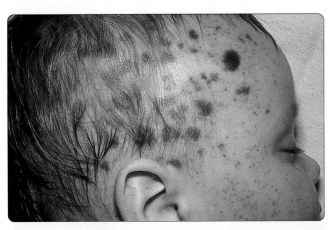

Fig 7.21 Intravascular purpura. A child with acute lymphocytic leukemia shows bruises of various sizes, which are typically found in individuals with low platelet counts.

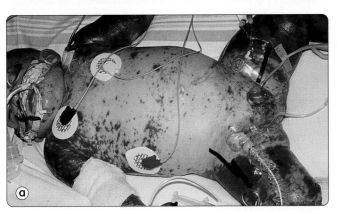

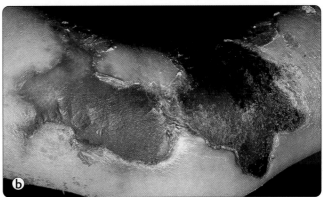

Fig 7.22 Disseminated intravascular coagulation. **(a)** Purpura fulminans developed in this infant with meningococcemia. Widespread bleeding into the skin was noted, particularly on the extremities. **(b)** A toddler with staphylococcal sepsis and DIC developed widespread cutaneous necrosis on the legs.

the face, ears, and trunk (Fig 7.23). Crops erupt episodically for 2–4 weeks, and individual lesions usually fade over 3–5 days. Confluent ecchymoses occasionally evolve from small lesions, and rarely necrosis and hemorrhagic bullae develop. Scalp edema and periarticular swelling (Schönlein purpura), and paroxysmal abdominal colic with melena or frankly bloody stools (Henoch purpura) may occur before, during, or after the rash. Vasculitis may also involve vessels in the kidneys, lungs, and central nervous system.

Recurrences occur in about half of patients for up to several months, but these episodes are usually mild. In most cases, the visceral disease is self-limiting. However, acute renal failure develops rarely and intussusception may complicate vasculitis in the bowel. More subtle renal disease may persist for years.

Leukocytoclastic vasculitis involves small, dermal blood vessels, usually postcapillary venules. Classic histologic findings include endothelial swelling, fibrin deposition within and around the vessels, neutrophilic infiltrate within the vessel walls, and nuclear dust (scattered nuclear fragments from neutrophils). Vascular destruction with hemorrhage may be prominent. Fresh biopsies demonstrate IgA and C3 deposition around the dermal blood vessels.

Although most children with HSP may be observed at home, patients with progressive renal disease or severe abdominal pain require hospitalization.

A normal blood count, platelet count, and coagulation studies help to differentiate HSP from intravascular forms of purpura. Identification of typical clinical findings and course, histopathology, and other screening studies (e.g. antinuclear antibodies [ANA], rheumatoid factor, precipitin antibodies) exclude lupus erythematosus and other connective tissue disorders.

Polyarteritis nodosa

Polyarteritis nodosa (PAN) is a leukocytoclastic vasculitis that involves small- and medium-sized arteries. A systemic form, which occurs extremely rarely in children, presents acutely with fever, weakness, abdominal pain, and cardiac failure. Despite treatment with high-dose corticosteroids and immunosuppressive agents, death may ensue quickly from renal failure, gastrointestinal bleeding, and bowel perforation. Cutaneous lesions, which include livedo reticularis, erythema, and purpura on the lower extremities, are not diagnostic.

Cutaneous PAN is more likely to come to the attention of the dermatologist. In this distinct variant, cutaneous findings

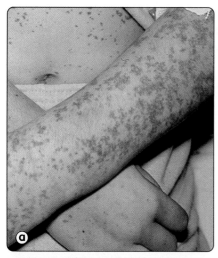
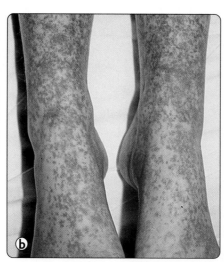
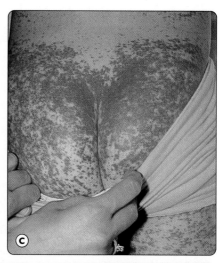
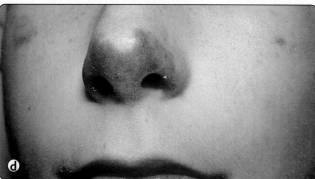
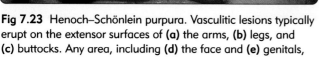
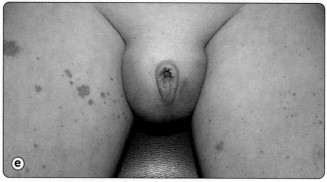

Fig 7.23 Henoch–Schönlein purpura. Vasculitic lesions typically erupt on the extensor surfaces of **(a)** the arms, **(b)** legs, and **(c)** buttocks. Any area, including **(d)** the face and **(e)** genitals, may be involved. Nonpitting edema of the face, chest, and genitals may be prominent as in the child shown in **(e)**.

predominate and the viscera are usually spared. Crops of painful nodules and annular plaques blossom on the arms and legs, particularly the hands and feet, and less commonly on the trunk, head, and neck (Fig 7.24). Urticaria, livedo, and cutaneous ulcerations may also develop. Episodes last for several weeks and tend to recur for years. Although severe systemic disease does not usually occur, fever and arthralgias frequently accompany flares in disease activity.

The diagnosis of cutaneous PAN is made by establishing the clinical pattern and histopathology, which demonstrates a leukocytoclastic vasculitis of medium-sized arteries. Patients usually respond quickly to prednisone, but resistant cases require methotrexate or azathioprine. Nodules localized to the palms and soles melt away with intralesional corticosteroids. Long-term monitoring is required to detect those children who develop severe systemic involvement.

The painful nodules of cutaneous PAN may be difficult to differentiate from erythema nodosum, cold panniculitis, and lupus panniculitis, particularly early in the course. Associated clinical findings and histopathology, however, are distinctive in these disorders.

Infectious vasculitis

Although overwhelming infection with a number of bacterial organisms may trigger rapidly fatal disseminated intravascular coagulation with widespread bleeding into the skin, mucous membranes, and viscera, many patients develop discrete vasculitic lesions. In fact, the presence of 0.5–2 cm diameter, angulated, pink-to-red, hemorrhagic macules, papules, pustules, and plaques is associated with a relatively good prognosis (Fig 7.25). Over several hours lesions become hemorrhagic and central necrosis with bulla formation or ulceration may

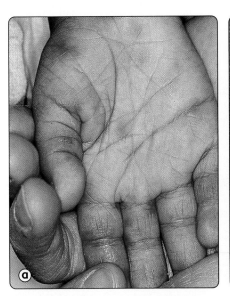
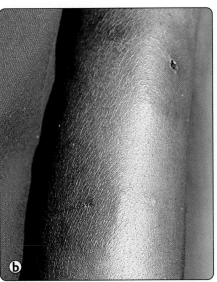
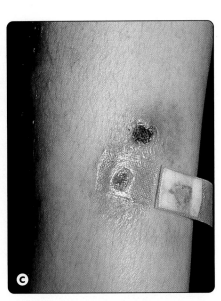

Fig 7.24 Polyarteritis nodosa. Over several days a 3-year-old girl developed painful nodules on the trunk, face, and extremities. **(a)** Lesions on the hands were associated with arthritis. **(b)** Some of the nodules on the legs developed central necrotic vesicles. **(c)** An 8-year-boy with chronic cutaneous polyarteritis nodosa complained of recurrent, painful, ulcerated nodules on his shins.

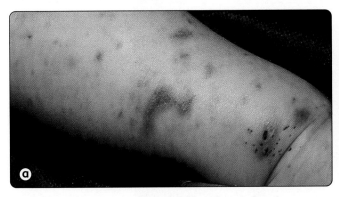
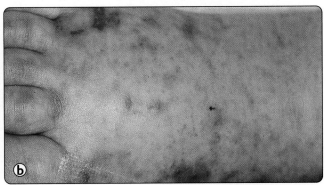

Fig 7.25 Infectious vasculitis. **(a)** Sharply angulated, purpuric, and necrotic papules developed on the extremities of a toddler with meningococcemia. He presented with meningitis and responded quickly to parenteral antibiotics.

(b) A similar rash appeared on the extremities of a 6-year-old boy with Rocky Mountain spotted fever. In both children vasculitic papules spread to the palms, soles, and (to a lesser extent) the trunk.

develop. Prompt recognition of this condition and the initiation of antibiotics and supportive care may be lifesaving.

Although the rash may be caused by hematogenous dissemination of the organism to the skin, many lesions result from immune complex deposition in dermal vessels. For example, Osler nodes (tender nodules on the finger or toe pads) and Janeway lesion (small, painless nodules on the palms and soles) probably represent an immune-mediated phenomenon (Fig 7.26a–c). *Neisseria meningitidis*, *Haemophilus influenzae* type B, *Streptococcus pneumoniae*, other *Streptococcus* spp., and *Staphylococcus aureus* have been cultured from blood and skin in normal hosts with infectious vasculitis (Fig 7.26d). Rocky Mountain spotted fever may produce a similar clinical picture, but the inflammation tends to be primarily lymphocytic. In immunosuppressed individuals these organisms, as well as opportunistic bacteria and fungi, must also be considered.

Ecthyma gangrenosum

Ecthyma gangrenosum, characterized by a punched-out ulceration with a central opalescent eschar and a hemorrhagic border, results from *Pseudomonas* septicemia (Fig 7.27). Lesions typically appear on the lower abdominal wall, thighs, and groin in leukemics, burn patients, and other debilitated individuals who have been on antibiotics. Although most patients are severely ill with multiple lesions, in some cases only one or several indolent ulcers are present. Other Gram-negative organisms, as well as fungi such as *Candida* and *Aspergillus* spp., may produce the same type of skin lesions.

The diagnosis can be made by searching for organisms in Gram stains obtained from pustules and necrotic ulcers. Identification of specific organisms from blood and tissue cultures is required to select the appropriate antibiotics. Skin biopsies show a necrotizing vasculitis with neutrophils and a variable number of bacteria within vessels. Aplastic patients may show minimal inflammation with large numbers of organisms.

Lymphocytic vasculitis

Rather than being a distinct entity, lymphocytic vasculitis represents a reaction pattern in the skin found in a number of disorders in which lymphocytic inflammation predominates. Lymphocytic vasculitis has been described in cutaneous drug reactions, vasculitic lesions of Sjögren syndrome, and as a late phase of leukocytoclastic vasculitis. Progressive pigmented purpuric dermatosis (PPPD) is the only disorder in which lymphocytic vasculitic occurs consistently.

The development of localized patches of petechiae and larger patches of purpura, particularly on the lower extremities, characterizes PPPD (Fig 7.28). Hemosiderin deposition

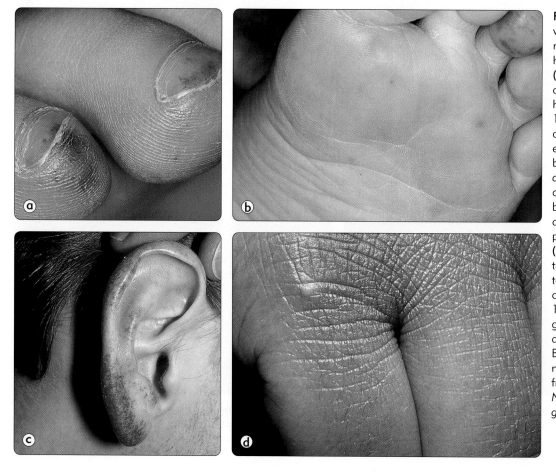

Fig 7.26 Infectious vasculitis. **(a)** Osler nodes, splinter hemorrhages, and **(b)** Janeway lesions appeared on the hands and feet of this 10-year-old boy with acute bacterial endocarditis caused by *Staphylococcus aureus*. **(c)** Another child with subacute bacterial endocarditis developed vasculitis papules on his ears. **(d)** This exquisitely tender pustule on the toe was the only cutaneous finding in a 16-year-old girl with gonococcal arthritis dermatitis syndrome. Blood cultures were negative, but cultures from the cervix grew *Neisseria gonorrhoeae*.

and postinflammatory hyperpigmentation lead to shades of brown, gold, and bronze as lesions evolve. Confluent patches may form a reticulated pattern. Although lesions are usually flat and asymptomatic, fine scale and lichenoid papules may be associated with mild pruritus.

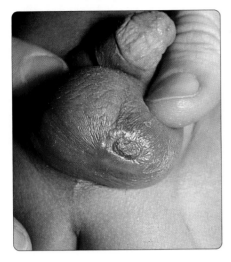

Fig 7.27 Ecthyma gangrenosum. An infant with an inherited immunodeficiency experienced recurrent episodes of Gram-negative septicemia. *Pseudomonas* grew from cultures obtained from blood and the necrotic, crusted ulcer on the scrotum.

Skin biopsies from active areas demonstrate lymphocytes around and within the walls of superficial dermal capillaries. Mild hemorrhage and hemosiderin deposition are also present.

Clinically and histologically, it may be impossible to differentiate PPPD from a drug reaction, and occasionally practitioners have reported children with large patches over the lower back or buttocks for suspected abuse. Unfortunately, no treatment has proved satisfactory, and lesions may persist for years. Systemic and topical corticosteroids may arrest progression temporarily.

Sweet syndrome

Sweet syndrome, also referred to as acute febrile neutrophilic dermatosis, is characterized by violaceous, 0.5–3 cm diameter nodules and plaques that erupt abruptly on the face and extremities (Fig 7.29). Recurrent crops of nodules that appear over 1–8 months are heralded by high fever, arthralgias, and occasionally periarticular swelling and arthritis. Necrotic vesicles and bullae may also form. Although Sweet syndrome is self-limiting, symptoms may be debilitating. Skin lesions, arthralgias, and fever usually melt away with systemic corticosteroids; however, recurrences are common when the medication is tapered.

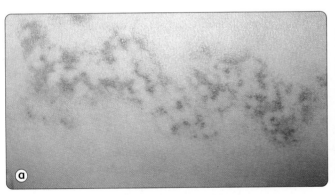

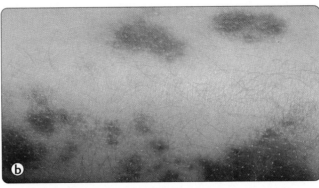

Fig 7.28 Progressive pigmented purpuric dermatosis.
(a) Reticulated hyperpigmented patches had slowly advanced across the leg of a 15-year-old girl for years. **(b)** Dark bronze macules on the leg of a 12-year-old boy were misdiagnosed as bruises. He had no history of trauma, and a skin biopsy showed the typical changes of progressive pigmented purpuric dermatosis.

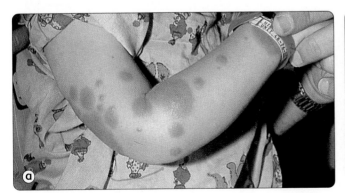

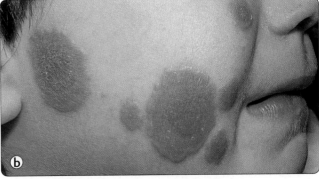

Fig 7.29 (a, b) Sweet syndrome. A 2-year-old girl developed fever, arthritis, leukocytosis, and widely disseminated, red-to-violaceous plaques and nodules, which demonstrated intense neutrophilic inflammation on skin biopsy. An extensive evaluation failed to reveal any underlying disease. Although she responded quickly to systemic corticosteroids, it took nearly a year to wean her because of frequent recurrences.

Although initially described in middle-aged women, a number of cases have been reported in infants and children. About 10% of adult cases are associated with myeloproliferative disorders, especially acute myelocytic or myelomonocytic leukemia. Children with this syndrome require a thorough physical examination and laboratory evaluation, including a blood count, peripheral smear, and bone marrow biopsy, to exclude any underlying disorder.

Sweet syndrome may be confused with EM, erythema nodosum, viral exanthems, HSP, infectious vasculitis, and PAN. Although Sweet syndrome may be suspected because of the cutaneous lesions and clinical course, skin biopsy of a fresh lesion demonstrates diagnostic findings, which include a dense, perivascular, neutrophilic infiltrate and intense edema in the upper dermis, some leukocytoclasia without true vasculitis, and in some cases subepidermal bullae formation.

Pyoderma gangrenosum

In pyoderma gangrenosum, painful pustules or nodules develop central necrosis and an enlarging ulcer with a hemorrhagic, purple, undermined, advancing border (Fig 7.30). Ulcers range in size from about 1 cm in diameter when they first appear to over 10 cm as they evolve. One or several lesions may occur, and any area, including the face, trunk, and extremities, may be involved. Pathergy, or the development of new lesions at sites of trauma, such as venipunctures, is a reliable diagnostic clue. An underlying systemic disease, such as inflammatory bowel disease, myelogenous leukemia, or rheumatoid arthritis, is associated with cutaneous lesions in half of the cases.

Skin biopsies show typical (but nondiagnostic) findings, which include a lymphocytic vasculitis at the advancing border and necrosis with abscess formation and reactive polymorphous inflammation that extends into the subcutaneous tissue.

Pyoderma gangrenosum usually responds to treatment of the underlying condition. Idiopathic cases can be treated with antibiotics, systemic corticosteroids, or dapsone. Resistant cases may require immunosuppressive agents such as azathioprine, methotrexate, or cyclosporine.

FIGURATE ERYTHEMA

A number of disorders are characterized by the development of annular plaques with a well-defined, advancing, red border and central clearing. Typical, but nondiagnostic, histologic findings include a tight, perivascular, mononuclear cell infiltrate in the superficial dermis with occasional extension to the mid and deep dermis. The overlying epidermis is normal or shows mild spongiosis. Erythema annulare centrifugum (EAC) and erythema chronicum migrans (ECM) are the most commonly recognized figurate erythemas in children.

Erythema annulare centrifugum

In EAC, one or multiple asymptomatic, expanding, annular or serpiginous, red plaques with well-defined raised borders and trailing scales on the inner aspect of the border occur (Fig 7.31). As lesions progress from less than 1 cm to over 20 cm in diameter over several weeks, new plaques may arise within the borders to produce concentric rings. The eruption typically spreads from the central trunk to the proximal extremities (centrifugal), and lesions continue to evolve for months to years.

Although EAC probably represents a hypersensitivity reaction to the same sort of phenomena that trigger urticaria and EM, a number of reports suggest a common association with chronic dermatophyte infection (e.g. tinea pedis, tinea cruris). Cases of EAC may erupt throughout childhood, but it occurs most commonly in adults. Annular erythema of infancy is undoubtedly a clinical variant of this disorder.

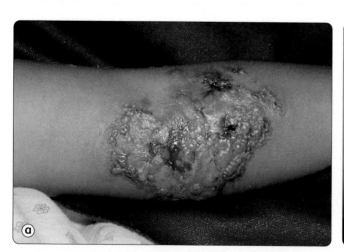

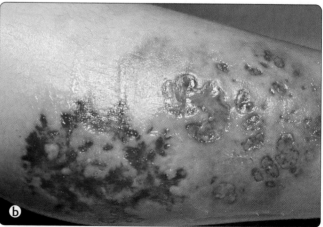

Fig 7.30 Pyoderma gangrenosum. **(a)** A 9-year-old boy developed a painful, expanding, crusted, necrotic plaque with an undermined border on his arm. An exhaustive medical evaluation was unrevealing until bone marrow biopsy demonstrated chronic myelogenous leukemia. **(b)** A similar plaque in a teenager with Crohn disease shows cribriform scarring as inflammation abates. Lesions in both children healed after aggressive treatment of the underlying disorders.

The persistence of individual lesions and lack of pruritus differentiate EAC from urticaria. The chronic course and absence of viral symptoms help to exclude an urticarial viral exanthem. Granuloma annulare may be excluded by the finding of epidermal changes (erythema and scale) in EAC. Although there are no specific laboratory tests for EAC, skin biopsy typically shows a tight, lymphocytic, perivascular infiltrate (coat-sleeve pattern) in the mid and deep dermis. Dermatitic changes may also be present in the epidermis.

When a fungal infection is identified, oral antifungal medications may result in clearing of the rash. Otherwise, no specific treatment is indicated.

Erythema chronicum migrans

In ECM, which marks the onset of Lyme disease, a single papule begins 3–30 days after a tick bite and expands quickly to form an enlarging, annular, red plaque with central clearing (Fig 7.32). New lesions may continue to evolve successively or in crops over several months. Plaques over 4 cm in diameter are typical, and some may exceed 30 cm. Mild, influenza-like symptoms, which include headache, sore throat, arthralgias, and malaise, are commonly associated with the skin rash. If untreated, resolution of skin lesions is followed several months later by a pauciarticular arthritis that involves the knees, elbows, and/or wrists in 50% of patients. In 15% of cases, neurologic abnormalities, including meningoencephalitis, neuropathy, or facial palsy, occur 2 weeks to 8 months after the tick bite. Cardiac symptoms, which appear in 5% of patients, may mimic rheumatic fever.

Lyme disease is caused by the spirochete *Borrelia burgdorferi*, which can be carried by *Ixodes dammini* and related ticks (Fig 7.32d). These ticks are widely distributed throughout the US and Europe, and in some places such as coastal New England and the Great Lakes States the infection has become endemic. The ticks are the size of a pin head, and up to 50% of patients do not recall the bite.

The incidence of Lyme disease is highest in children, but all ages are affected. Although the diagnosis is usually made clinically, new, more reliable serologic tests may aid in differentiation of the annular plaques of ECM from urticaria, viral exanthems, erythema marginatum, and EAC. Skin biopsy specimens obtained from the expanding border or the center of lesions may demonstrate spirochetes with the use of special silver stains. Otherwise, the histopathologic findings are not diagnostic and show changes typical of insect-bite reactions.

Any individual in an endemic area who develops an annular eruption, especially if it is associated with viral symptoms and a tick bite, should be treated to reduce the risk of arthritis and other late complications. Although treatment recommendations vary, a 3-week course of doxycycline 100 mg twice a day is the choice for older children and adults, and amoxicillin at a dose of 25–50 mg/kg/day with a maximum of 2 g daily given in three divided doses is recommended for children younger than 8 years old. Children allergic to penicillin may be treated with 30 mg/kg of erythromycin up to 250 mg three times a day.

Avoiding tick-infested areas or wearing protective clothing reduces the risk of exposure. Tick repellents containing diethyltoluamide are also effective. However, excessive use of diethyltoluamide, particularly in infants and young children, has been associated with neurotoxic reactions. Low-concentration lotions (Skedaddle® 7.25% and OFF® 10%) are as effective as traditional repellents with concentrations over 50% and have a much better safety profile. Tick inspections after hikes and camping trips and removal of ticks within 24–48 hours of attachment also reduce transmission of the spirochete.

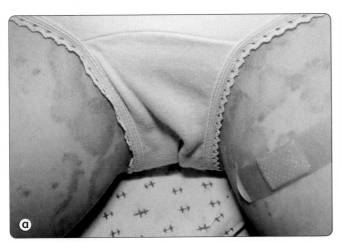

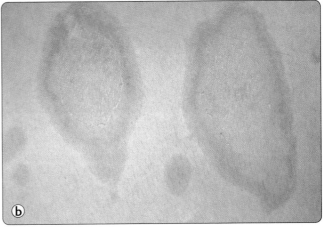

Fig 7.31 Erythema annulare centrifigum. **(a)** Symmetric, annular, red plaques slowly expanded on the anterior thighs of a 10-year-old girl. **(b)** Another child with large lesions on the trunk demonstrates the bright red border with fine trailing scale and central clearing

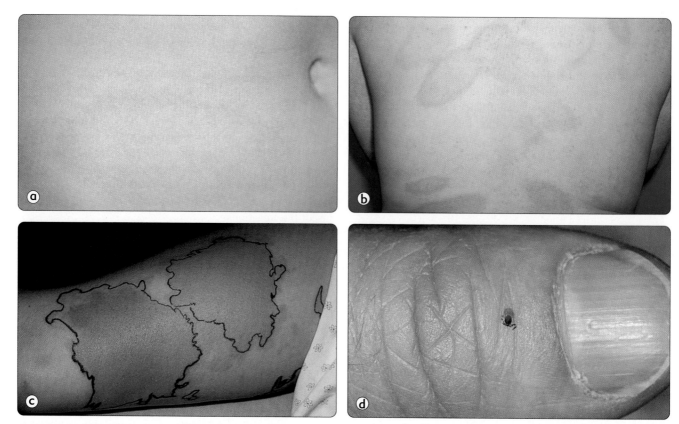

Fig 7.32 Erythema chronicum migrans. **(a)** A solitary, indurated, light-pink plaque with central clearing grew over several weeks from a small, red papule at the site of a tick bite. The lesion, as well as associated arthralgias and intermittent low-grade fever, resolved within 48 hours of starting oral amoxicillin. **(b)** In some patients, multiple papules and plaques appear as the organism disseminates. **(c)** In this 12-year-old girl, two solid, dark-red patches were initially diagnosed and treated as cellulitis. **(d)** The spirochete is transmitted from animals to humans by the tiny *Ixodes dammini* and related tick vectors.

PANNICULITIS

Panniculitis refers to a group of disorders in which an inflammatory process involves the fat lobules, intervening fat septae, or both. Clinically, patients present with deep-seated, poorly defined, tender, violaceous nodules. The overlying epidermis is usually intact, although it may be taut and shiny. If necrosis develops, ulcerations may occur.

Erythema nodosum

Erythema nodosum (EN) is the most common panniculitis to appear in children, usually in adolescents. Typically, painful, red, subcutaneous nodules and plaques, 1–5 cm in diameter, erupt on the shins, but lesions may also involve the arms and thighs, and rarely the trunk and face (Fig 7.33). Nodules usually fade over several weeks, but recurrences are frequent. In some cases, crops recur for months.

Over 100 years ago the development of EN with tuberculosis was recognized. More recently, EN has been associated with a number of infections, including viral pharyngitis, streptococcal pharyngitis, histoplasmosis, coccidioidomycosis, and other deep fungi and atypical mycobacteria. Noninfectious inflammatory conditions, such as sarcoidosis, inflammatory bowel disease, and lupus erythematosus, may trigger the reaction.

The finding of a septal panniculitis without fat necrosis is characteristic of EN. Early in the course neutrophilic inflammation is common. Later, lymphocytes, histiocytes, and giant cells predominate. Vessels show endothelial cell swelling, inflammation in the vascular walls, and hemorrhage.

In most children EN is self-limiting and treatment, when necessary, is tailored to the underlying disorder. Leg elevation and nonsteroidal anti-inflammatory agents may help to reduce the pain.

Cold panniculitis

In infants and young children, cold injury results in crystallization and rupture of fat cells and subsequent inflammation. Persistent, indurated, red nodules and plaques appear most commonly on the cheeks, but the trunk and extremities may also be involved (Fig 7.34). Ulceration and atrophy do not usually develop, and nodules resolve without treatment in several weeks to several months.

Although the cause is not known, the increased saturation of fatty acids in the subcutaneous fat of infants compared with adults makes their fat more prone to solidification at low temperatures.

Fat necrosis of the newborn is a variant of cold panniculitis that occurs within the first month of life. Several circumscribed lesions appear on the trunk and proximal extremities in an otherwise healthy infant. Nodules heal without scarring, but transient depression of the skin surface occurs frequently and ulceration on occasion.

Cold injury may also produce sclerema of the newborn. In this process, widespread, woody induration of the skin develops in a severely ill infant. This process probably results as a complication of multisystem failure and associated cooling of the skin and fat from decreased cutaneous perfusion. In skin biopsies from these infants, edema of the fibrous septae is found with no necrosis of fat cells. Fat necrosis of the newborn and cold panniculitis in older infants and children are associated with necrosis of fat cells and granulomatous inflammation.

Morphologically, cold panniculitis may be confused with bacterial cellulitis (Fig 7.35). However, in cellulitis the indurated plaques are warm, tender, and progressive, and the patients are febrile and of toxic appearance. Other nodular erythemas, such as polyarteritis nodosa and EN are usually differentiated by the clinical course and skin biopsy findings when necessary.

Lupus panniculitis

In lupus panniculitis, persistent, purple, painless nodules, 1–5 cm in diameter develop on the face, extremities, and buttocks (Fig 7.36). Although these lesions usually occur in a child with other signs of systemic lupus erythematosus (SLE), they may be the first or only manifestation of the disease. Individual lesions may persist for months to years, and ulceration and

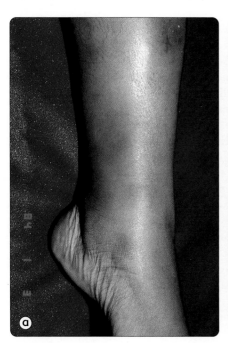
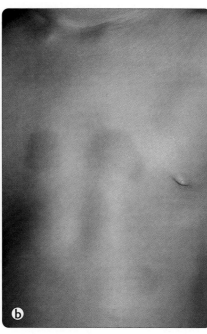

Fig 7.33 Erythema nodosum. (a) Tender, deep-seated nodules appeared on the shins of a 16-year-old girl 2 weeks after starting birth-control pills. The lesions resolved when the medication was discontinued. (b) An 18-month-old boy developed (biopsy proved) erythema nodosum on the chest and abdomen following a cold. The nodules resolved without therapy over several weeks.

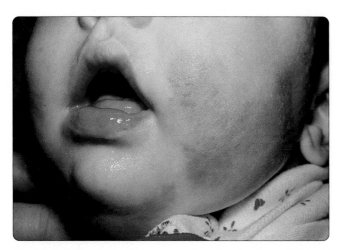

Fig 7.34 Cold panniculitis appeared on the cheeks and chin of this 6-month-old infant 1 day after he was given an ice-filled teething ring.

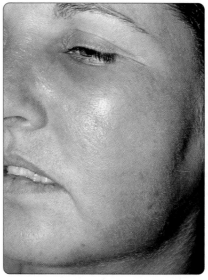

Fig 7.35 Facial cellulitis/erysipelas. A painful, indurated, red plaque spread within several hours across the cheek of this 17-year-old girl. She also had a fever and tender cervical adenopathy, which resolved on parenteral penicillin.

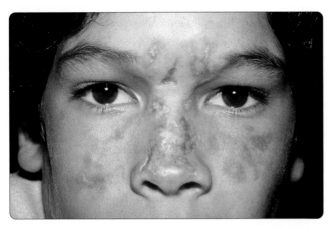

Fig 7.36 Lupus panniculitis. A 13-year-old boy presented with chronic, recurring, deep-seated nodules and plaques, which healed with punched-out scars.

scarring occur frequently. Unfortunately, lupus panniculitis is often resistant to treatment with antimalarial drugs, and the use of systemic corticosteroids and immunosuppressive agents should probably be guided by systemic symptoms.

Histopathology is nonspecific and shows lymphohistiocytic inflammation within the fat lobules and hyalinization of fat cells. Inflammation and vasculitis may also occur in the fat septae.

PHOTOSENSITIVITY

Photosensitivity is a term used to describe a group of conditions marked by abnormal reactions to light. Sunburn is a phototoxic reaction that results from exposure to naturally occurring, short-wavelength, ultraviolet (UV) B light. Longer wavelength (UVA) light is only weakly phototoxic; however, all individuals deliberately or accidentally exposed to high-enough doses of topical or oral UVA-photosensitizing agents may also develop burns. In photoallergic reactions, susceptible patients, who are exposed to certain photosensitizing chemicals or drugs, develop an immunologically mediated rash which is activated by light. A number of genetic and metabolic disorders are associated with photosensitivity, and the recognition of cutaneous findings may be a clue to diagnosis. Photodermatoses include several specific conditions that have unusual reactions to light. In some of these dermatoses, the action spectrum, or the wavelengths that trigger the skin findings, have been described. Finally, other diseases may be exacerbated by light. The recognition of this phenomenon may be important in managing these conditions.

Phototoxic and photoallergic reactions
Exposure of the skin to sunlight results in a number of biologic reactions. Small amounts of UVB activate the conversion of 7-dehydrocholesterol into vitamin D_3. Large amounts of UV light produce erythema and swelling, known as sunburn (Fig 7.37). Intense reactions may result in the development of blistering burns on sun-exposed surfaces. Healing is marked by

desquamation, thickening, and hyperpigmentation of the skin.

Although UVB is 100 times more erythemogenic than UVA, the large quantity of UVA ($1,000 \times$ UVB) that reaches the ground contributes substantially to sunburn (10–15%). On overcast days, when 15–20% of UVB is absorbed and scattered by the cloud cover, the role of UVA is even greater. The minimum dose of light required to produce a discrete area of sunburn is referred to as the minimal erythema dose (MED). The MED tends to increase with increasing skin types. Individuals with skin type 1 always burn and never tan. These people have blonde or red hair, blue eyes, and often demonstrate freckling in sun-exposed sites. Skin type 2 denotes individuals who always burn at first, but sometimes tan after repeated sun exposure. Type 3 people occasionally burn, but tan readily. Olive-complected individuals who always tan fall into type 4. Types 5 and 6 include members of darkly pigmented races.

Factors that potentiate the development of sunburn include increasing elevation above sea level, wind, low humidity, and applications that result in thinning of the epidermis, such as peeling agents (topical retinoids, salicylic acid, lactic acid). Damage to DNA is the initiating event in the development of the erythema response. The subsequent production of inflammatory mediators (e.g. prostaglandins, histamine) triggers the clinical response. Factors that interfere with normal DNA repair mechanisms (hereditary defects in DNA repair enzymes or antimetabolites, such as methotrexate) result in an exaggerated or prolonged erythema response.

Wrinkling, elastosis, lentigines, and other 'age'-related changes in the skin result from long-term exposure to sunlight; the majority of most individual's lifetime exposure occurs during childhood. It has been estimated that the incidence of nonmelanoma skin cancers (basal cell carcinoma and squamous cell carcinoma) could be reduced by 75–80% if people used sun-protective clothing, sunscreens (chemicals that absorb UV light), and sunblocks (agents that reflect sunlight) from early childhood. Although most sunscreens (e.g. *p*-aminobenzoic acid, its esters, and cinnamates) provide good

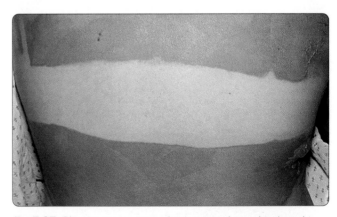

Fig 7.37 Phototoxic reaction. A severe sunburn developed in sun-exposed areas after this teenager applied a topical photosensitizing cream to her skin and spent the day outdoors. Note the areas of sparing under her bathing suit.

coverage against UVB, only parsol absorbs adequately in the UVA range. The sun-protective factor (SPF) of a product is determined by calculating the ratio of the MED of unprotected skin to the MED of sunscreen-protected skin. In infants, who should not be left in the sun, sunscreens are only rarely necessary. Parents of ambulatory children, particularly individuals with light pigmentation, should be given aggressive counseling about sun protection. People with skin types 1–2 must use sunscreens with an SPF of 15–30, whereas darker pigmented individuals may be safe with lower SPFs, particularly after gradually increasing sun exposure has produced protective darkening of the skin.

Unlike phototoxicity, photoallergic reactions involve an immunologic response in a small number of individuals who are sensitized to certain chemicals or drugs in the presence of sunlight. In many cases, a Type IV delayed hypersensitivity reaction results in the development of an eczematous dermatitis in a sun-exposed distribution, rather than a sunburn. A number of medications have been implicated in the production of both phototoxic and photoallergic reactions. Some of the most common photosensitizers are furocoumarins, nalidixic acid, dyes, salicylanilides, fragrances, p-aminobenzoic acid, phenothiazines, sulfonamides, tetracyclines, thiazides and related sulfonamide diuretics, and nonsteroidal anti-inflammatory agents. Patients on these drugs must be warned to protect themselves against the risk of photosensitivity.

Rarely, photoactivated, eczematous reactions persist for months or years. A persistent light reaction usually evolves from a previous photocontact allergic dermatitis, but oral medications have been implicated as well. In actinic reticuloid, the chronic dermatitis often spreads to involve covered sites, the lesions become lichenified and nodular, and skin biopsies may show lymphoma-like infiltrates in addition to a chronic dermatitis. In these patients, the dermatitis may be reproduced on normal patches of skin by exposure to UVA, UVB, and sometimes visible light, and MEDs at various wavelengths of UV light are markedly decreased. Some patients with atopic dermatitis note a flare of disease activity in sun-exposed sites.

These individuals may be differentiated from patients with photoactivated eczematous reactions by the absence of exposure to photosensitizing drugs and topical agents, negative photopatch tests, and an abnormal MED to UVB only.

Photodermatoses
Polymorphous light eruption
Several photoinduced dermatoses may be identified by distinctive clinical and histologic findings. Polymorphous light eruption (PMLE) is the most common childhood photodermatosis, accounting for over 75% of photoinduced rashes. In PMLE, crops of red macules, papules, vesicles, or plaques typically erupt on exposed areas several hours to several days after intensive sun exposure in the early spring (Fig 7.38). The morphology of lesions varies from patient to patient. However, the rash tends to be monomorphous in a given individual. PMLE appears most commonly in girls and women under 30 years old and may recur each spring for years. Although the rash usually progresses for several weeks, complete regression occurs within 3–4 weeks, despite continued light exposure. In fact, phototherapy (psoralen-UVA) has been used to trigger the reaction deliberately and treat or 'harden' the skin in a controlled setting to avoid inconvenient expression of the rash. PMLE is most common in temperate or northern climates, where the 'hardening' of the skin tends to wane during the winter months. In the sunbelt states and tropics, where sun exposure occurs all year round, the rash is less common and often spares the face and 'V' of the neck, which are most prominently exposed.

The histopathology of PMLE typically shows an intense, lymphocytic, perivascular infiltrate in the upper and mid dermis. Dermal edema may also be prominent. Differential diagnosis from lupus erythematosus may be difficult clinically and histologically. The histology of lupus usually demonstrates inflammation at the dermal–epidermal junction and the dermal infiltrate often surrounds both adnexal structures and vessels. However, early in the course of lupus the histology may be nonspecific, clinical findings may be confined to the skin, and serologic studies may be negative.

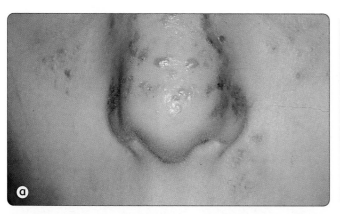

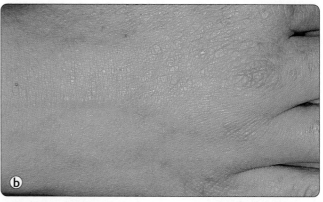

Fig 7.38 Polymorphous light eruption. **(a)** Red papules and vesicles erupted on the face of a 14-year-old girl after a trip to the beach in the spring. She had experienced this phenomenon every spring for the previous 5 years. **(b)** An 8-year-old girl developed a mildly pruritic, papular rash on the tops of her hands and face after a spring picnic. In both girls the rashes peaked within several weeks and healed despite continuing sun exposure.

Solar urticaria

Although urticaria following sun exposure may be caused by medications or associated with systemic illness, such as lupus or porphyria, a rare group of otherwise healthy individuals develops hives within minutes of sun exposure. Although the lesions may become quite itchy and extensive, symptoms usually abate with continued light exposure. Various wavelengths of light, including UV and visible radiation, have been associated with hives.

In many cases, solar urticaria is caused by a Type I IgE-mediated reaction, and lesions result from the release of histamine and other vasoactive substances. In time, inflammatory mediators are depleted and lesions subside. Unfortunately, antihistamines only partially suppress solar urticaria. However, persistent light exposure can be maintained with phototherapy to keep the reaction under control.

Genetic disorders

A number of inherited and metabolic disorders are associated with photosensitivity. In xeroderma pigmentosum, Bloom syndrome, Cockayne syndrome, and Rothmund–Thomson syndrome, light alone triggers an abnormal reaction in the skin and subsequent acute and chronic changes. Disorders that result in pigment dilution, such as albinism, phenylketonuria, and other aminoacidopathies, markedly increase sensitivity to phototoxic reactions. In congenital porphyrias, porphyria cutanea tarda, and Hartnup disease, endogenous metabolites function as potent photosensitizers (Fig 7.39). In many of these disorders the clinical findings provide the key to diagnosis.

Photoexacerbated disorders

Many disorders are triggered or aggravated by sunlight. For instance, although careful exposure to sun may result in improvement of psoriasis and repigmentation in vitiligo, sunburn often produces Koebner phenomenon and results in exacerbation of both disorders (Fig 7.40). Sun exposure, particularly sunburn, is also known to exacerbate acne vulgaris,

acne rosacea, EM, viral exanthems, pemphigus and other bullous disorders, lichen planus, lupus erythematosus, pityriasis alba, and herpes labialis.

COLLAGEN VASCULAR DISEASE

Collagen vascular disorders present with a myriad of confusing and overlapping cutaneous findings. Although the clinical picture and laboratory markers help to define a specific entity, often the practitioner is unable to make a definitive diagnosis. A number of autoantibody systems have been identified in these diseases. Antibodies target vascular endothelium and epithelial basement membrane zone structures, which results in cutaneous and visceral inflammation. In the skin, inflammation produces distinctive reaction patterns.

Lupus erythematosus

Lupus is a chronic multisystem disorder that can affect any organ system. Although SLE was considered to be progressive, often with a fatal outcome, as recent as 25 years ago, the aggressive use of systemic corticosteroids and immuno-suppressive agents has greatly improved the prognosis. Early intervention requires immediate recognition of variable and sometimes subtle signs and symptoms. Cutaneous findings may suggest the diagnosis.

The most common variant of lupus in childhood is SLE. Although the incidence is only 1/200,000 in childhood, nearly 25% of all cases begin before the age of 20 years. In young children, boys are affected almost as often as girls. However, in adolescence, when the incidence begins to rise, girls account for 80–90% of cases. Other forms of lupus, which are uncommon in childhood, include benign cutaneous or discoid lupus, lupus panniculitis, subacute cutaneous lupus, and neonatal lupus (see Fig. 2.89).

Discoid lupus lesions are the most common skin rash found in childhood SLE. This eruption is characterized by red, coin-shaped plaques 0.5–5 cm in diameter, with central

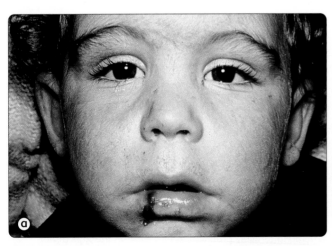

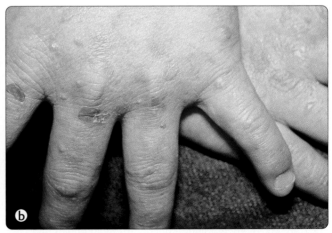

Fig 7.39 Congenital erythropoietic porphyria. Severe photosensitivity from accumulation of cutaneous porphyrins results in recurrent blistering and scarring in sun-exposed areas.

(a) Note scarring, erosions, and hirsutism on his face and (b) scarring with milia formation on his hands.

atrophy and hypopigmentation, and peripheral hyperpigmentation (Fig 7.41). Adherent scale, follicular plugging, and telangiectasias, especially in areas of atrophy, may be prominent. Although these plaques may develop on any area, sunexposed sites, which include the face (in a malar distribution), scalp, ears, neck, upper trunk, and extensor surfaces of the arms are most commonly involved. Discoid lesions may be the sole cutaneous finding in SLE. However, when discoid lesions occur without systemic disease, the disorder is referred to as benign cutaneous or discoid lupus erythematosus (DLE). About 15–20% of patients with DLE eventually go on to develop SLE. These patients must be counseled and followed

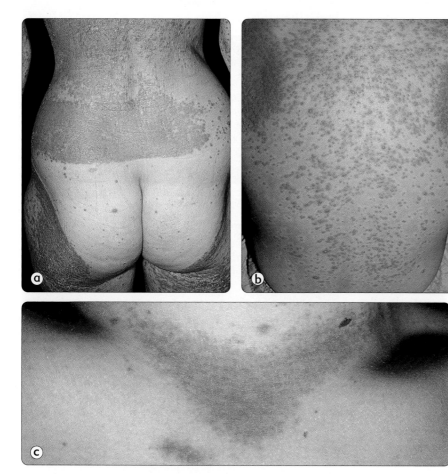

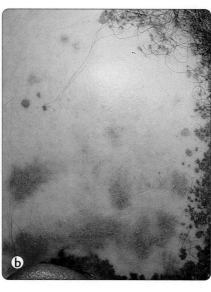

Fig 7.40 Photoexacerbated conditions. (a) This young woman with psoriasis developed recurrent skin lesions in sun-exposed areas after a sunburn (Koebner phenomenon). (b) Photoexacerbation was evident in this child with varicella. The bathing trunk area was relatively spared. (c) For this woman, vasculitic plaques of Henoch–Schönlein purpura erupted in sun-exposed sites.

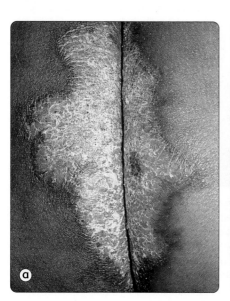

Fig 7.41 Discoid lupus erythematosus. (a) An atrophic, scaly, red plaque with a hyperpigmented border in the gluteal cleft showed histologic changes typical of lupus. (b) Atrophy, depigmentation, scarring alopecia, and telangiectasias persisted in an old lesion.

accordingly. Discoid plaques may progress and heal with extensive scarring. Topical corticosteroids, systemic corticosteroids, and antimalarial drugs are the mainstay of therapy, depending on the severity of the systemic disease. Topical retinoids have been used to remodel scars and treat hyperpigmentation when lesions go into remission.

Other cutaneous findings in SLE include red, edematous, malar rashes, diffuse, annular, psoriasis-like plaques in sun-exposed areas (subacute cutaneous lupus erythematosus), scarring and nonscarring scalp hair loss, nail fold telangiectasias, livedo reticularis, and palpable purpura that results from small vessel vasculitis (Fig 7.42). Severe Raynaud phenomenon with digital infarcts may also develop. Mucous membranes can be involved, with nasal and oral ulcerations and painful erosions on the lip.

In addition to cutaneous features, the most common presenting complaints in SLE are fevers and arthralgias. Other common findings include pulmonary disease (pleuritis, pneumonitis – 66%), cardiac manifestations (pericarditis, myocarditis, endocarditis – 50%), lupus nephritis (60%), and central nervous system disease (50%).

Serologic findings may be very useful in establishing the diagnosis (Fig 7.43). Almost 100% of patients with SLE have a positive ANA. The rate of positivity varies, however, with the substrate used for the test. In the past, a subset of SLE patients were identified as ANA negative. Many of these patients have subsequently tested positive using Hep 2 cells, which are derived from a human tumor line, as a substrate. Although there is no direct correlation between ANA titers and disease activity, patients with high-titer ANAs tend to have active SLE. A number of other antibodies are also found in lupus patients and may correlate with certain aspects of disease activity. One of these antibody systems, Ro (SSA) and La (SSB), which is directed against a small, cytoplasmic ribonuclear protein, is associated with photosensitivity, neonatal lupus, and subacute cutaneous lupus erythematosus. Ro and La are also found in Sjögren syndrome in the absence of SLE. Patients with photosensitivity should be counseled about sunscreens, protective clothing, and judicious sun exposure. Occasionally, systemic disease can be triggered by excessive sun exposure.

The symptoms of juvenile rheumatoid arthritis (JRA) may suggest the diagnosis of lupus (Fig 7.44). However, the rash of JRA is urticarial and evanescent, peaking with fever spikes. Unlike the destructive arthritis of JRA, the arthritis in lupus is often transient and does not impair function. Many of the other reactive erythemas may share features with lupus. However, the diagnosis of lupus is dependent on clearly defined criteria.

Dermatomyositis

Dermatomyositis (DM) accounts for only 5% of pediatric collagen vascular disease. However, cutaneous lesions are distinctive and mark the onset of nonsuppurative inflammation in the muscle. Unlike the adult variant, DM in childhood is self-limiting and not associated with underlying malignancy. Unfortunately, calcinosis cutis, which follows the disease, can be debilitating.

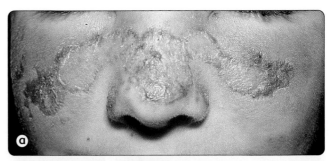

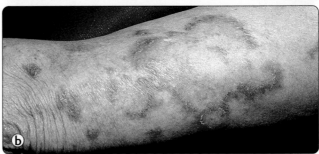

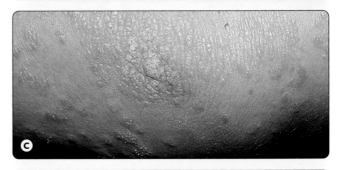

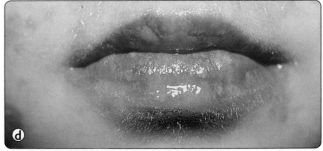

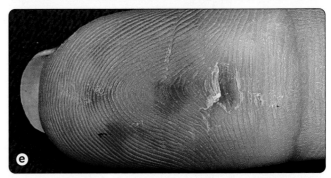

Fig 7.42 Lupus erythematosus. **(a)** A 13-year-old girl with systemic lupus erythematosus developed malar erythema, edema, and erosions associated with a flare of nephritis after spending a day in the sun at the beach. Other lesions typical of lupus include **(b)** annular, scaly patches and plaques, **(c)** psoriasis-like plaques, **(d)** erosions on the oral mucosa and vermilion border, and **(e)** Raynaud phenomenon with digital infarcts.

	Designation	Subtype	Antigen	Frequently associated disease states
Antinuclear antibodies	dsDNA		Double-stranded DNA	Lupus erythematosus, nephritis
	ssDNA		Single-stranded DNA	Lupus erythematosus, other nonrheumatic diseases
	ENA		Extractable nuclear antigen	Subtypes as below
		Sm	RNAase-resistant glycoprotein (U1, U2, U4, U5, and U6 small ribonucleoproteins)	Lupus erythematosus, nephritis
		RNP	RNAase-sensitive ribonucleoprotein (U1 small ribonucleoprotein)	Lupus erythematosus, discoid lupus erythematosus; mixed connective tissue disease, Raynaud phenomenon
		Leukocyte specific		Rheumatoid arthritis, Felty syndrome
	SSC (RAP)		Trypsin-sensitive protein	Rheumatoid arthritis
	RANA			Rheumatoid arthritis
	NANA		Nucleolar ANA	Systemic sclerosis
	PM-1 (Mi)		Trypsin-sensitive protein	Polydermatomyositis
	DNP		DNA-histone	Drug-induced lupus erythematosus; rheumatoid arthritis; lupus erythematosus
	Centromere		Kinetochore	Calcinosis cutis, Raynaud phenomenon, esophageal dysfunction, sclerodactyly, telangiectasia (CREST) syndrome
	Centriole		Centriole	Sclerosis–Raynaud phenomenon
	Scl-70		Nonhistone nuclear protein	Systemic sclerosis, CREST syndrome
Anticytoplasmic antibodies	ssRNA		Single-stranded RNA	Systemic sclerosis
	Ro (SSA)		Acidic glycoprotein	Lupus erythematosus, photosensitivity, Sjögren syndrome
	Ribosomal		Ribosome	Lupus erythematosus
	La (SSB)		RNA-protein	Lupus erythematosus, Sjögren syndrome

Antinuclear and anticytoplasmic antibodies in collagen vascular disorders

Fig 7.43 Antinuclear and anticytoplasmic antibodies in collagen vascular disorders. (Adapted from Dahl MV, *Clinical Immunology*. Yearbook Medical Publishers, Chicago, 1988, pp. 243.)

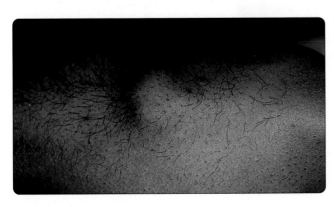

Fig 7.44 Rheumatoid nodule. This adolescent girl developed rheumatoid factor positive rheumatoid arthritis and systemic lupus erythematosus. The painless nodules appeared on her forearms.

Most cases of childhood DM occur between 4 and 12 years of age. As in lupus, there is a 2:1 female predominance. There is no known inheritance pattern or racial predisposition.

Cutaneous findings may precede myositis for over a year, and the onset of signs and symptoms is usually insidious. Conversely, progressive, symmetric proximal muscle weakness may precede the rash by months. Patients often complain of easy fatigability with routine tasks such as brushing teeth, combing hair, and climbing steps. Muscle tenderness may be accompanied by anorexia, malaise, and fever. Dysphagia, dysphonia, and dyspnea occur in 10% of patients and signal palatal, esophageal, and thoracic involvement.

Nearly 75% of children with DM develop a diagnostic rash. Periorbital findings include a periorbital dermatitis, with or without edema, which gives a violaceous hue and is known as heliotrope (Fig 7.45). A psoriasis-like rash involves the extensor surfaces of the elbows, knees, and knuckles (Fig 7.46). When over the distal interphalangeal joints these changes are referred to as Gottron papules. A malar rash reminiscent of lupus is variably present. Periungual and facial telangiectasias may become prominent. Atrophy, fibrosis, hypopigmentation, and hyperpigmentation progress gradually, which results in poikiloderma like salt and pepper.

Up to 50% of children with DM develop dystrophic calcification in skin and muscle, probably secondary to necrosis and scarring of the involved tissues (Fig 7.47). In some patients, painful, chronic ulceration of calcified nodules, recurrent cellulitis, and progressive contractures continue to limit recovery, even after active inflammation resolves. Complications may also occasionally result from gastrointestinal, cardiac, and pulmonary involvement. Treatment consists of aggressive use of systemic corticosteroids and physical therapy to preserve muscle function. In severe cases, methotrexate or other immunosuppressives may be required. Persistent, widespread telangiectasias and calcinosis cutis are resistant to therapy.

Clinical diagnosis is usually confirmed by detecting elevated muscle enzymes, typical electromyographic findings, and muscle biopsy. In DM, as in lupus, the inflammatory process targets blood vessels in the involved tissues. Skin biopsies from the heliotrope rash, Gottron papules, and the psoriasiform dermatitis demonstrate perivascular and dermal–epidermal junction changes indistinguishable from those of lupus.

Scleroderma

Although scleroderma is uncommon, accounting for only 5% of collagen vascular disease in childhood, the most common variant, localized scleroderma or morphea, can be very subtle and is probably underdiagnosed.

Localized morphea can present in a plaque, linear, guttate, or generalized pattern (Fig 7.48). Sclerotic plaques with an ivory-white center and an advancing lilac-colored border characterize scleroderma. During the course hyperpigmentation may also be marked. In the most common form one or several lesions from 1 to 10 cm in diameter appear on the trunk. In generalized morphea, similar widespread lesions develop on the trunk and extremities. Occasionally, multiple, small, oval lesions reminiscent of lichen sclerosis et atropicus erupt on the upper trunk in the guttate variant. Morphea can also progress in a linear pattern, particularly on the scalp, face, and extremities. Coup de sabre describes a subset of linear morphea cases in which a furrow extends vertically from the scalp across the forehead and down the face. Involvement of the underlying soft tissue and bone may result in severe disfigurement. Over months to years, lesions heal with softening of the involved areas and atrophy. In children, cutaneous disease with no systemic symptoms is not associated with progression to systemic sclerosis.

Laboratory findings in localized scleroderma are not specific or prognostic. Occasionally, eosinophilia is present on a complete blood count, and rheumatoid factor may be elevated. In 10–15% of cases, ANAs are present. Skin biopsies from new

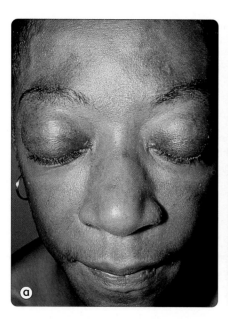

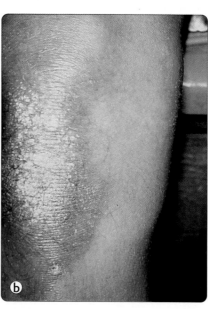

Fig 7.45 Dermatomyositis. **(a)** Heliotrope. A young women with dermatomyositis presented with violaceous erythema and edema of the upper eye lids. **(b)** A 10-year-old boy with a psoriasis-like dermatitis on the elbows and knees for 6 months developed rapidly progressive proximal muscle weakness.

lesions or from the advancing borders of established lesions show lymphocytic inflammation between collagen bundles and around blood vessels in the deep dermis, which extends into the subcutis. Some areas of fat may be replaced by newly formed collagen. In late sclerotic plaques, thick, homogeneous collagen extends from the dermal–epidermal junction into the subcutaneous tissue. Adnexal structures appear to be enveloped in collagen, and little if any inflammatory infiltrate remains.

Unfortunately, therapy has been disappointing. The use of penicillamine, even in severe localized disease, is controversial. Short courses of high-dose corticosteroids (1–2 mg/kg/day) may help to shut off rapidly progressive linear morphea when it endangers important structures. Physical therapy may be necessary when lesions extend across joints.

Progressive systemic sclerosis

Progressive systemic sclerosis (PSS) is rare in childhood, and clinically the course is similar to that of adult cases. Raynaud phenomenon is present in 90% of patients and may precede the onset of systemic disease by years. Classic findings in the skin include tightening of the skin associated with woody induration, edema, and pigmentary changes. Life-threatening disease in the gastrointestinal tract, musculoskeletal system, heart, lungs, and kidneys may result from PSS. Most patients with PSS develop ANAs, and nearly 50% have antinucleolar antibodies. A number of other antibody systems are also present in some cases of PSS and may have special prognostic value.

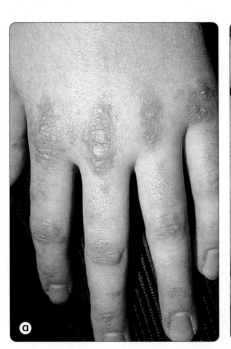

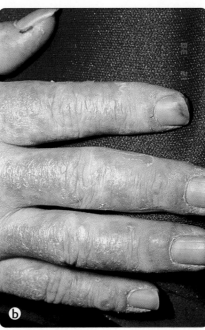

Fig 7.46 Gottron papules **(a)** in a child with dermatomyositis are contrasted with **(b)** a psoriasis-like dermatitis on the hands of a patient with systemic lupus erythematosus. Note the sparing of the knuckles in lupus.

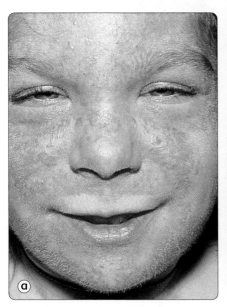

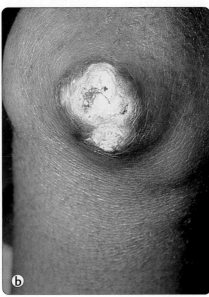

Fig 7.47 Dermatomyositis. **(a)** Despite resolution of cutaneous inflammation and myositis with systemic corticosteroids, telangiectasias progressed on the face of this 6-year-old girl. **(b)** Extensive cutis calcinosis, particularly over bony prominences, resulted in chronic, painful, draining ulcers and cellulitis in this 12-year-old boy with burned-out dermatomyositis. Note the white, chalk-like calcium deposits at the base of an ulcer on his knee.

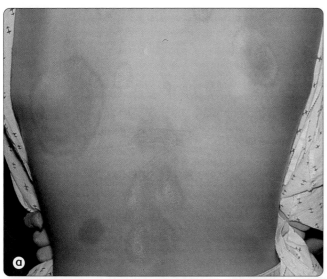

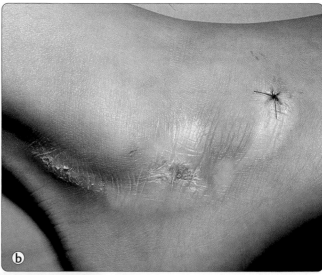

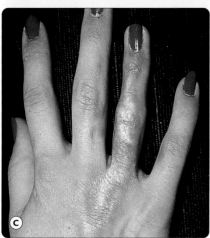

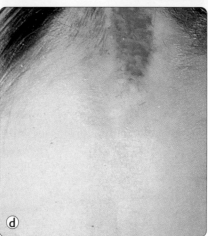

Fig 7.48 Scleroderma. **(a)** Multiple, fibrotic plaques with central pigmentary changes and peripheral erythema slowly enlarged on the back of an adolescent girl. **(b)** An atrophic, fibrotic, hypopigmented plaque extended around the ankle of a 10-year-old girl for 2 years. Fortunately, she did not experience functional impairment. **(c)** Linear morphea produced fibrosis and atrophy of the soft tissue of this young woman's right fourth finger. **(d)** An unusual variant of morphea that affects the scalp, coup de sabre (stroke of the saber), extends from the midfrontal scalp down the forehead to the nasal bridge.

Lichen sclerosis et atrophicus

Lichen sclerosis et atrophicus (LSA) occurs most commonly in postmenopausal women. However, about 10% of cases appear in children under 7 years old. Although the cause is unknown, the association with morphea suggests an immunologic basis.

The anogenital area is the most common site of involvement. Typically, small, white, flat-topped papules arise on the cutaneous and mucous membrane surfaces of the labia, perineum, and perianal area. Confluent, white, atrophic patches may extend symmetrically in a figure-of-eight pattern around the vagina and rectum (Fig 7.49). Scaling, vesiculation, and hemorrhage may be prominent, particularly after accidental trauma or rubbing and scratching from pruritus. A mild, watery discharge may be present. In some patients, extragenital patches on the trunk and extremities predominate (Fig 7.50). In these lesions, follicular dimpling caused by hyperkeratosis with follicular plugging is characteristic. Truncal patches also share clinical and histologic features with morphea, and lesions typical of both entities have been described simultaneously in the same patients.

Histopathologic findings are often diagnostic. In addition to scale and follicular plugging, thinning of the mid epidermis,

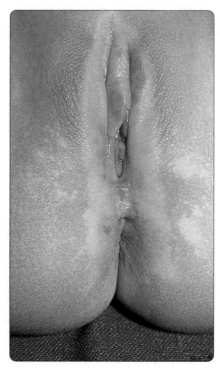

Fig 7.49 Lichen sclerosis et atrophicus. A pruritic, atrophic, eroded, hypopigmented patch involved the anogenital skin and mucous membranes in this 5-year-old girl.

hydropic degeneration of the basal layer, edema and homogenization of the upper dermis, and a band-like lymphohistiocytic infiltrate beneath the zone of homogenization are observed.

Clinically, LSA must not be confused with child abuse, candidiasis, or streptococcal perianal or vaginal dermatitis. Cultures may be obtained to exclude bacterial and herpetic infections. The symmetric pattern and characteristic morphology of LSA also help to eliminate child abuse as a serious consideration. In vitiligo, which may also present in a symmetric pattern in the anogenital area, the skin is completely normal except for depigmentation (Fig 7.51). Inflammatory bowel disease may present with vaginal and perianal nodules, sinus tracts, and ulcers (Fig 7.52). Other symptoms of gastrointestinal disease may be absent. Skin biopsies in these cases demonstrate granulomas typical of Crohn disease. Primary bullous dermatoses may also present a diagnostic dilemma. If the clinical presentation is not distinctive, a skin biopsy with direct immunofluorescence may be necessary to make the diagnosis.

Necrobiosis lipoidica

In necrobiosis lipoidica, reddish–yellow, indurated plaques typically appear on the shins in diabetics (Fig 7.53). As the lesions expand from less than 1 cm to 4 cm in diameter or larger over months, the center of the plaque becomes shiny and atrophic. Telangiectasias extend from the center. Although lesions may remain stable and occasionally heal without treatment, most persist or slowly progress, and minor trauma may result in chronic, painful ulcerations. Some patients improve with topical or intralesional corticosteroids injected into the expanding red border.

About 75% of patients with necrobiosis lipiodica are female and over half have diabetes mellitus (necrobiosis lipoidica diabeticorum). In some cases, necrobiosis lipiodica precedes the onset of clinical diabetes by years. Although the cause is unknown, investigators have suggested that some sort of vascular insult triggered by diabetes initiates the necrobiotic changes in collagen. Histologically, granulomatous inflammation is observed around altered and degenerating collagen, which extends in large bands into the deep reticular dermis. The overlying epidermis is atrophic and ulceration may be present. Thickening of vascular walls, endothelial cell proliferation, and occasionally vascular occlusion are seen throughout the dermis. The yellow color is imparted by deposition of lipid around necrobiotic collagen.

Necrobiosis lipoidica is usually differentiated from granuloma annulare, which does not develop epidermal changes. In some patients, fibrotic or atrophic plaques in scleroderma or LSA mimic necrobiosis. The clinical course and skin biopsy findings, however, are distinctive. One third of juvenile diabetics develop diffuse, nonpitting, waxy edema of the hands during the first two decades of life (Fig 7.54). Although this process may be associated with progressive joint contractures, distinctive cutaneous lesions, atrophy, and pigmentary changes do not occur. Histology demonstrates increased dermal collagen, which is thought to be caused by increased glycosylation of the proteins in the collagen matrix and by dermal fibroblast proliferation.

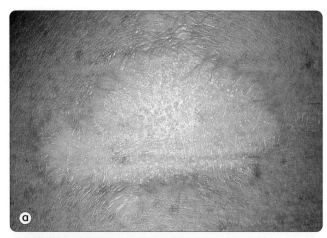

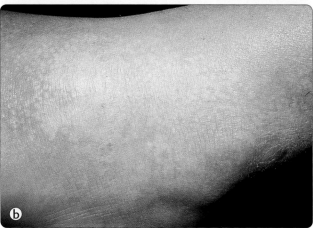

Fig 7.50 Lichen sclerosis et atrophicus. Atrophic, hypopigmented, scaly papules coalesced into confluent patches on **(a)** the trunk and **(b)** extremities of a 10-year-old girl.

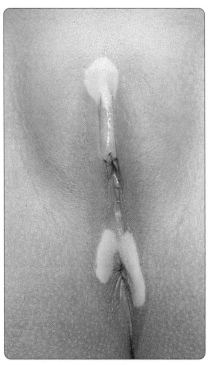

Fig 7.51 Vitiligo developed around the vagina and anus of a 2-year-old girl, mimicking the pattern of lichen sclerosis et atrophicus.

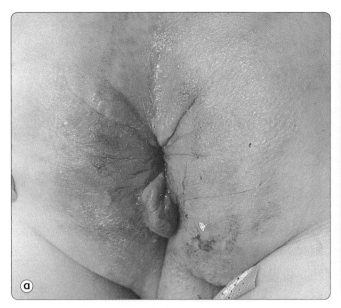

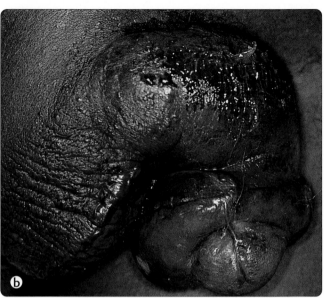

Fig 7.52 Inflammatory bowel disease. **(a)** A 2-year-old girl was treated for chronic diaper dermatitis and candidiasis for months before the diagnosis of Crohn disease was considered. A biopsy of the perianal skin showed granulomas.

(b) This 10-year-old boy had nontender swelling of the penis for almost a year before the diagnosis of Crohn disease was made. Granulomas were noted on biopsy of his penis and colon.

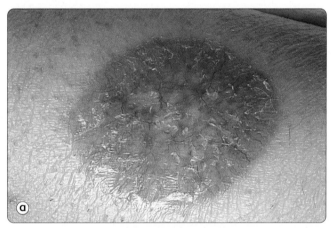

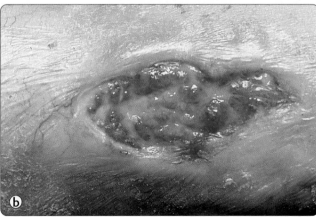

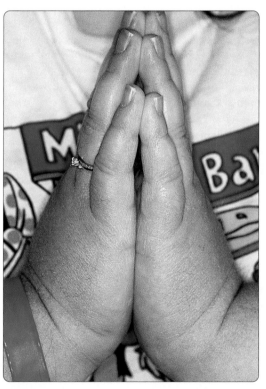

Fig 7.53 Necrobiosis lipoidica. **(a)** A plaque on the shin of a 17-year-old diabetic demonstrates the typical red border and yellow, shiny, atrophic center with telangiectasias.
(b) This patient developed a chronic, painful ulcer after repeated trauma. The ulcer healed after several months of treatment with occlusive dressings.

Fig 7.54 Prayer sign. This 16-year-old Type I diabetic developed progressive, waxy, nonpitting edema of her hands, associated with joint contractures.

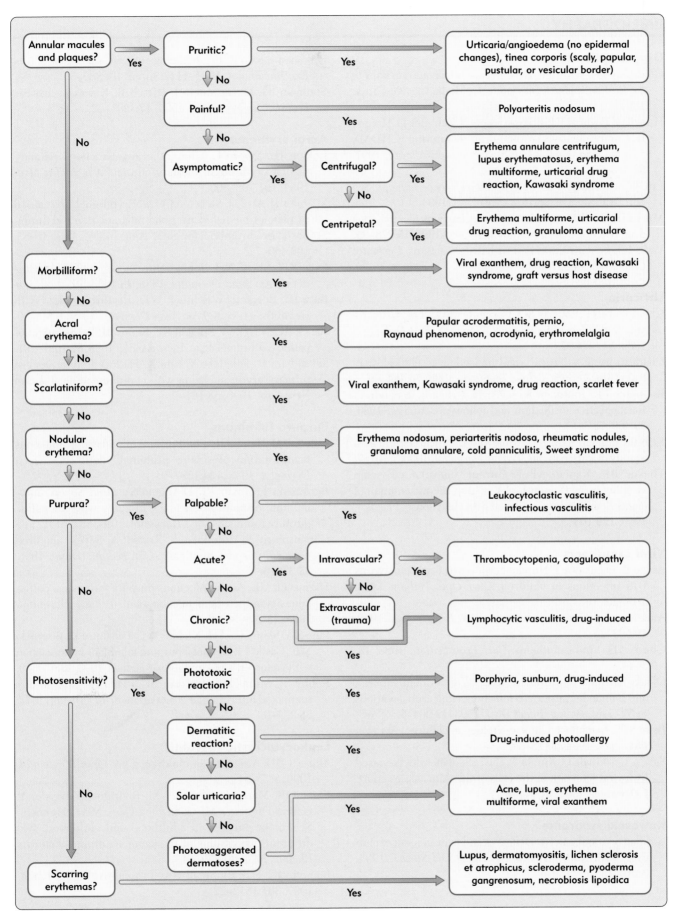

Algorithm for evaluation of reactive erythema.

BIBLIOGRAPHY

Drug eruptions

Goldstein SM, Wintroub BU. *Adverse cutaneous reactions to medication, a physician's guide.* CoMedia Inc, New York, 1994.

Hunziker T, Kunzi UP, Braunschweig S, Zehnder D, Hoigne R. Comprehensive hospital drug monitoring (CHDM): adverse skin reactions, a 20 year survey. *Allergy.* 1997, **52**:388–93.

Litt JZ, Pawlak WA. *Drug eruption reference manual*, 3rd edn. Wal-zac Enterprises, Cleveland, 1994.

Merk HF, Hertl M. Immunologic mechanisms of cutaneous drug reactions. *Semin Cutan Med Surg.* 1996, **15**:228–35.

Parks ET. Lesions associated with drug reactions. *Dermatol Clin.* 1996, **14**:327–37.

Urticaria

Champion RH, Roberts SO, Carpenter RG, *et al.* Urticaria and angioedema. A review of 554 cases. *Br J Dermatol.* 1969, **81**:588–97.

Charlesworth EN. Urticaria and angioedema: a clinical spectrum. *Ann Allergy Asthma Immunol.* 1996, **76**:484–99.

Kauppinen K, Juntunen K, Lanki H. Urticaria in children. Retrospective evaluation and follow-up. *Allergy.* 1984, **39**:469–72.

Legrain V, Taieb A, Sage T, Maleville J. Urticaria in infants: a study of forty patients. *Pediatr Dermatol.* 1990, **7**:101–7.

Thakur BK, Kaplan AP. Recurrent 'unexplained' scalp swelling in an 18-month-old: an atypical presentation of angioedema causing confusion with child abuse. *J Pediatr.* 1996, **129**:163–5.

Viral exanthems

Asano Y, Yoshikawa T. Human herpesvirus 6 and parvovirus B19 infections in children. *Curr Opin Pediatr.* 1993, **5**:14–20.

Anderson LJ. Human parvovirus B19. *Pediatr Ann.* 1990, **19**:509–16.

Cherry JD. Viral exanthems. *Curr Prob Pediatr.* 1983, **13**:5–44.

Okada K, Ueda K, Kusuhara K, *et al.* Exanthem subitum and human herpesvirus 6 infection: clinical observations in 57 cases. *Pediatr Infect Dis J.* 1993, **12**:204–8.

Ryan ME, Leichter J. Clinical virology in children. *Am Fam Physician.* 1994, **50**:78–84.

Sata T, Urishibata O, Kurata T. The rash of measles is caused by a viral infection in the cells of the skin: a case report. *J Dermatol.* 1994, **21**:741–5.

Kawasaki syndrome

Gidding SS, Shulman ST. Diagnosis and management of children with Kawasaki disease. *Heart Dis Stroke.* 1994, **3**:210–15.

Pelkonen P, Salo E. Epidemiology of Kawasaki disease. *Clin Exp Rheumatol.* 1994, **1112**(Suppl. 10):S83–5.

Shulman ST, DeInocencio J, Hirsch R. Kawasaki disease. *Pediatr Clin North Am.* 1995, **42**:1205–22.

Acral erythema

Lokich JL, Moore C. Chemotherapy-associated palmar–plantar erythrodysesthesia syndrome. *Ann Intern Med.* 1984, **101**:798–800.

Michiels JJ, Abels J, Steketee J, *et al.* Erythromelalgia caused by platelet-mediated arteriolar inflammation and thrombosis in thrombocytopenia. *Ann Intern Med.* 1985, **102**:466–71.

Page EH, Shear NH. Temperature-dependent skin disorders. *J Am Acad Dermatol.* 1988, **18**:1003–19.

Ratz JL, Bergfeld WF, Steck WD. Erythromelalgia with vasculitis: a review. *J Am Acad Dermatol.* 1979, **1**:443–50.

Rauck RL, Naveira F, Speight KL, Smith BP. Refractory idiopathic erythromelalgia. *Anesth Analg.* 1996, **82**:1097–101.

Sakakibara R, Fukutake T, Kita K, Hattori T. Treatment of primary erythromelalgia with cyproheptadine. *J Auton Nerv Syst.* 1996, **58**:121–2.

Purpura fulminans

Auletta MJ, Headington JT. Purpura fulminans. A cutaneous manifestation of severe protein C deficiency. *Arch Dermatol.* 1988, **124**:1387–91.

Bergmann F, Hoyer PF, D'Angelo SV, *et al.* Severe autoimmune protein S deficiency in a boy with idiopathic purpura fulminans. *Br J Haematol.* 1995, **89**:610–4.

Chuansumrit A, Hotrakitya S, Kruavit A. Severe acquired neonatal purpura fulminans. *Clin Pediatr (Phila).* 1996, **35**:373–6.

Darmstadt GL. Acute infectious purpura fulminans: pathogenesis and medical management. *Pediatr Dermatol.* 1998, **15**:169–83.

Pipe SW, Schmaier AH, Nichols WC, Ginsburg D, Bozynski ME, Castle VP. Neonatal purpura fulminans in association with factor VR506Q mutation. *J Pediatr.* 1996, **128**:706–9.

Robby SJ, Mihm MC, Colman RC, *et al.* The skin in disseminated intravascular coagulation. *Br J Dermatol.* 1973, **88**:221–9.

Leukocytoclastic vasculitis

Athreya BH. Vasculitis in children. *Curr Opin Rheumatol.* 1996, **8**:77–84.

Blanc OR, Martinez-Taboada VM, Rodriguez-Valverder V, Garcia-Fuentex M, Gonzalez-Gay MA. Henoch–Schönlein purpura in adulthood and childhood: two different expressions of the same syndrome. *Arthritis Rheum.* 1997, **40**:859–64.

Jennette JC, Falk RJ. Small-vessel vasculitis. *N Engl J Med.* 1997, **337**:1512–22.

Jessop SJ. Cutaneous leucocytoclastic vasculitis: a clinical and aetiological study. *Br J Dermatol.* 1995, **34**:942–5.

Salisbury FT. Henoch–Schönlein purpura. *Pediatr Dermatol.* 1984, **1**:195–208.

Sharieff GQ, Francis K, Kuppermann N. Atypical presentation of Henoch–Schönlein purpura in two children. *Am J Emerg Med.* 1997, **15**:375–7.

Polyarteritis nodosa

Jones SK, Lane AT, Golitz LE, Weston WL. Cutaneous periarteritis nodosa in a child. *Am J Dis Child.* 1985, **139**:920–2.

Kumar L, Thapa BR, Sarkar B, Walia BN. Benign cutaneous polyarteritis nodosa in children below 10 years of age – a clinical experience. *Ann Rheum Dis.* 1995, **54**:134–6.

Ozen S, Besbas N, Saatci U, Bakkaloglu. Diagnostic criteria for polyarteritis nodosa in childhood. *J Pediatr.* 1992, **120**:307–14.

Siberry GK, Cohen BA, Johnson B. Cutaneous polyarteritis nodosa. Report of cases in children and review of the literature. *Arch Dermatol.* 1994, **130**:884–9.

Ecthyma gangrenosum

Doriff GI, Geimer NF, Rosenthal DR, *et al. Pseudomonas* septicemia. Illustrated evolution of its skin lesion. *Arch Intern Med.* 1971, **128**:591–5.

Secord E, Mills C, Shah B, Tunnessen WW Jr. Picture of the month. Ecthyma gangrenosum. *Am J Dis Child.* 1993, **147**:795–6.

Progressive pigmented purpuric dermatosis

Kano Y, Hirayama K, Orihara M, Shiohara T. Successful treatment of Schamberg disease with pentoxifylline. *J Am Acad Dermatol.* 1997, **36**:827–30.

Newton RC, Raimer SS. Pigmented purpuric eruptions. *Dermatol Clin.* 1985, 3:165–9.

Price ML, Jones EW, Calnan CD, MacDonald DM. Lichen aureus: a localized persistent form of pigmented purpuric dermatitis. *Br J Dermatol.* 1985, **112**:307–14.

Sweet syndrome

Boatman BW, Taylor RC, Klein LE, Cohen BA. Sweet syndrome in children. *South Med J.* 1994, **87**:193–6.

Hazen PG, Kark EC, Davis BR, *et al.* Acute febrile neutrophilic dermatosis in children: report of two cases in male infants. *Arch Dermatol.* 1983, **119**:998–1002.

Itami S, Nishioka K. Sweet syndrome in infancy. *Br J Dermatol.* 1980, **103**:449–51.

Levin DL, Esterly NB, Herman JJ, Boxall LB. The Sweet syndrome in children. *J Pediatr.* 1981, **99**:73–8.

Seidel D, Huguet P, Lebbe C, Donadieu J, Odievre M, Labrun P. Sweet syndrome as the presenting manifestation of chronic granulomatous disease in an infant. *Pediatr Dermatol.* 1994, **11**:237–40.

Pyoderma gangrenosum

Gilman AL, Cohen BA, Wrbach AH, Blatt J. Pyoderma gangrenosum a manifestation of leukemia in children. *Pediatrics.* 1988, **81**:846–8.

Hayani A, Steuber CP, Mahoney DH, Levy ML. Pyoderma gangrenosum in childhood leukemia. *Pediatr Dermatol.* 1990, **7**:296–8.

Leon JT, Atherton MT, Byrne JP. Neutrophilic dermatoses: pyoderma gangrenosum and Sweet syndrome. *Postgrad Med J.* 1997, **73**:65–8.

Figurate erythema

Berger BW. Lyme disease. *Semin Dermatol.* 1993, **12**:357–62.

Bressler GS, Jones RE. Erythema annulare centrifugum. *J Am Acad Dermatol.* 1981, 4:597–602.

Gerber MA, Shapiro ED, Burke GS, Parcells VJ, Ball GL. Lyme disease in southeastern Connecticut. Pediatric Lyme disease study group. *N Engl J Med.* 1996, **335**:1270–4.

Sahn EE, Maize JC, Silver RM. Erythema marginatum: an unusual histopathologic manifestation. *J Am Acad Dermatol.* 1989, **21**:145–7.

Shapiro ED. Lyme disease in children. *Am J Med.* 1995, **98(4A)**:69S–73S.

Panniculitis

Crowson AN, Magro CM. Idiopathic perniosis and its mimics: a clinical and histologic study of 38 cases. *Hum Pathol.* 1997, **28**:478–84.

Koransky JS, Esterly NB. Lupus panniculitis (profundus). *J Pediatr.* 1981, **98**:241–4.

Labbe L, Maleville J, Taieb A. Erythema nodosum in children: a study of 27 patients. *Pediatr Dermatol.* 1996, **13**:447–50.

Rotman H. Cold panniculitis in children. *Arch Dermatol.* 1966, **94**:720–4.

Shuval SJ, Frances A, Valderramo E, Bonajura VR, Ilowite NT. Panniculitis and fever in children. *J Pediatr.* 1993, **122**:372–8.

Ter Poorten JC, Herbert AA, Ilkiw R. Cold panniculitis in a neonate. *J Am Acad Dermatol.* 1995, **33**:383–5.

White WL, Wieselthier JH, Hitchcock MG. Panniculitis: recent developments and observations. *Semin Cutan Med Surg.* 1996, **15**:278–99.

Photosensitivity

Allen JE. Drug induced photosensitivity. *Clin Pharmacol.* 1993, **12**:580–7.

Donauho C, Wolf. Sunburn, sunscreen, and melanoma. *Curr Opin Oncol.* 1996, 8:159–66.

Fotiades J, Soter NA, Lim HW. Results of evaluation of 203 patients for photosensitivity in a 7.3 year period. *J Am Acad Dermatol.* 1995, **33**:597–602.

Gonzalez E, Gonzalez S. Drug photosensitivity, idiopathic photodermatoses, and sunscreens. *J Am Acad Dermatol.* 1996, **35**:871–85.

Harris A, Burge SM, George SA. Solar urticaria in an infant. *Br J Dermatol.* 1997, **136**:105–7.

Stern RS, Weinstein MC, Baker SG. Risk reduction for non-melanoma skin cancer with childhood sunscreen use. *Arch Dermatol.* 1986, **122**:537–45.

Taylor CR, Sober AS. Sun exposure and skin disease. *Ann Rev Med.* 1996, **47**:181–91.

Connective tissue disease

Buckley D, Barnes L. Childhood subacute cutaneous lupus erythematosus associated with a homozygous complement 2 deficiency. *Pediatr Dermatol.* 1995, **12**:327–30.

Christianson HB, Dorsey CS, O'Leary PA, Kierland RRL. Localized scleroderma: a clinical study of 235 cases. *Arch Dermatol.* 1956, **74**:629–39.

Chung HT, Huang JL, Wang HS, Hung PC, Chow ML. Dermatomyositis and polymyositis in childhood. *Acta Paediatr Sin.* 1994, **35**:407–14.

George PM, Tunnessen WW Jr. Childhood discoid lupus erythematosus. *Arch Dermatol.* 1993, **124**:613–17.

Ilowite NT. Childhood systemic lupus erythematosus, dermatomyositis, scleroderma, and systemic vasculitis. *Curr Opin Rheumatol.* 1993, **5**:644–50.

Lee LA, Weston WL. Cutaneous lupus erythematosus during neonatal and childhood periods. *Lupus.* 1997, **6**:132–8.

Lehman TJ. Systemic and localized scleroderma in children. *Curr Opin Rheumatol.* 1996, **8**:576–9.

Nelson AM. Localized forms of scleroderma, including morphea, linear scleroderma, and eosinophilic fasciitis. *Curr Opin Rheumatol.* 1996, **8**:473–6.

Rockerbie NR, Woo TY, Callen JP, Giustina T. Cutaneous changes of dermatomyositis precede muscle weakness. *J Am Acad Dermatol.* 1989, **20**:629–32.

Sansome A, Dubowitz V. Intravenous immunoglobulin in juvenile dermatomyositis – four year review of nine cases. *Arch Dis Child.* 1995, **72**:25–8.

Yokota J. Mixed connective tissue disease in childhood. *Acta Paediatr Jpn.* 1993, **35**:472–9.

Lichen sclerosis et atrophicus

Loening-Baucke V. Lichen sclerosis et atrophicus in children. *Am J Dis Child.* 1991, **145**:1058–61.

Meffert JJ, Davis BM, Grimwood RE. Lichen sclerosis. *J Am Acad Dermatol.* 1995, **32**:393–416.

Meuli M, Briner J, Hanimann B, Sacher P. Lichen sclerosis et atrophicus causing phimosis in boys: a prospective study with 5-year followup after complete circumcision. *J Urol.* 1994, **152**:987–9.

Sahn EE, Bluestein EL, Oliva S. Familial lichen sclerosis et atrophicus in childhood. *Pediatr Dermatol.* 1994, **11**: 160–3.

Necrobiosis lipoidica

Kavanagh GM, Novelli M, Hartog M, Kennedy CT. Necrobiosis lipoidica – involvement of atypical sites. *Clin Exp Dermatol.* 1993, **18**:543–4.

Kelly WF, Nicholas J, Adams J, Mahmood R. Necrobiosis lipoidica diabeticorum: association with background retinopathy, smoking, and proteinuria. A case controlled study. *Diabet Med.* 1993, **10**:725–8.

Ullman S, Dahl MV. Necrobiosis lipoidica. *Arch Dermatol.* 1977, **113**:1671–3.

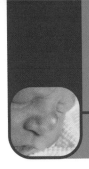

Chapter Eight

Disorders of the Hair and Nails

INTRODUCTION

Diseases of the hair and nails are an important part of pediatric dermatology. Both hair and nails are composed of keratin, produced by the hair follicle and nail matrix. Some diseases are specific to these structures, while others affect the skin and other organ systems as well. In many cases, important diagnostic clues to skin and systemic disease can be found in related abnormalities of the hair and nails.

HAIR DISORDERS

Embryology and anatomy

Hair follicles first appear on the face of the developing fetus at the end of the first trimester. They develop as a down-budding of the epidermis in association with proliferating mesenchyme, which eventually becomes the dermal papilla. The development of scalp and body hair follicles is delayed until about the fourth month. By 17 weeks, emergent hair shafts are found covering the face and at 18 weeks they are over the scalp. The growth of hair shafts occurs in a cephalocaudal direction. No new hair follicles develop, or are follicles destroyed after birth. However, the hair density decreases somewhat as the body surface area increases.

In the premature infant, the scalp, forehead, and trunk are covered by variable amounts of fine, soft, long, lightly pigmented lanugo hair (Fig 8.1). Lanugo is usually shed *in utero* at 7–8 months of gestation. A second covering of subtle lanugo is shed shortly after birth and replaced by short, fine, lightly pigmented vellus hair. Terminal hair is thicker and more darkly pigmented, and usually grows on the scalp, eyebrows, and eyelashes before puberty and the sites of sexual hair after puberty.

At term, most infants have full scalp coverage with normal terminal hair. However, shortly before birth or up to 4 months postnatally, infants undergo a period of brisk shedding when the infantile pattern shifts to a normal adult pattern of hair growth (Fig 8.2). In blondes and red heads the process is often complete before birth, and the hair is sparse at delivery. Shedding may be delayed in dark-haired individuals and may occur rapidly during early infancy. Parents should be reassured that this is a normal physiologic process.

The normal hair cycle consists of a number of components (Fig 8.3). When the hair enters anagen, or the active growth phase, the hair follicle enlarges into the deep dermis, where it surrounds the developing dermal papilla.

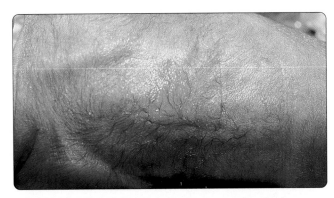

Fig 8.1 Lanugo hair. A 31-week premature infant had extensive lanugo hair that covered most of the back. At term, this hair is usually shed before delivery.

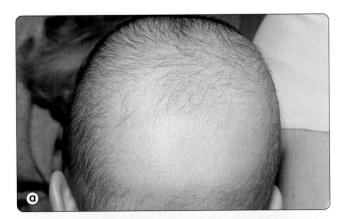

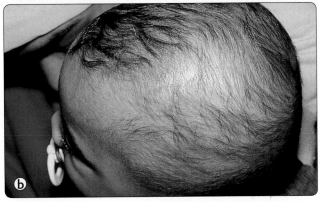

Fig 8.2 Physiologic hair shedding. (a, b) These infants demonstrate the physiologic hair shedding that occurs in dark-haired babies at 3–5 months of age. In (a), note the band of exaggerated alopecia, probably brought on by trauma, that girdles the occiput.

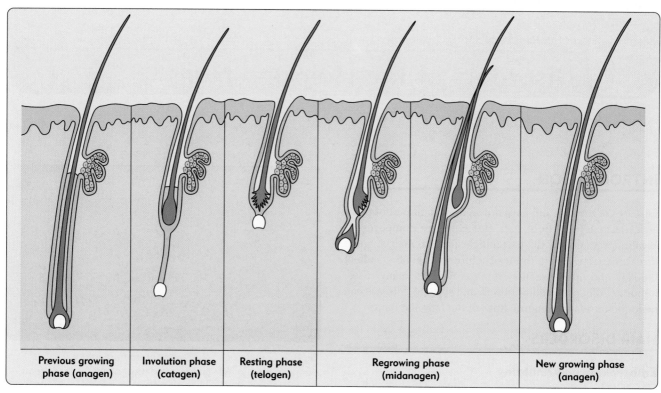

Fig 8.3 Normal hair cycle.

Previous growing phase (anagen)	Involution phase (catagen)	Resting phase (telogen)	Regrowing phase (midanagen)	New growing phase (anagen)

Fig 8.4 Selected hair anomalies.

Selected hair anomalies	
Alopecia (localized)	**Hirsutism (generalized)**
Harmartomatous nevi	Berardinelli lipodystrophy syndrome
Pigmented nevi	Cerebro-oculofacio skeletal syndrome
Halo scalp ring	Coffin–Siris syndrome
Incontinentia pigmenti	Fetal hydantoin syndrome
Aplasia cutis congenita	Frontometaphyseal dysplasia
	Mucopolysaccharidoses
Hirsutism (localized)	Leprechaunism
	Marshall–Smith syndrome
Congenital pigmented nevus	Trisomy 18
Congenital smooth muscle and pilar hamartoma	Schinzel–Giedion syndrome
	Fetal alcohol syndrome
Alopecia (generalized)	**Hair shaft anomalies**
Hypohidrotic ectodermal dysplasia	
Congenital hemidysplasia with ichthyosiform	Pili torti (twisted hair)
erythroderma and limb defects (CHILD) syndrome	Björnstad syndrome
Clouston syndrome	Trichothiodystrophy
Cockayne syndrome	Menkes syndrome
Dyskeratosis congenita	Monilethrix (beaded hair)
Hallermann–Streiff syndrome	Trichorrhexis nodosa
Hay–Wells syndrome	Argininosuccinicaciduria
Homocystinuria	Trichorrhexis invaginata (bamboo hair)
Menkes syndrome	Netherton syndrome
Oculodentodigital syndrome	Kinky hair
Progeria	Trichodento-osseous syndrome
Trichorhinophalangeal syndrome	Uncombable hair syndrome
Trichothiodystrophy	Woolly hair nevus
Cartilage–hair hypoplasia	
Papillon–Lefèvre syndrome	
Acrodermatitis enteropathica	

Matrix cells proliferate and migrate into the upper part of the bulb to form the hair shaft. The length of anagen is genetically determined and varies by anatomic location. Anagen in the scalp varies from 2 to 3 years. Catagen is a transitional phase, which lasts about 3 weeks, during which matrix cell growth ceases and the end of the hair bulb shrinks, forms a club shape, and rises up the hair follicle. Finally, during telogen, the hair is attached to the upper portion of the hair follicle for 3–4 months before being shed. Telogen hairs are pushed out by the new anagen hair shafts that arise from the base of the follicle.

In the newborn, scalp hair growth is synchronous, with all hairs in a given area in the same phase of the hair cycle. Between 4 months and about 2 years of age, the normal dyssynchronous pattern becomes established. In this adult pattern, approximately 85–90% of hairs in any given location are in anagen, 10–15% in telogen, and fewer than 1% in catagen.

Congenital and hereditary disorders

The normal pattern of hair growth and shaft morphology may be disturbed in a number of hereditary disorders and congenital syndromes (Fig 8.4).

Localized patches of alopecia may be associated with perinatal trauma or hamartomatous malformations (Fig 8.5). In halo scalp ring, transient hair loss or permanent scarring results from local edema and vascular compromise produced by trauma to the scalp during labor. Scarring alopecia is a frequent complication of aplasia cutis congenita and incontinentia pigmenti, in which localized vasospasm, thrombosis, or vasculitis results in necrosis and ulceration of the skin. A

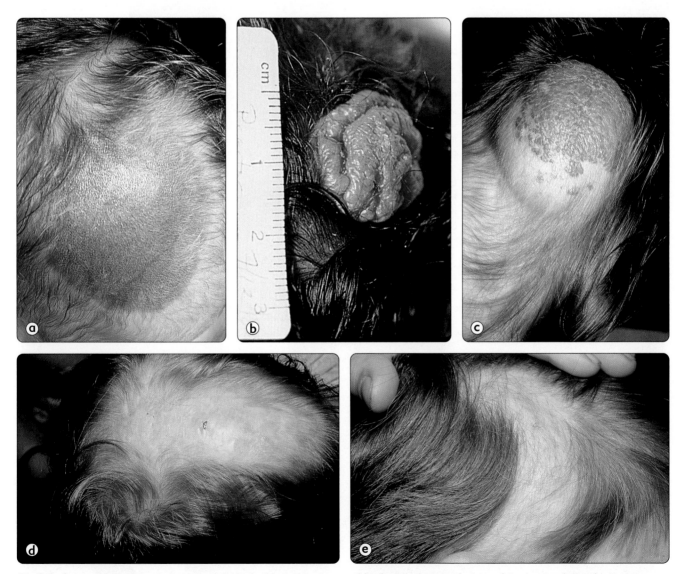

Fig 8.5 Congenital localized alopecia. **(a)** Marked hair thinning was present in a congenital pigmented nevus on the scalp. At 12 months of age, the hair overlying the nevus was sparse, dark, long, and coarse. **(b)** An area of complete alopecia was noted at birth in a cerebriform nevus sebaceous. **(c)** A 1-year-old infant had sparse hair overlying an involuting hemangioma on the scalp. **(d)** A patch of permanent, scarring alopecia extended across the mid-scalp of a child with amniotic band syndrome. **(e)** An arcuate patch of sparse hair above the ear marked the site of an epidermal nevus in an adolescent boy.

number of nevi, such as hemangiomas, epidermal nevi, pigmented nevi, and connective tissue nevi, may also interrupt normal hair-growth patterns.

Generalized sparse or abnormal hair growth suggests an inherited hair-shaft anomaly or genodermatosis (Figs 8.6 and 8.7). Monilethrix is a relatively common developmental hair defect that results in brittle, beaded hair (Fig 8.8). The condition is autosomal dominant, and clinical manifestations usually appear after 2–3 months of age, when vellus hairs are replaced by abnormal, beaded hairs. Although the scalp is most severely affected, hair on any area of the body may be involved. The condition persists throughout life, but may improve in adolescence or adulthood.

Care must be taken not to confuse monilethrix with pili torti, another structural defect in which the hair shaft is twisted on its own axis (Fig 8.9). Pili torti may be localized or generalized and also appears with the first terminal-hair growth of infancy. Pili torti may occur as an isolated hair defect or in association with a multisystem disorder, such as Menke syndrome (an inherited disease of copper metabolism which also affects the central nervous, cardiovascular, and skeletal systems).

In the ectodermal dysplasia syndromes, a heterogeneous group of genodermatoses, sparse hair is associated with dysmorphic facies and abnormalities of other structures, which include nails, sweat glands, and teeth (Fig 8.10). In the

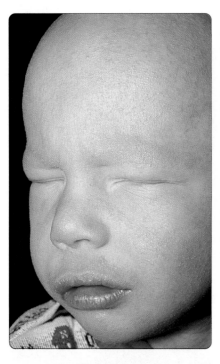

Fig 8.6 Ulerythema of the eyebrows and cheeks. In this variant of keratosis pilaris, inflammation of the pilosebaceous structures is associated with progressive alopecia and atrophy of the involved hair follicles. This may occur as an isolated disorder of keratinization or in association with other anomalies.

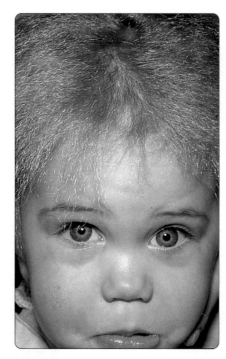

Fig 8.7 Uncombable hair syndrome is characterized by light blond, frizzy, unruly hair that does not lie flat on the scalp, which makes combing almost impossible. Diagnosis may be made by identifying the triangular-shaped hairs with longitudinal grooves along the hair shaft using light microscopy. Although some cases appear to be autosomal dominant, most are sporadic.

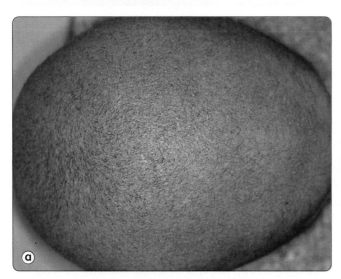

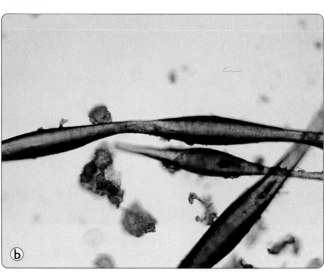

Fig 8.8 Monilethrix. **(a)** Short, broken hairs give the appearance of diffuse alopecia. **(b)** Microscopically, periodic narrowing of the hair shafts are seen. Hairs are brittle and break off at constricted points near the scalp.

hypohidrotic variants, early diagnosis may be lifesaving by preventing fatal hyperthermia, which may develop during otherwise self-limited childhood infections.

Trichothiodystrophy is a distinctive hair-shaft defect of autosomal-recessive inheritance characterized by increased fragility, splitting of the hair, low sulfur content, and alternating light-and-dark transverse bands on polarizing microscopy. Clinically, the hair is sparse, dull, and brittle. Multisystem features, including progeria-like appearance, mental retardation, growth retardation, hypogonadism, photosensitivity, cataracts, and other neurologic abnormalities, have been reported with trichothiodystrophy.

Children with congenital hair disorders require a careful medical and neurodevelopmental evaluation. Family history aids in establishing a pattern of inheritance. Hairs are examined microscopically to detect specific anomalies.

Acquired alopecia

Acquired alopecias may be differentiated by the presence or absence of clinical scarring. In nonscarring processes, inflammation may be clinically evident, subtle, or absent. Nonscarring disorders may be further subdivided by the presence of localized or diffuse involvement.

Scarring alopecia

A number of inflammatory disorders may involve the hair follicle primarily or by spread from contiguous skin (see Figs 7.41b and 7.48d). In lichen planus and lupus of the scalp, hair structures are usually involved early in the course of the disease. Folliculitis decalvans, a noninfectious folliculitis, also produces slowly but relentlessly enlarging areas of cicatricial alopecia. Physical agents, which include allergens, irritants (acids and alkalis), thermal burns, and blunt trauma may cause necrosis of the skin and nonspecific scarring. Examples include alkali burns from hair-grooming products, surgical scars, and radiation-induced injuries.

Patients with scarring alopecia deserve a careful examination of the skin, nails, and mucous membranes to identify clues for diagnosis. When the cause is not readily apparent, a skin biopsy is considered. A delay in diagnosis and treatment may result in widespread patches of disfiguring scarring alopecia.

Nonscarring alopecia

Most hair loss in children occurs without scarring. Clinically, the practitioner can differentiate between nonscarring alopecia associated with inflammation (erythema, scale, vesicles, pustules, etc.) and those disorders in which the scalp appears otherwise normal. The most common cause of inflammatory alopecia in children is tinea capitis. On the contrary, the scalp usually appears normal in telogen and anagen effluvium, alopecia areata, and traumatic hair loss.

Tinea capitis

Tinea capitis is the most common cause of hair loss in children between the ages of 2 and 10 years (Fig 8.11). For unknown reasons, this form of ringworm is endemic among black school children, although it is occasionally found in whites.

A variety of clinical presentations of tinea capitis occur. In some children, mild redness and scaling of the scalp, reminiscent of seborrhea, are seen in areas of partial alopecia. In other cases, widespread hair breakage caused by endothrix, or invasion of the hair shaft by the fungus, creates a 'salt-and-pepper' appearance, with short, residual hairs poking up as black dots on the surface of the scalp. Occasionally, scalp lesions are annular, like patches of tinea corporis. In some children, sensitization to the infecting organism results in erythema, edema, and pustule formation. As the pustules rupture and the area weeps, thick, matted, yellow crusts form, which simulates impetigo. Less commonly, intense inflammation causes the formation of raised, tender, boggy, plaques studded with pustules, known as kerions. Large, and

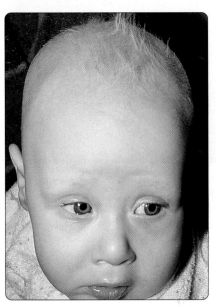

Fig 8.9 Menke syndrome. This child presented with lightly pigmented skin, blue eyes, sparse hair that demonstrated pili torti, seizures, and loss of developmental landmarks. Copper and ceruloplasmin levels in the serum were low.

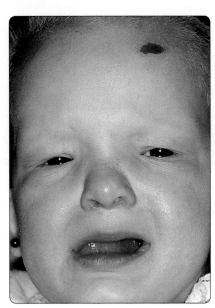

Fig 8.10 Hypohidrotic ectodermal dysplasia. This toddler demonstrates the typical findings of sparse hair, absent eyebrows and lashes, absent teeth, prominent forehead and supraorbital ridges, pointed chin, and mid-facial hypoplasia.

occasionally painful, occipital, postauricular, and preauricular adenopathy occurs with inflammatory tinea. Unless treated promptly and aggressively with oral antifungal agents and, in severe cases, oral corticosteroids, kerions may heal with scarring and permanent hair loss. Incision and drainage are not indicated, as loculations are small and septae thick.

Fungal infection of the scalp is readily confirmed by a potassium hydroxide (KOH) preparation of infected hairs.

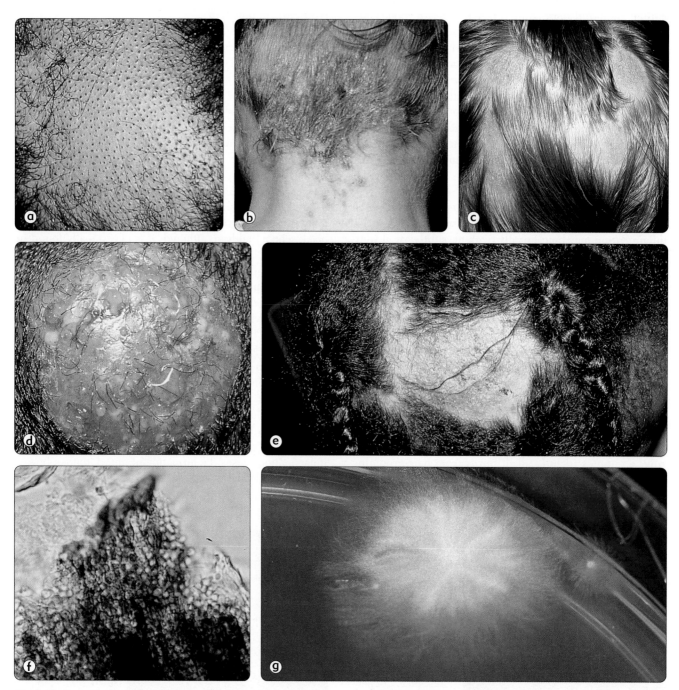

Fig 8.11 Tinea capitis. **(a)** Infiltration of the hair shafts has resulted in widespread breakage of the hair at the scalp, to produce a 'salt-and-pepper' appearance known as black dot ringworm. **(b)** Superficial papules and pustules have ruptured and produced a weeping, crusted patch that simulates impetigo. **(c)** Multiple, crusted patches developed in this child with tinea caused by *Microsporum canis*. **(d)** A boggy mass has formed as a result of an intense, inflammatory response known as a kerion. **(e)** A 10-year-old girl developed scarring alopecia after successful treatment of a large kerion with a 2-week course of prednisone and 4 months of griseofulvin. **(f)** Microscopic appearance of hair shafts infected with fungi. Note the tight packing of fungal arthrospores that cause hair-shaft fragility and breakage (KOH mount for endothrix). **(g)** On Sabouraud medium, *Trichophyton tonsurans* produces a folded thallus with a suede-like surface, which varies in color from cream–white to grayish or brownish buff. The undersurface of the colony may be reddish brown and dark pigment may diffuse into the medium.

The best hairs for examination are those that are broken off at the surface. A good specimen may be obtained by scraping hairs and scale onto a glass slide with a #15 blade. A toothbrush may be used to brush hairs and scale from large areas of the scalp directly onto fungal medium for culture. Before 1970, most cases of tinea capitis in the US were caused by *Microsporum* species, which fluoresce bright blue–green under Wood light. Unfortunately, this screening tool is of little value today, because the endothrix infection produced by *Trichophyton tonsurans* does not fluoresce.

However, oral griseofulvin administered over 2–4 months is effective. Although this usually eradicates infection, the risk of reinfection is high. Recurrent infection prompts a careful examination and possible culture of other family members to identify untreated cases. Concurrent use of selenium sulfide 2.5% shampoo or ketoconazole shampoo may help minimize the risk of recurrence and of spread to siblings and classmates.

Ketoconazole is approved in the US as an alternative for children with tinea capitis and a history of griseofulvin allergy. However, clinical studies show that it is less effective and, unlike griseofulvin, patients on ketoconazole require regular blood counts and liver profiles. Two new oral antifungals, terbinafine and itraconazole, appear to be effective and safe in treating tinea capitis. Moreover, they tend to remain in hairs long after the drug is discontinued, which enables relatively short courses of therapy. Unfortunately, liquid preparations are not yet available, and they are not approved for use in children in the US.

Although most children who present with scalp pustules have tinea capitis, bacterial folliculitis should also be considered, particularly if pustules are small, superficial, not associated with hair loss, and appear at the base of hairs under tension along parts in the hair. This disorder, termed impetigo of Bockhart, is easily treated by regular shampooing and loosening of the hair (Fig 8.12). Occasionally, an oral antibiotic is required. Seborrhea may be difficult to differentiate from tinea. However, in seborrhea, scaly patches are usually symmetric and only mildly pruritic. A black schoolchild with patches of scalp 'seborrhea' warrants a KOH preparation and fungal culture to exclude tinea.

Alopecia areata

Alopecia areata is a form of asymptomatic, localized alopecia that presents with round patches of complete hair loss anywhere on the body, including the scalp, eyebrows, lashes, extremities, and trunk (Fig 8.13). Occasionally, hair loss

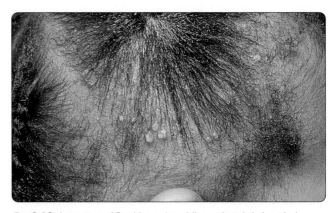

Fig 8.12 Impetigo of Bockhart. A toddler with tightly braided plaits developed follicular pustules in the area of greatest traction.

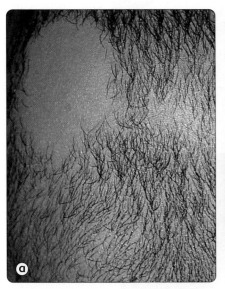
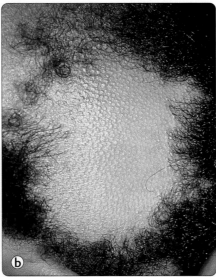
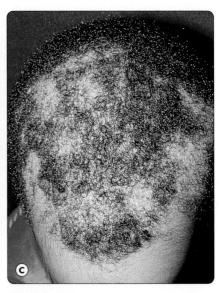

Fig 8.13 Alopecia areata. **(a)** Multiple, round patches of alopecia continued to progress despite treatment with griseofulvin for presumed tinea capitis. Cultures for fungus were negative, and the lesions of alopecia areata waxed and waned for years before resolving. **(b)** A round patch of alopecia, with no scale or inflammation, appeared on the scalp of this 10-year-old boy. The shiny, complete alopecia is typical of alopecia areata. **(c)** This 5-year-old boy with diffuse, moth-eaten alopecia developed alopecia totalis over several weeks.

progresses to involve the entire scalp (alopecia totalis) and body (alopecia universalis). The insult that triggers alopecia areata is unknown, but probably immunologic in origin. Although clinical signs of inflammation are absent, skin biopsies from sites of active disease show perifollicular, lymphocytic inflammation as well as deposition of antibody and immune complexes.

Clues to diagnosis include the absence of inflammation and scaling in involved areas of the scalp and the presence of short (3–6 mm), easily epilated hairs at the margins of the patch. Under magnification, these hair stubs resemble exclamation points, as the hair shaft narrows just before its point of entry into the follicle. Another finding in many patients with alopecia areata is Scotch-plaid pitting of the nails, which consists of rows of pits that cross in a transverse and longitudinal pattern.

The course of alopecia areata is unpredictable. In adolescents and young adults hair loss usually resolves without permanent alopecia over months to years. In infants and young children, particularly when alopecia is diffuse, the prognosis is more guarded. Treatment includes safe measures that do not carry risk of systemic toxicity. Topical corticosteroids, local irritants (e.g. tar preparations, anthralin [dithranol]), topical minoxidil, topical sensitizers (e.g. diphencyclopropenone), and ultraviolet light therapy have been used with some success. Although oral corticosteroids may induce hair regrowth, no investigator has ever demonstrated that these medications change the prognosis of alopecia areata. Consequently, their use should be restricted to short courses in selected patients with widespread, rapidly progressive disease.

Traumatic hair loss

Alopecia caused by breakage of the hair shaft often results from an acquired structural defect of the hair, and is easily diagnosed by microscopic examination. The most common defect is trichorrhexis nodosa, which can develop at any age as brittle, short hairs that are perceived by the patient as non-growing. By gently pulling, it can be demonstrated that many hairs are easily broken. Microscopically, the distal ends of the hairs are frayed, resembling a broom (Fig 8.14). Other hairs may have nodules that resemble two brooms stuck together. The fragility is caused by damage to the outer cortex of the hair shaft, which results in the loss of structural support.

Without this support the weaker, fibrous medulla frays, like an electrical cord with broken insulation. This disorder is most common in blacks, arising from the trauma of combing tightly curled hairs. It may also occur after repeated trauma to the cortex from hair straighteners, hot combs, bleaches, and permanent waves. Since the growth of the hair shaft is normal, the disorder is self-limited, and normal hairs regrow when the source of damage is eliminated.

Traction alopecia

Traction alopecia is a form of traumatic alopecia common in young girls and women whose hairstyles, such as ponytails, plaits, and braids, maintain a tight pull on the hair shafts (Fig 8.15). This traction causes shaft fractures, as well as follicular damage. If prolonged, permanent scarring alopecia can result.

Hair pulling

Hair pulling is a common disorder seen in toddlers, children of school age, and adolescents; it mimics many other forms of alopecia (Fig 8.16). It presents with bizarre patterns of hair loss, often in broad, linear bands on the vertex or sides of the scalp, where the hair is easily twisted and pulled out. Rarely, the entire scalp, eyebrows, and eyelashes are involved. The most important clue is to find short, broken-off hairs along the

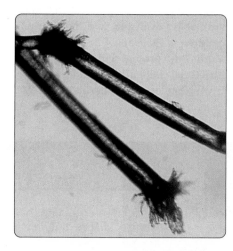

Fig 8.14 Trichorrhexis nodosa ('split ends') is a brittle hair-shaft defect, usually caused by overmanipulation of the hair or chemical use. The frayed broom appearance is typical.

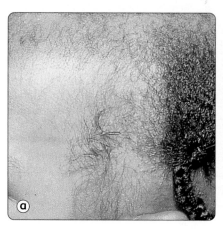

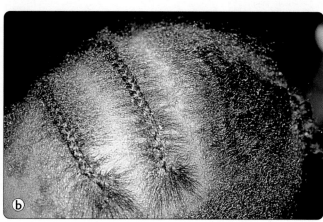

Fig 8.15 Traction alopecia. Alopecia is most prominent at **(a)** the periphery of the scalp and **(b)** along the parts in the hair. These areas are under the most traction.

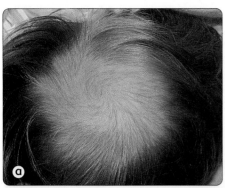

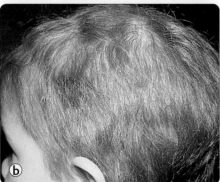

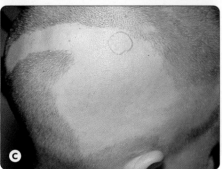

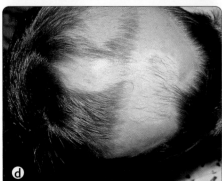

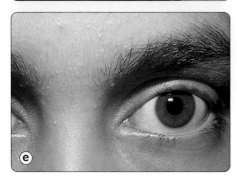

Fig 8.16 Hair pulling.
(a) Alopecia from hair pulling is found most commonly on the occiput.
(b) Hairs broken off and regrowing at various lengths may produce a moth-eaten appearance.
(c, d) Bizarre patterns that defy anatomic landmarks are typical. In **(c)** a short hair cut failed to camouflage the alopecia.
In **(d)** note the rectangular area of regrowth in the mid scalp, which followed 1 month of covering with an occlusive dressing.
(e) Eyebrow and eyelash involvement may be difficult to differentiate from alopecia areata.

scalp, with stubs of different lengths in adjacent areas. This is caused by repetitive pulling and/or twisting of the hair, which fractures the longer shafts. Once broken, the hairs are too short to be rebroken until they grow longer.

Hair pulling is often confused with alopecia areata. However, in hair pulling patches of hair loss are not completely bald, and the hair shafts are usually difficult to remove from the scalp. In addition, no associated nail abnormalities occur. Skin biopsy of the scalp from an area of recent hair pulling may demonstrate large numbers of catagen hairs, perifollicular hemorrhage, and trichomalacia or small, wavy, ghost-like hairs adjacent to normal hairs.

Although hair pulling may occur in children with severe obsessive–compulsive psychiatric disease, many cases are associated with habitual behavior or situational stress (Fig 8.17). Parents and children may deny vigorously that the hair loss could be caused by the child, and thus the diagnosis rests on a high index of suspicion and recognition of the clinical findings. In young, habitual hair twirlers, positive reinforcement of socially acceptable alternative behaviors may succeed in extinguishing hair pulling.

Other forms of deliberate and accidental physical, thermal, and chemical injury to the hair shaft and scalp can also cause alopecia. Examples include child abuse and pressure necrosis of the skin (Fig 8.18).

Telogen and anagen effluvium

Telogen effluvium is the most common form of noninflammatory, nonscarring, diffuse hair loss to occur in children (Fig 8.19). In this form of alopecia, some sort of systemic insult, such as severe illness, high fever, surgery, or certain drugs, triggers an abnormally high number of anagen hairs to switch over to telogen. This is followed 3–5 months later by diffuse, brisk, shedding of telogen hairs. Although quite distressing, telogen effluvium is temporary and rarely produces more than 50% hair loss. In fact, the hair loss marks the end of the process as new anagen hairs replace those being shed. In some children, telogen loss occurs repeatedly after

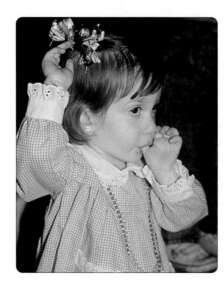

Fig 8.17 Hair pulling occurs frequently as a habitual behavior. At bedtime and naptime, this happy, healthy toddler pulls and twirls her hair and sucks her thumb.

recurrent ear infections and upper respiratory infections. Even in these cases, the prognosis for full recovery is excellent. Neither treatment nor laboratory studies are usually required. Early in the course, diagnosis may be confirmed by examination of hairs pulled from the scalp, which should demonstrate an increased percentage of telogen hairs. Parents are also reminded that hair grows only about 1 cm each month, so that the return to hair length pretelogen effluvium may take many months.

In anagen effluvium, sudden loss of growing hairs is caused by abnormal cessation of the anagen phase. Various toxins and antimetabolites trigger this diffuse process, which may involve up to 90% of scalp hairs over several days to several weeks. The extent of hair loss is determined by the toxicity of the agent, and by the dose and length of exposure. In anagen effluvium, the hair shafts taper and lose adhesion to the follicle.

This type of alopecia is most common after systemic chemotherapy. Patients may be identified by the few remaining long telogen hairs scattered throughout the scalp. Other toxins, which include lead, arsenic, thallium, and X-ray irradiation, may also cause anagen loss. Full hair regrowth usually occurs when the toxic agent is discontinued.

Anagen effluvium must not be confused with loose anagen syndrome, an autosomal-dominant disorder characterized by actively growing hairs that are loosely anchored to the follicle and easily and painlessly pulled from the scalp. Although the typical patients described are blonde girls between 2 and 5 years old, children of both sexes and dark hair color may be affected. These children demonstrate short, variably sparse scalp hair and rarely require haircuts. A hair pull shows dystrophic anagen hairs with darkly pigmented, misshapen hair bulbs, and absence of the internal and external root sheaths. There is no known therapy, but many patients improve during adolescence. Although the relationship between loose anagen syndrome and alopecia areata is unknown, recently the disorders have been reported in the same patients.

Generalized changes in the color and/or texture of the hair may also accompany a number of medical disorders (e.g. hypothyroidism, hyperthyroidism), the use of certain medications (e.g. antimalarials), and nutritional deficiencies (e.g. zinc, copper, protein; Fig 8.20).

Acne

Acne vulgaris

Acne vulgaris, a disorder of the pilosebaceous apparatus, is the most common skin problem of adolescence (Fig 8.21). Lesions may appear on the face as early as 8 years of age, but they usually begin to develop during the second decade of life with the onset of puberty. Other areas with prominent sebaceous hair follicles, including the upper chest and back, may become involved.

The exact pathogenesis of acne is unknown. However, abnormalities in follicular keratinization are thought to produce the acne lesion that develops earliest, the microcomedone. In time, microcomedones may grow into

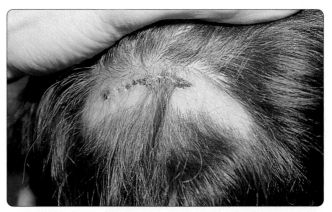

Fig 8.18 An 11-year-old boy developed pressure necrosis of the skin on the occiput and a linear patch of alopecia several days after liver transplant surgery. The area of injury conformed to the shape of a rubber doughnut, on which his head had been placed at the beginning of surgery.

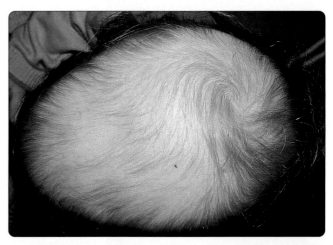

Fig 8.19 Telogen effluvium. An otherwise healthy 6-year-old developed diffuse thinning of scalp hair 3 months after febrile illness. After a 6-week period of brisk shedding, his hair regrew to normal thickness.

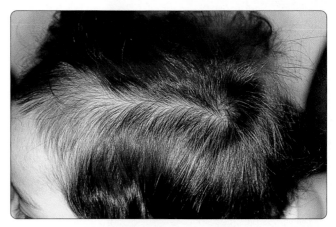

Fig 8.20 Flag sign. A light pigmented band of hair appeared on the scalp of this 6-year-old girl with cystic fibrosis after several months of inadequate pancreatic enzyme replacement. When her medication was adjusted the hair pigment returned to normal, and the light band of hair continued to grow outward.

clinically apparent, open comedones (blackheads; Fig 8.21a) and closed comedones (whiteheads; Fig 8.21b). The entire process is fueled by androgens, which stimulate sebaceous-gland differentiation and growth, and the production of sebum. The proliferation of *Propionibacterium acnes* in non-inflammatory comedones, and the rupture of comedone contents into the surrounding dermis, may trigger the development of inflammatory papules, pustules and cysts (Fig 8.21c–e). Cystic acne is characterized by nodules and cysts scattered over the face, chest, and back (Fig 8.21f). This variant frequently leads to disfiguring scarring.

Although therapy must be individualized, patients with mild-to-moderate comedonal and/or inflammatory acne respond well to a combination of topical retinoids (tretinoin, adapalene), benzoyl peroxide, antibiotics, and azaleic acid.

Moderate-to-severe papulopustular acne warrants the use of oral antibiotics in combination with topical agents. Oral 13-*cis*-retinoic acid (isotretinoin) is reserved for patients with severe, scarring, cystic acne recalcitrant to conservative measures.

Fortunately, acne is usually self-limited, and winds down in late adolescence and early adult life. However, some middle-aged adults continue to require aggressive treatment for stubborn disease.

Evaluation of a patient with acne includes a careful medical and family history and physical examination. Although no special laboratory studies are usually necessary, signs and symptoms of precocious puberty, hyperandrogenism, or ovarian dysfunction warrant further investigation. A history of severe acne in a first-degree relative also serves as a warning for potentially serious disease.

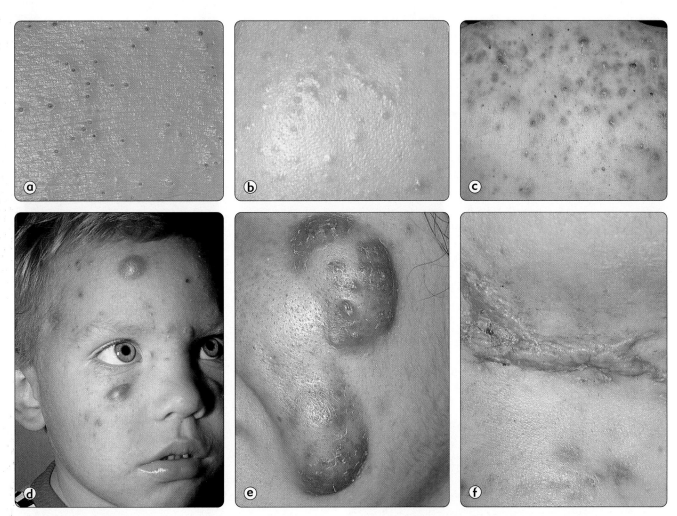

Fig 8.21 Acne. **(a)** Open comedones (blackheads) dot the forehead of this 16-year-old boy. **(b)** Closed comedones (whiteheads) cover the forehead of this 14-year-old girl. **(c)** Red papules, pustules, comedones, and cysts with scarring extended over the upper trunk of this 16-year-old boy. His nodulocystic acne went into remission after treatment with 13-*cis*-retinoic acid (isotretinoin). **(d)** Papules, pustules, and cysts spread over the face, neck, and scalp of this toddler. He also responded well to 13-*cis*-retinoic acid. Both of his parents had scars from previous cystic acne. **(e)** Large, communicating cysts erupted on the cheeks and chin of this 15-year-old girl during the first trimester of her pregnancy. Although she improved somewhat with intralesional corticosteroids, the severe cystic acne, which some clinicians refer to as pyoderma faciale, did not settle down until several months after she delivered. **(f)** Old sinus tracts and scars on the neck were the only remaining findings in an adolescent boy with a history of cystic acne treated with 13-*cis*-retinoic acid.

Acneiform reactions differ from classic acne vulgaris by the presence of uniform lesions in a widespread distribution, which may extend to involve the arms, legs, and lower trunk (Fig 8.22). Endogenous corticosteroids (e.g. Cushing syndrome), prednisone, anabolic steroids, isoniazid, anticonvulsants, and lithium may trigger acneiform eruptions. When the medication dose cannot be decreased or discontinued, traditional management with topical and oral acne preparations may help.

Acne vulgaris may be confused with bacterial or fungal folliculitis (Fig 8.23). In folliculitis, pustules predominate and the distribution is often restricted to areas of occlusion. Gram stains, KOH preparations, and cultures also help to differentiate folliculitis from acne. Occasionally, an acne patient on long-standing antibiotics develops an acute worsening of acne in association with a Gram-negative folliculitis. This probably results from selection of a resistant Gram-negative organism. Pustules usually resolve with an alternative antibiotic or 13-*cis*-retinoic acid.

Acne rosacea is differentiated from acne vulgaris by the presence of red papules, pustules, cysts, and extensive telangiectasias, but the absence of comedones (Fig 8.24). Rosacea occurs most commonly in middle age, but some patients date the onset of lesions to adolescence or early adulthood.

Hidradenitis suppurativa

Hidradenitis suppurativa may develop in association with cystic acne or as a separate entity (Fig 8.25). Hidradenitis is

Fig 8.22 Acneiform eruption. Uniform pustules on an inflamed base cover the trunk and proximal extremities of this 14-year-old boy who was placed on high-dose corticosteroids to manage inflammatory bowel disease. The eruption resolved when the corticosteroids were tapered.

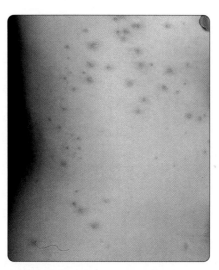

Fig 8.23 Hot-tub folliculitis. Painful, red papules and pustules erupted (in a bathing suit distribution) on this teenage girl 24 hours after lounging in a neighbor's hot tub. *Pseudomonas* grew from pus obtained from one of the lesions. Fortunately, she remained well, and the folliculitis resolved over 3 days without treatment.

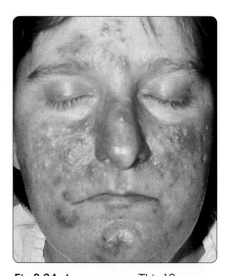

Fig 8.24 Acne rosacea. This 19-year-old demonstrates the classic rash with red papules, pustules, cysts, and telangiectasias.

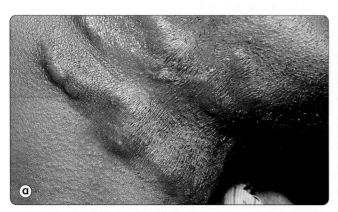

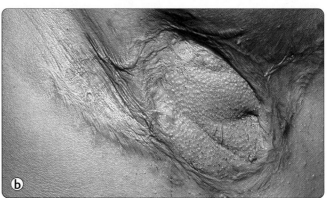

Fig 8.25 Hidradenitis suppurativa. (a) An adolescent boy with severe involvement of the axillae underwent extensive surgery with (b) an excellent result. Note the painful cysts and communicating sinus tracts in (a).

a severe, noninfectious inflammatory process that involves apocrine, follicular structures in the axilla, groin, suprapubic, and perianal areas. As with acne, hyperkeratosis of the follicular epithelium is probably the initiating event. In the acute form tender, red pustules and deep-seated nodules become fluctuant and discharge pus. Over time many patients develop chronic draining abscesses, sinus tracts, and severe scarring. Early in the course, hidradenitis improves with oral antibiotic therapy. Chronic disease responds only somewhat to antibiotics, 13-*cis*-retinoic acid, and systemic corticosteroids. Severe cases heal only after surgical excision of apocrine glands, scars, and sinus tracts in affected areas.

Hypertrichosis and hirsutism

Hypertrichosis refers to localized patches of increased hair growth, whereas hirsutism is a term used to describe excessive hair growth, usually in children and women, in an adult male pattern (Fig 8.26).

Congenital hypertrichosis has been noted in pigmented nevi and other cutaneous hamartomas. Generalized increase in hair at birth may occur as a normal physiologic variant. However, unusual patterns or persistence beyond early infancy prompt a careful evaluation for potentially serious hereditary aberrations (e.g. hypertrichosis lanuginosa, Cornelia de Lange syndrome).

Acquired, localized hypertrichosis occurs frequently in Becker nevi (hairy epidermal nevus) and patches of chronic physical trauma, chemical irritation, or thermal injury. The application of topical corticosteroids or androgens may also stimulate localized hair growth. Widespread hypertrichosis may appear in hypothyroidism, porphyria, and following the use of certain medications, such as phenytoin, cyclosporine, and minoxidil.

Hirsutism may appear as a physiologic variant in an otherwise healthy child. However, an endogenous or exogenous source of androgens must be excluded. Cushing, adrenogenital, and Stein–Leventhal syndromes may present with hirsutism. Endocrinologic evaluation is guided by careful history and physical examination.

NAIL DISORDERS

As with hair disorders, abnormalities of the nails may provide a clue to the diagnosis of multisystem hereditary or acquired disease. Patients may also seek the advice of practitioners for nail problems because of pain or cosmetic concerns.

Embryology and anatomy

Nails are first delineated as a fold in the skin of the developing fetus at 10–11 weeks. By the fifteenth week, the nail plate has already begun to keratinize, well before other epidermal structures. At birth the nail is fully formed.

The major part of the nail comprises the hard nail plate, which arises from the matrix beneath the proximal nail fold (Fig 8.27). The pink color of the nail bed is derived from the

extensive plexus of vessels that lies beneath the normally transparent nail plate. A white, crescent-shaped lunula, which extends from under the proximal nail fold, represents the distal portion of the nail matrix. As the nail plate emerges from the matrix, its lateral borders are enveloped by the

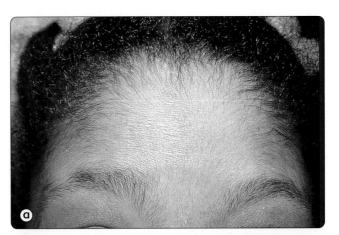

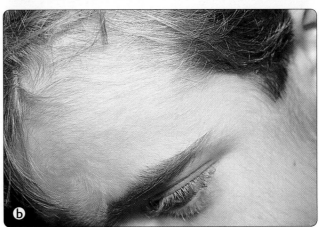

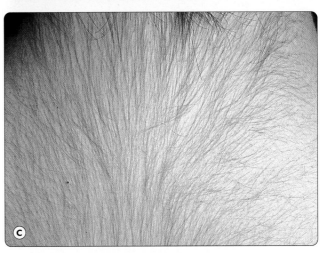

Fig 8.26 Hypertrichosis. **(a)** Excessive hair was noted at birth on the face of this 2-year-old girl with microcephaly, hypertelorism, developmental delay, and other dysmorphic features. A 10-year-old liver transplant recipient receiving cyclosporine developed generalized hypertrichosis demonstrated here on **(b)** the face and **(c)** back of the neck.

lateral nail folds. The skin that underlies the free end of the nail is referred to as the hyponychium, which connects the nail bed with the adjacent skin on the tips of the digits. Abnormalities in any part of the nail anatomy may result in characteristic clinical findings.

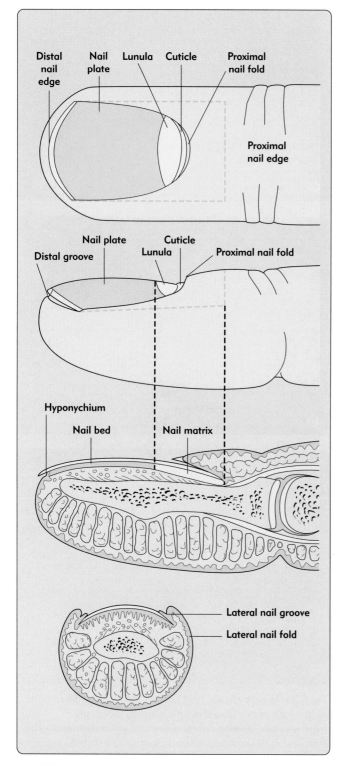

Fig 8.27 Anatomy of the nail.

Congenital and hereditary disorders

Absence, hypoplasia, or dysplasia of the nails may occur as an isolated phenomenon or as part of an ectodermal dysplasia or other genodermatosis (Fig 8.28).

Isolated malformations

Clubbing and spooning (koilonychia) of the nails may occur as autosomal-dominant abnormalities with no other anomalies (Fig 8.29). Although congenital ingrown toenails may result from congenital malalignment of the great toenails (and resolve only with surgical realignment), a self-limiting variant has also been described (Fig 8.30). In the spontaneously regressing type, the ingrown nail may result from trauma or paronychia.

Ectodermal dysplasias

In pachonychia congenita, an autosomal-dominant disorder with variable penetrance, hyperkeratosis of the nail bed, which develops in the first few months of life, is followed by vertical thickening and elevation of the nail plate with yellow–brown discoloration (Fig 8.31). Minor trauma may induce painful separation of the nail plate from the nail bed and bleeding. Hyperhidrosis of the palms and soles, as well as callosities and blistering, is common. Other findings include leukokeratosis of the oral mucosae (not associated with malignant degeneration), thickening of the tympanic membranes that results in deafness, leukokeratosis of the cornea, and cataracts. Hyperkeratotic papules on the extensor surfaces of the extremities, dermoid cysts, and steatocystoma multiplex have also been reported.

Dyskeratosis congenita may be confused with pachonychia congenita. However, in dyskeratosis congenita, which may be gender linked, autosomal dominant, or autosomal recessive, the nail plate is thinned with longitudinal ridging and pterygium formation (Fig 8.32). In dyskeratosis congenita, poikiloderma with reticulated pigmentation, telangiectasias, and atrophy is most prominent on the neck and trunk. Leukoplakia of the oral mucosae may be associated with the development of squamous cell carcinoma and other malignancies of the gastrointestinal tract. Pancytopenia occurs in 50% of affected individuals during their second and third decades and resembles Fanconi anemia. Hypoplasia of the nails may also be a feature of hidrotic ectodermal dysplasia and Coffin–Siris syndrome.

Genodermatoses and systemic disease

Nail–patella syndrome is an autosomal-dominant disorder that presents with congenital absence or hypoplasia of the nails and patellae (Fig 8.33). Glomerulonephritis occurs in a small percentage of cases and is rarely fatal. Heterochromia of the iris, keratoconus, and cataracts have also been reported.

Periungual fibromas, which arise from the proximal nail groove, are a common finding in patients with tuberous sclerosis. Although the fibromas do not appear until later childhood or adult life, they may provide the first clue to diagnosis in individuals who are otherwise mildly affected.

Fig 8.28 Selected nail anomalies.

Selected nail anomalies	
Anonychia	**Koilonychia (spoon nails)**
Deafness, onycho-osteodystrophy, mental retardation (DOOR) syndrome Nail–patella syndrome Hallermann–Streiff syndrome Coffin–Siris syndrome Klein syndrome	Mal de Meleda keratoderma Monilethrix Nail–patella syndrome Incontinentia pigmenti Trichothiodystrophy
Hereditary ectodermal dysplasias	**Drug-induced malformations**

(Variable findings in which alopecia, dental defects, nail defects, or anhidrosis occur in combination with one sign affecting other structures of epidermal origin)	Phenytoin, trimethadione, paramethadione
	  Hyperpigmentation
	  Hypoplasia
	Warfarins
	  Hypoplasia
	Fetal alcohol syndrome
	  Hypoplasia

Chromosomal anomalies	**Miscellaneous disorders with nail dystrophy**
Monosomies 4p, 9p Trisomies 3q partial, 7q, 8, 8p, 9p, 13, 18, 21 Turner syndrome Noonan syndrome Group G-ring chromosome	Epidermolysis bullosa Acanthosis nigricans Acrodermatitis enteropathica Diabetes Gingival fibromatosis Hyper-IgE syndrome Hyperuricemia Lesch–Nyhan syndrome Tuberous sclerosis
Hyperplastic nails	
Palmar–plantar keratodermas Ichthyosis Pachonychia congenita Group G-ring chromosome	

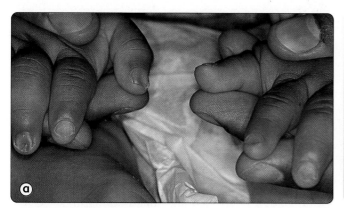

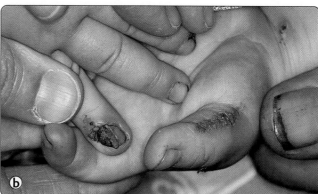

Fig 8.29 Congenital nail dystrophy. (a) Koilonychia was noted at birth in this infant whose mother had similar nails.

(b) An extensive epidermal nevus involved this infant's left thumb and right fifth fingernail.

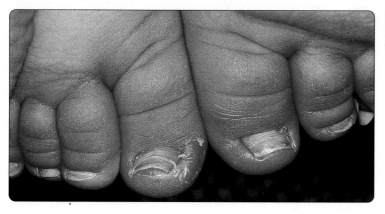

Fig 8.30 Congenital ingrown nails. This infant had involvement of both great toe nails, which improved without treatment by 6 months of age.

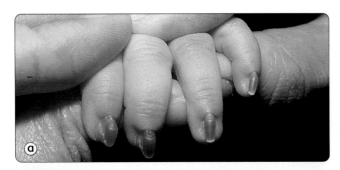

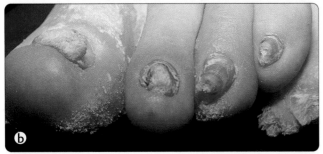

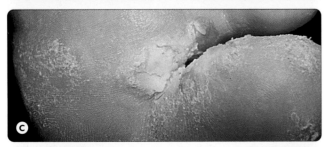

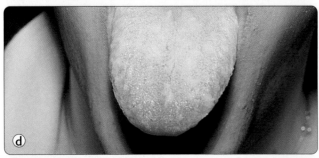

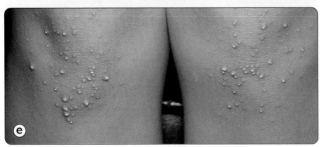

Fig 8.31 Pachonychia congenita. **(a)** At 3 months of age all 20 of this child's nails showed early changes of pachonychia with yellowing and pinched-up hyperplasia. **(b, c)** His father had marked involvement of all nails, as well as painful callosities on the dorsal and plantar aspects of the feet. **(d)** Leukokeratosis without a risk of malignant degeneration usually appears in infancy or early childhood and may involve the tongue, gingivae, and oral mucosae. **(e)** Hyperkeratotic papules on the extensor surfaces of the extremities are also common, particularly over the knees and elbows.

Congenital hypoplasia of the nails in infants with intrauterine exposure to anticonvulsants, alcohol, warfarins, or other teratogens prompts a thorough evaluation for other drug-induced stigmata.

Acquired nail disorders
Paronychia

Paronychia is a common childhood disorder. It presents as a red, tender swelling of the proximal or lateral nail fold. In the acute form, exquisite pain, sudden swelling, and abscess formation around one nail are caused by bacterial invasion after trauma to the cuticle (Fig 8.34). Chronic paronychia may involve one or several nails. There is usually a history of frequent exposure to water (dishwasher's or thumb-sucker's paronychia). Tenderness is mild, and a small amount of pus may sometimes be expressed. In chronic cases, the nail may be discolored and dystrophic (Fig 8.35). The causative organisms are *Candida* species, usually *C. albicans*.

Acute paronychia responds quickly to drainage of the abscess and warm tap-water soaks. Occasionally, oral anti-staphylococcal antibiotics are required. Chronic lesions resolve with topical antifungal agents and avoidance of water. Parents of toddlers must be reassured that recurrent

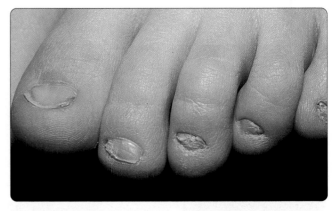

Fig 8.32 Dyskeratosis congenita. Unlike pachonychia congenita, the nails are usually thin, fragile, and hypoplastic.

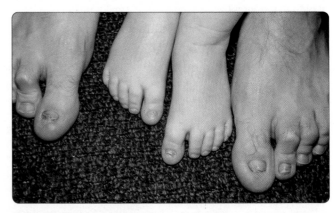

Fig 8.33 Nail–patella syndrome. Both father and son had hypoplastic patellae and dystrophic, hypoplastic nails.

candidal paronychia eventually heals without scarring when thumb sucking ends. Intermittent, chronic use of antifungal creams in young children is effective and safe.

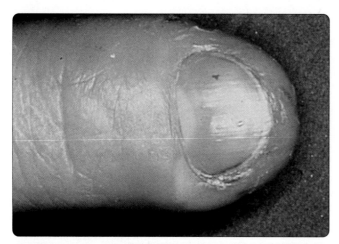

Fig 8.34 Paronychia. An acute, staphylococcal paronychia developed after this child picked at a hangnail.

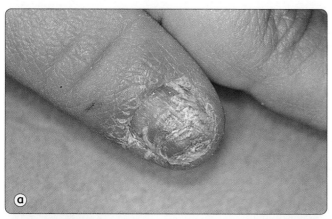

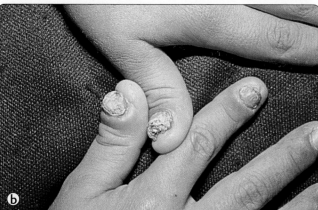

Fig 8.35 Chronic paronychia. **(a)** A chronic, candidal paronychia recurred for over a year on the finger of an otherwise healthy toddler. Note the erythema at the base of the nail and loss of the cuticle. **(b)** All 20 nails were discolored and hyperplastic in this 8-year-old boy with chronic mucocutaneous candidiasis. The chronic paronychia and nail dystrophy resolved on long-term treatment with oral ketoconazole.

Nail dystrophy

Nail dystrophy (distortion and discoloration of normal nail-plate structure), may result from any traumatic or inflammatory process that involves the nail matrix, nail bed, or surrounding tissues. Although onychomycosis, the result of dermatophyte fungal infection, is the most common cause of nail dystrophy in adults, it is unusual in children before puberty (Fig 8.36). Dystrophic nails occur frequently as a complication of trauma (Fig 8.37) or underlying dermatoses, such as psoriasis, atopic dermatitis, and lichen planus (Figs 8.38–8.40).

Trauma to the nail may cause a subungual hematoma, which results in a brown–black discoloration. This is particularly likely following crush injuries. Usually, the diagnosis is simple, unless trauma is subtle. Although most hematomas resolve without treatment, large, painful collections of blood may be drained by drilling a small hole in the nail plate using a sterile, large-bore needle or a hot, sterile paper clip. This relieves pain and reduces the risk of infection. Dark pigmentation at the base of the great toenail, caused by jamming the toe into the end of the shoe at a sudden stop, is called 'turf toe' and also results from subungual hemorrhage (Fig 8.41). This must be differentiated from melanoma and melanonychia (Fig 8.42). Hemorrhage may be identified by the presence of purple–brown pigment in the distal nail and normal proximal outgrowth of the nail. In melanonychia, gray–brown streaks of pigment of varying width extend longitudinally from the proximal nail fold of one or several nails. Although this finding is common in darkly pigmented individuals, it may occur in individuals of any race at any age. Irregular or changing pigment streaks may require a nail biopsy to confirm their innocent nature and exclude melanoma.

Nail biting, grooming, and chronic manipulation of any sort may also result in nail dystrophy. Repeated trauma to

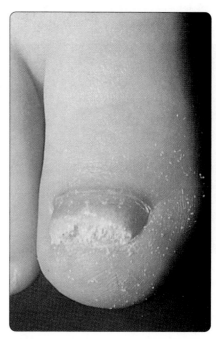

Fig 8.36 Onychomycosis. This 4-year-old boy developed a single dystrophic toenail, which grew *Trichophyton rubrum* on fungal culture. His father had chronic athlete's foot.

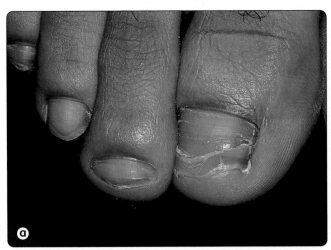

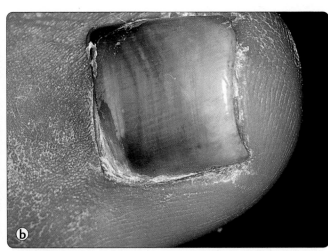

Fig 8.37 Traumatic nail dystrophy. **(a)** Onychoschizia (transverse splitting of the nail at the distal free edge) occurred in both great toenails as a result of recurrent trauma from

basketball in this high-school athlete. **(b)** Another adolescent athlete developed chronic *Pseudomonas* infection in a dystrophic great toenail.

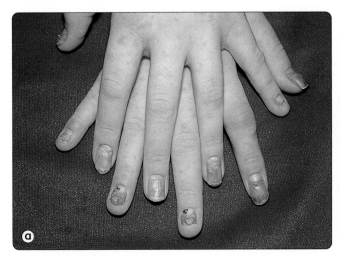

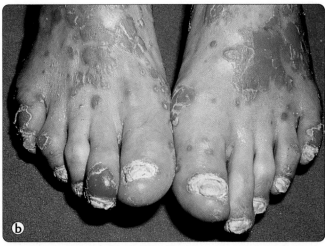

Fig 8.38 Psoriatic nails. Psoriasis produced **(a)** typical pitting and onycholysis in this adolescent with plaque psoriasis and

(b) yellow, friable, flaking nails in another child with severe psoriatic arthritis.

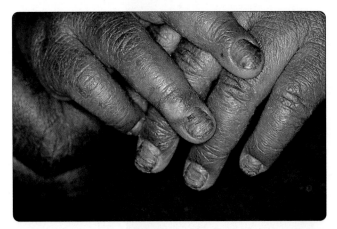

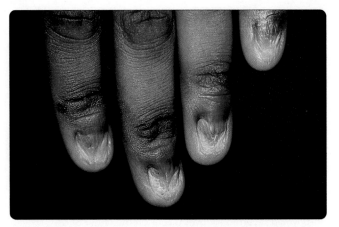

Fig 8.39 Atopic nails. Multiple, transverse ridges and splitting of the nails developed in an atopic patient with generalized skin disease, which included severe hand involvement.

Fig 8.40 Lichen planus. An adolescent girl demonstrates the characteristic nail changes in lichen planus, which include onychorrhexis (longitudinal splitting) and pterygeum formation (forward growth of the skin at the proximal nail fold, which results from scarring).

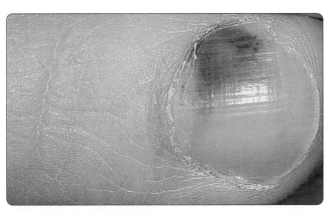

Fig 8.41 Traumatic subungual hematoma. Discoloration as a result of traumatic hemorrhage under the toenail is common in children and athletic adults. It is a result of repeated jamming of the toe into the end of the shoe while running or stopping suddenly (turf toe).

the cuticle may produce leukonychia (transverse white lines) and median nail dystrophy (central longitudinal ridging; Fig 8.43).

Twenty nail dystrophy (trachonychia) is a disorder of otherwise healthy children of school age and is characterized by yellowing, pitting, increased friability, and other dystrophic changes that progresses over 6–18 months to involve most or all of the nails. Although the course is variable, in many cases the dystrophy resolves without scarring over a period of several years. This disorder probably includes a number of conditions that cannot be differentiated unless other cutaneous findings appear.

Nail dystrophy may accompany other skin disorders and help with their diagnosis. For example, alopecia areata is associated with characteristic Scotch-plaid pitting of the nails (Fig 8.44). Psoriasis in the nail matrix results in scattered pits that are larger, deeper, and less numerous than those

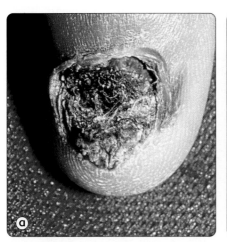
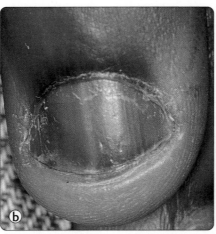
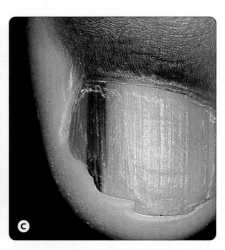

Fig 8.42 (a) In this patient with an acral melanoma, which arose in the nail matrix or nail bed, the nail has become dystrophic and the nail bed is infiltrated with pigmented, malignant cells.

(b, c) In melanonychia, neat, hyperpigmented streaks extend vertically across the nail from the proximal nail fold. This can appear in **(b)** a diffuse pattern or **(c)** in narrow bands.

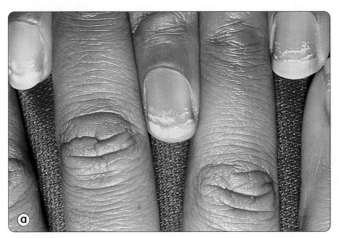
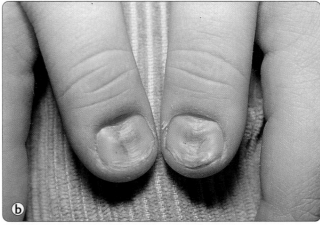

Fig 8.43 (a) Leukonychia consists of punctate lesions or transverse white lines that grow out along the nail plate and frequently result from trauma to the nail at the cuticle.

(b) Median nail dystrophy developed in this teenage boy, who admitted to chronically picking at his nails.

found in alopecia areata. Psoriasis of the nail bed, especially under the distal nail, causes separation of the nail plate from the underlying skin (onycholysis) and oil-drop discoloration with heaped-up scaling (see Fig 8.38). Onycholysis alone, without pits or discoloration, may be caused by trauma, infection, nail-polish hardeners, or phototoxic reactions to drugs such as tetracycline.

Nail changes and systemic disease

Finally, nail findings may provide a clue to the diagnosis of underlying medical disorders (Fig 8.45). For example, clubbing may be associated with chronic pulmonary disease or congenital heart disease with a right-to-left shunt. Splinter hemorrhages in the nail bed are a physical sign of bacterial endocarditis (see Fig 7.25a). Cyanosis of the nail beds in Raynaud phenomenon and periungual telangiectasias may support a diagnosis of collagen vascular disease. Thickened, yellow, slow-growing nails (yellow nail syndrome) occurs in chronic pulmonary disease and lymphedema. Koilonychia has been reported in hemochromatosis and iron deficiency. Half-and-half nails, in which the proximal nail appears white and the distal nail red, probably results from edema and changes in blood flow in the nail bed, and has been associated with uremia, heart failure, and cirrhosis. Uniform, transverse, white lines and/or grooves in the nail that move distally with nail growth result from growth arrest because of systemic illness, medications, or toxins. These lesions, known as Beau lines, have been reported with acute childhood infections, surgery, chemotherapy, and flares of systemic disorders.

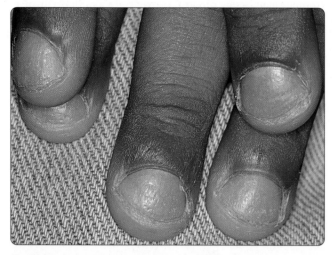

Fig 8.44 Scotch-plaid pitting, transverse rows of regularly spaced pits, was associated with alopecia areata in this teenager.

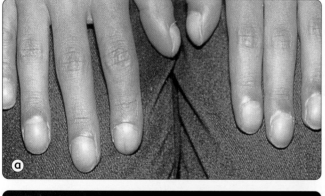

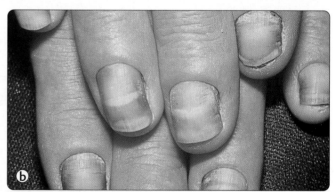

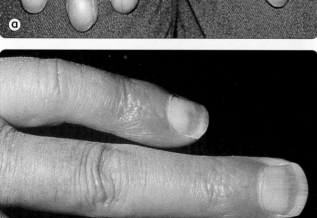

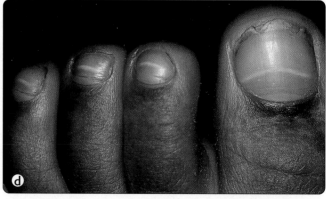

Fig 8.45 Nail changes and systemic disease. **(a)** Clubbing may occur as an isolated, inherited defect or a complication of chronic lung or heart disease. **(b)** Yellow nail syndrome with chronic yellowing and slow growth of all nails was noted in this patient with Hodgkin disease. **(c)** Half-and-half nails (proximal nail bed white and distal nail bed red) were a marker for uremia in this 14-year-old girl with chronic renal failure. **(d)** White, transverse bands and ridging (Beau lines) appeared in all nails of this 12-year-old boy several months after a sickle cell crisis that required hospitalization.

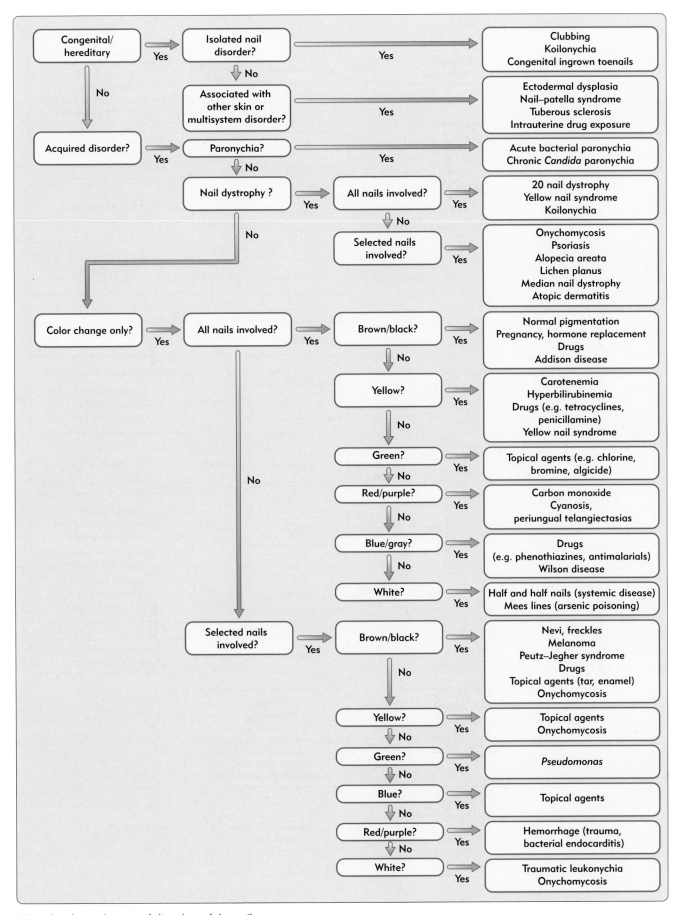

Algorithm for evaluation of disorders of the nails.

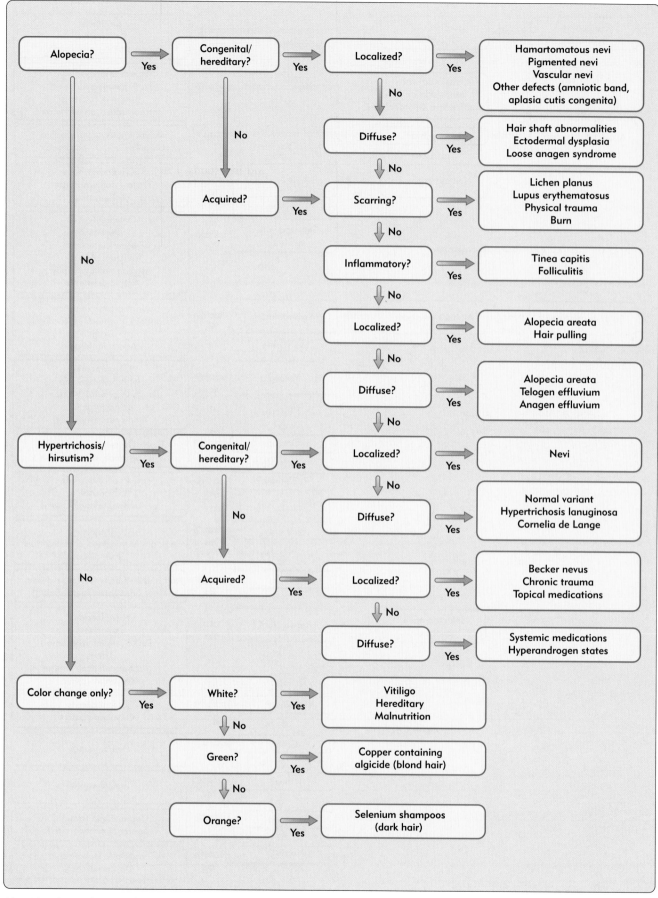

Algorithm for evaluation of disorders of the hair.

BIBLIOGRAPHY

Hair disorders

Baden HP. *Diseases of the hair and nails.* Yearbook Medical Publishers, Chicago, 1987.

Barth JH. Normal hair growth in children. *Pediatr Dermatol.* 1987, 4:173–84.

Caserio R, Hordinsky. Disorders of hair. *J Am Acad Dermatol.* 1988, **19**:895–903.

Frieden IJ. Genetic hair disorders. In: Alper JC (ed.), *Genetic disorders of the skin.* Mosby Year Book, St Louis, 1990, pp. 209–21.

Hurwitz S. Hair disorders. In: Schachner LA, Hansen RC (eds.), *Pediatric dermatology,* 2nd edn. Churchill Livingstone, New York, 1995, pp. 583–615.

Itin PH, Pittelkow MR. Trichothiodystrophy: review of sulfur-deficient brittle hair syndromes and association with the ectodermal dysplasias. *J Am Acad Dermatol.* 1990, **22**:705–17.

Levy ML. Disorders of the hair and scalp in children. *Pediatr Clin North Am.* 1991, **38**:905–19.

Rook A, Dawber R. *Diseases of the hair and scalp.* Blackwell Scientific, Oxford, 1982.

Skelsey MA, Price VH. Noninfectious hair disorders in children. *Curr Opin Pediatr.* 1996, 8:378–80.

Sperling LC. Hair anatomy for the clinician. *J Am Acad Dermatol.* 1991, **25**(Suppl. 1, Pt 1):1–17.

Tosti A, Peluso AM, Miscali C, Venturo N, Patrizi A, Fenti PA. Loose anagen hair. *Arch Dermatol.* 1997, **133**:1089–93.

Uno H. The histopathology of hair loss. *Curr Concepts (Upjohn).* 1988, 3–47.

Whiting DA. The diagnosis of alopecia. *Curr Concepts (Upjohn).* 1990, 3–41.

Whiting DA. Structural abnormalities of the hair shaft. *J Am Acad Dermatol.* 1987, **16**:1–25.

Nail disorders

Baran R, Dawber RPR. *Diseases of the nails and their management.* Blackwell Scientific, Oxford, 1984.

Barnett JM, Scher RK, Taylor SC. Nail cosmetics. *Dermatol Clin North Am.* 1991, **38**:921–40.

Cohen JL, Scher RK, Pappert AS. Congenital malalignment of the great toenails. *Pediatr Dermatol.* 1991, **8**:40–2.

Daniel CR, Scher RK. Nail changes secondary to systemic drugs and ingestants. *J Am Acad Dermatol.* 1987, **17**: 1012–6.

Kechijian P, Salasche S. Biology and disorders of nails. In: Arndt KA, LeBoit PE, Robinson JK, Wintroub BU (eds), *Cutaneous medicine and surgery.* WB Saunders, Philadelphia, 1996, pp. 1295–306.

Léauté-Labrèze C, Bioulac-Sage P, Taich A. Longitudinal melanonychia in children, a study of 8 cases. *Arch Dermatol.* 1996, **132**:167–9.

Norton LA. Genetic nail disorders. In: Alper JC (ed.), *Genetic disorders of the skin.* Mosby Year Book, St Louis, 1990, pp. 195–208.

Pappert AS, Scher RK, Cohen JL. Nail disorders in children. *Pediatr Clin North Am.* 1991, **38**:921–40.

Scher RK, Norton LA, Daniel CR. Disorders of the nails. *J Am Acad Dermatol.* 1986, **15**:523–8.

Silverman R. Nail and appendageal abnormalities. In: Schachner LA, Hansen RC (eds.), *Pediatric dermatology,* 2nd edn. Churchill Livingstone, New York, 1995, pp. 615–60.

Telfer NR. Congenital and hereditary nail disorders. *Semin Dermatol.* 1991, **10**:2–6.

surface erosions and ulcerations that may heal with

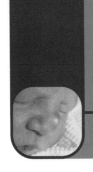

Chapter Nine

Factitial Dermatoses

INTRODUCTION

Factitial is defined as 'artificial' or 'not natural'. In dermatology, factitial disease usually refers to a group of specific psychodermatoses. However, in this chapter the definition is expanded to include a number of entities that do not fit neatly into other chapters. After a discussion of disorders with psychiatric implications, the cutaneous findings of child abuse are reviewed. The chapter concludes with sections on graft-versus-host reaction and acquired immunodeficiency syndrome (AIDS); diseases that have been, at least in part, created by human agency.

PSYCHODERMATOLOGY

Secondary psychiatric disorders, as well as psychophysiologic disorders, are common in pediatric practice. Fortunately, primary psychiatric disorders and neurologic and other organic disorders that mimic psychiatric disease (pseudopsychiatric disorders) are infrequent in children.

Secondary psychiatric disorders

Localized skin conditions, which involve cosmetically important areas such as the head and neck, or chronic, widespread rashes may be distressing enough to trigger secondary psychiatric disorders. In this group of diseases, disfigurement results in low self-esteem, social phobia, and paranoia. In severe cases major depression may result. Common skin problems associated with secondary psychiatric disorders include psoriasis, cystic acne, alopecia areata, vitiligo, portwine stains, and large, pigmented nevi.

Disfiguring lesions in infants and young children are a source of parental stress. However, if the lesions are treated before a critical period in psychologic development, long-term sequelae may be avoided. Although these critical periods are not well defined, many pediatricians agree that, if possible, treatment should be completed before patients begin school. For instance, facial pigmented nevi may be excised before kindergarten, and pulsed-dye laser treatment of portwine stains may begin shortly after birth. Treatment of chronic, recurrent disorders, such as psoriasis and vitiligo, is scheduled to minimize school absence and is focused on eradicating the lesions that are most visible or symptomatic. In adolescents, even mild acne may trigger a great deal of anxiety, which can be controlled by physician counseling and appropriate medical management. Cystic acne is treated early and aggressively to avoid permanent scarring.

Periodic reassurance from the practitioner provides adequate support for many patients. Others may find participation in support-oriented groups, such as the National Vitiligo Foundation and the National Portwine Stain Foundation, particularly helpful. However, when normal relationships with family and friends are disrupted, psychiatric consultation and counseling may be necessary.

Psychophysiologic disorders

Psychophysiologic disorders are also common in children. This term refers to a group of genuine dermatologic conditions that are triggered or exacerbated by emotional stress. Examples include atopic dermatitis, psoriasis, acne, hives, and hyperhidrosis.

Recognition of psychologic factors is key to successful treatment of these disorders. Some patients may require specific stress-reduction measures in addition to standard dermatologic therapy. Biofeedback training may help in disorders such as hyperhidrosis and atopic dermatitis, in which stress or anxiety can trigger a worsening of symptoms within minutes.

Primary psychiatric disorders

In this category of psychodermatoses, the skin becomes the focus of a primary psychosis. In most cases, either no true dermatologic disorder is present or minor findings are misinterpreted by the patient in accordance with his or her psychopathology. Although subtle symptoms may develop in childhood, most cases become manifest in adolescence or young adulthood.

Individuals with obsessive–compulsive disorder may develop trichotillomania. Unlike innocent hair pulling, trichotillomania is not self-limiting and requires long-term psychiatric and medical therapy. In a related condition, acne excoriée, patients pick and gouge trivial acne lesions on the face to produce erosions and ulcerations that may heal with scarring (Fig 9.1). Acne excoriée usually occurs in young women.

In monosymptomatic, hypochondriacal psychosis, patients develop a false fixation that there is a serious disturbance in their skin. The most common presentation is delusions of parasitosis, in which the individual is convinced that the skin is infested with imaginary mites, worms, or insects. Other examples include delusions of bromosis (foul odor) and dysmorphosis (abnormal or ugly appearance). These patients have little insight into their disease, and usually refuse consultation with psychiatrists. Unfortunately, the prognosis is guarded, and symptoms may persist indefinitely. Recent studies indicate that a large proportion of patients improve with pimozide, an antipsychotic drug of the diphenylbutyl-piperidione group.

A subset of patients with self-induced skin disease, usually teenagers, develop lesions in association with situational stress. (Figs 9.2–9.4). Disordered family dynamics, school phobia, lost love, and other acute or chronic psychosocial problems may result in this form of attention-seeking behavior. When this diagnosis is suspected, lesions may be covered with occlusive dressings for several weeks to see if healing occurs. When confronted, the patients usually admit to the self-injurious behavior. Counseling and improvement in the situation often result in an end to the lesions.

Pseudopsychiatric disorders

When patients develop bizarre symptoms with few or confusing clinical findings, a psychiatric source is often considered. However, careful attention to the course of symptoms and development of skin lesions may give a clue to the true dermatologic diagnosis.

Dermatitis herpetiformis (DH) is a good example of a pseudopsychodermatosis. In DH, persistent, intense pruritus and subsequent excoriations, which obliterate the primary vesiculobullous lesions, make diagnosis difficult. Unless DH is considered and confirmed by skin biopsy, the patient may be mistakenly referred to psychiatry for evaluation of 'neurotic' excoriations. Scabies, folliculitis, urticaria, and other pruritic dermatoses may also be misdiagnosed as psychogenic pruritus.

Occasionally, children with temporal lobe seizures present with pseudodelusions of parasitosis. Complaints of bizarre sensations in the skin also prompt a search for medication overdosage (e.g. diphenhydramine) or illicit drug exposure.

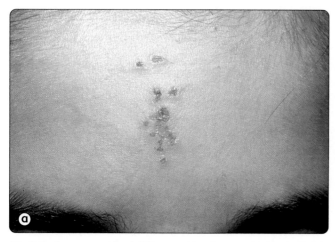
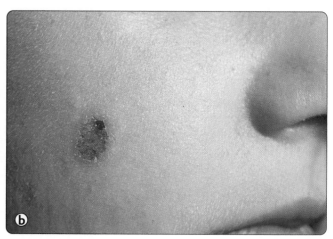

Fig 9.1 Acne excoriée. A 17-year-old girl compulsively picked at subtle comedones, which created punched out ulcerations on **(a)** her forehead and **(b)** her cheeks.

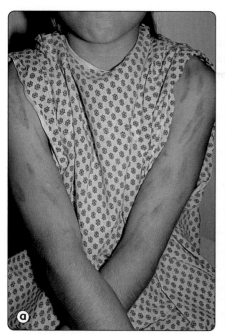
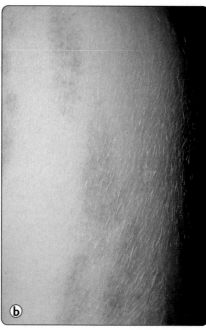

Fig 9.2 Factitial dermatitis. **(a, b)** An emotionally disturbed adolescent developed symmetric, linear bruises on her arms. During counseling, she admitted to producing the lesions with a coin.

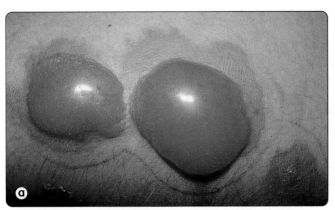

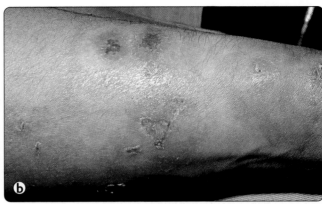

Fig 9.3 Factitial dermatitis. **(a)** A 15-year-old boy would periodically return from the woods behind his house with large, tense, bullous lesions on his arms. **(b)** Under close observation in the hospital, the lesions healed within several days. Later in therapy he admitted to applying a caustic liquid to the skin.

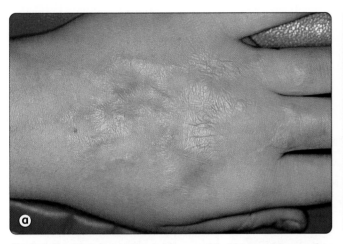

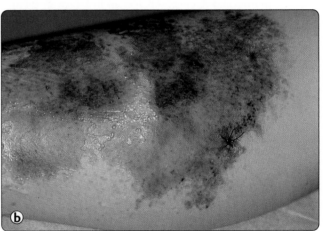

Fig 9.4 Factitial dermatitis. A 12-year-old girl has evidence of **(a)** old scarring and **(b)** new necrotic crusts on her leg from the application of a solvent to the skin. The fresh lesions healed under an occlusive dressing, which was left in place for 3 days.

CHILD ABUSE AND NEGLECT

Although the true incidence of child abuse is unknown, over 2,000,000 children are estimated to be abused or neglected in the US every year, which results in over 40,000 severely injured children and 4000 deaths. In many cases, affected children have been evaluated by practitioners who failed to recognize signs and symptoms that suggested the true diagnosis. Frequently, cutaneous findings provide clues to acute or chronic abuse.

Risk factors

Nearly two-thirds of children who suffer child abuse are under 3 years of age. Premature, disabled, and foster children are also more likely to be abused. About 10% of cases involve sexual abuse, of which girls are victims three times as often as boys. Parental risk factors include a personal history of child abuse, poor socialization, and limited ability to deal with stress. Although families living in poverty have increased exposure to stresses that may result in abuse and neglect, families of all socioeconomic levels may be affected. Alcoholism, addiction, and mental illness are often contributing factors. Families that move frequently and fail to develop support systems in the community are at particular risk.

Historical clues

When the history of how the injury occurred is vague or incompatible with the physical findings, abuse is included in the differential diagnosis. Inconsistencies in the history when parents are interviewed separately and changes in the history when it is taken by different health practitioners increase the index of suspicion.

Delay between the time of the injury and the visit to the clinician, inappropriate lack of concern for the injury, and abnormal interaction between the parent and child also raise suspicion.

A review of the primary care or emergency room medical records may reveal a large number of visits for accidental injuries, repeated fractures, and ingestions. Delayed immunizations and health maintenance visits may also serve as a warning. In infants and young children, poor growth or weight gain may be a sign of emotional abuse or neglect.

Clinical findings

Every child suspected of being abused deserves a thorough physical examination. Care must be taken to peruse the entire skin surface, including the anogenital area, mucous membranes, and scalp. All findings must be documented in the chart. Photographs of suspicious lesions are labeled and dated. The incident must be reported to the appropriate authorities, including Children's Protective Services or Social Services, and the police if necessary. Although the practitioner should play the role as an advocate for the family, the primary responsibility is to the safety of the child.

Cutaneous lesions

The distribution and shape of skin lesions may provide a clue to diagnosis. Innocent, play-induced bruises usually appear over bony prominences. Bruises suggestive of abuse occur on the inner and outer thighs, ears, groin, genitals, cheeks, and torso (Fig 9.5). Thumb prints on the chest and finger prints on the back of a seizing or floppy infant point to the diagnosis of

the so-called shaken-baby syndrome, in which shaking results in subdural hematoma with retinal hemorrhages.

Bruises appear purple and blue for the first 3–5 days and then change through greenish-yellow hues to faded brown at 10 days. Multiple bruises of varying ages suggest an ongoing problem, and the parents' history may not be compatible with the evolution of lesions.

In many cases the configuration of bruises may conform to the imprint of the object used to induce injury. Linear lesions result from a wooden stick or metal wire. Circumferential bruises or erosions on the arms, legs, or neck may be caused by rope or wire ligatures (Fig 9.6). Lamp cords (omega-shaped loops), belts ('U'-shaped cuts), belt buckles, and hands often inflict identifiable lesions (Fig 9.7).

Human bites also have a characteristic appearance. Animal-induced injuries usually produce puncture wounds or tear the skin, while human bites cause crush injuries. Small bite marks may be inflicted by siblings. However, widths of greater than 4 cm occur with bites from adults.

Although burns are fairly common accidental injuries, the shape and distribution of lesions, inconsistent history, and delay in seeking medical care may point to deliberate injuries (Fig 9.8). Burns from hot-water immersion are a common

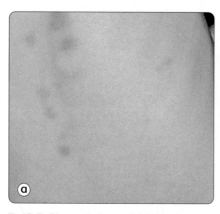
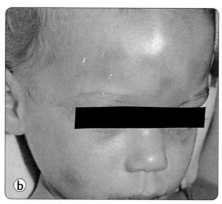
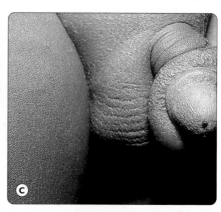

Fig 9.5 Physical abuse. **(a)** Multiple ecchymoses are evident over the back of this child who presented poorly nourished, but with normal coagulation studies. **(b)** The same patient with multiple bruises on the face and forehead. **(c)** This toddler developed edema of the foreskin after a beating with a belt. Note the belt-buckle mark on the right thigh.

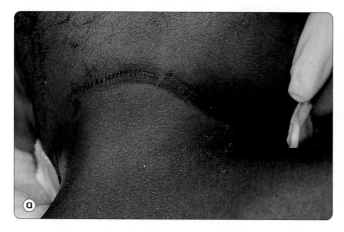
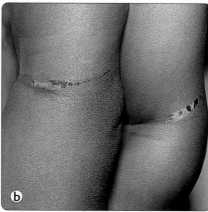

Fig 9.6 Physical abuse. These toddlers had rope tied around **(a)** the neck and **(b)** legs, which produced circumferential bruising and erosions.

presentation for abuse. Symmetric lesions on the hands, feet, and diaper area are typical (Figs 9.9 and 9.10). Frustration with toddlers during toilet training is a common complaint. The top of the feet and hands may be more severely involved, because the skin on the palms and soles is thicker and may be relatively protected when the extremities are held against the bottom of the sink or tub. Burns from metal objects usually demonstrate the shape of the object (Fig 9.11). A triangular-shaped injury may occur after branding from a hot iron. A child held against a hot, metal grate may show criss-crossing horizontal and vertical marks. Cigarette burns leave punched-out ulcers with dry, purple crusts (Fig 9.12). They can be differentiated from impetigo by their uniform size and dry, nonexpanding base. Repeated burns may result in lesions at various stages of healing. Some lesions may become impetiginized. Widespread, untreated impetigo and poor hygiene are also signs of child neglect.

Sexual abuse

Patients evaluated immediately after sexual assault often demonstrate evidence of physical and genital injury. Bruises on the head, neck, torso, and thighs are commonly present. Genital examination may show erythema, bruises, or lacerations (Fig 9.13). In cases of molestation or incest, which usually occur chronically in a family setting, physical signs are subtle or absent. Patients may present with chronic vaginitis, healed scars in the anogenital area, a patulous introitus, or reflex relaxation of the anal sphincter on perineal stimulation. About 10–15% of these children show evidence of sexually transmitted diseases at the time of diagnosis. Consequently, evaluation includes culturing of the oral pharynx, rectum, and vagina for gonorrhea and chlamydiosis, and a serologic test for syphilis. Children who have been sexually assaulted require a thorough examination and collection of forensic data in a medical setting equipped for the special needs of this evaluation.

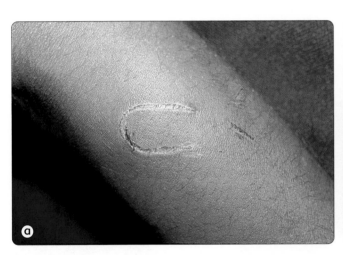

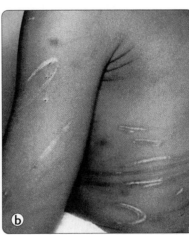

Fig 9.7 Physical abuse. The shape of lesions often gives a clue to the object used to inflict injury. **(a)** The end of a belt produced the 'U'-shaped cut on the leg of this 5-year-old boy.
(b) Multiple scars produced by prior whipping with a looped cord are seen in this child.

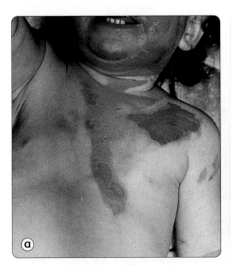

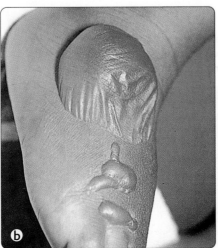

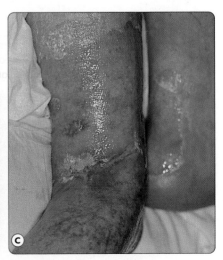

Fig 9.8 Accidental scald. **(a)** A 2-year-old accidentally spilled a teacup filled with hot water onto her face, neck, and chest. Note the irregular, asymmetric, but well-demarcated borders of the burn. **(b)** The accidental splash-and-droplet pattern of blistering is typical of an accidental spill on this toddler, who grabbed a hot cup of tea from the table while sitting on his grandmother's lap. **(c)** A 12-year-old girl with myelomeningocele and decreased sensation in the lower extremities accidentally dipped her feet into scalding water while preparing to take a bath.

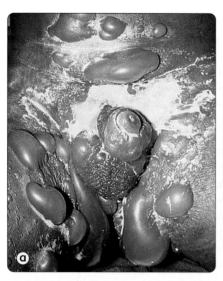

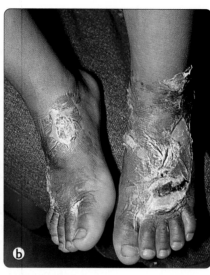

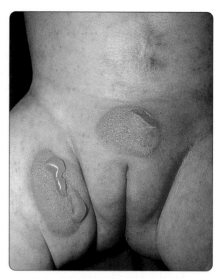

Fig 9.9 Hot water immersion burns. **(a)** First- and second-degree burns on the penis, thighs, and inguinal and suprapubic areas of a toddler who was held under a hot-water spigot. His sacrum and buttocks were spared. **(b)** Symmetric, healing, hot-water burns on the top of the foot of another toddler. Note the sharp line of demarcation at the ankle and sparing of the sole.

Fig 9.10 Caustic burn. A babysitter was applying a caustic liquid to patches in this child's diaper area. The morphology and course of lesions was not consistent with the history provided by the babysitter. Note the old scar on the abdomen.

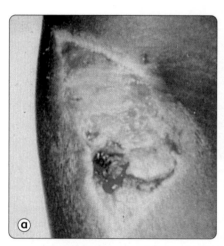

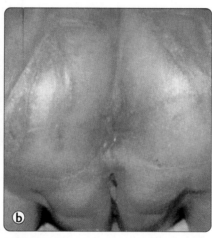

Fig 9.11 Hot-metal burns. **(a)** The pattern of this full-thickness burn to the arm reflects that a hot iron was used on this patient. **(b)** This infant received multiple, linear, full-thickness burns when she was forced to sit on the hot grill of a space heater.

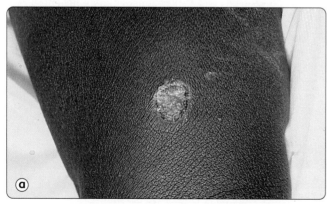

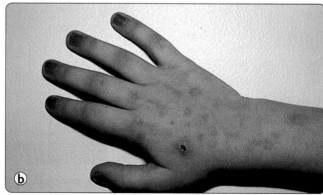

Fig 9.12 Cigarette burns. **(a)** A fresh cigarette burn occurred when this 6-week-old allegedly walked into a lighted cigarette. Note the dry, yellow eschar in the center, with purplish peeled-back scale at the border. **(b)** Cigarette burns in various stages of healing are present on the hand and wrist of this abused 5-year-old child.

Occasionally, dermatologic disease can simulate the findings of sexual abuse (see Figs 4.21 and 7.52). Bullous pemphigoid and chronic, bullous dermatosis of childhood have been misdiagnosed as sexually transmitted herpetic infection. Candidiasis and inflammatory bowel disease with genital involvement may also mimic sexual abuse.

Other findings in abuse

Multiple, unexplained fractures of various ages that involve the long bones and ribs of an infant or young child is a *sine qua non* of child abuse. Often, the bony injuries are noted as an incidental finding when the child is brought to the practitioner for a single injury or some other, unrelated problem. When child abuse is suspected a complete skeletal survey is obtained to assess the full extent of the injuries. Blunt objects may cause intra-abdominal injuries, which include duodenal hematomas, small intestinal or mesenteric tears, and lacerations of the liver and spleen. These children may require hospital admission until their safety at home is assured. About 50% of children who are returned to the same environment are eventually killed by the abusive adult.

Innocent mongolian spots must not be mistaken for bruises. Past documentation in the child's medical record or observation over several days reveals the proper diagnosis.

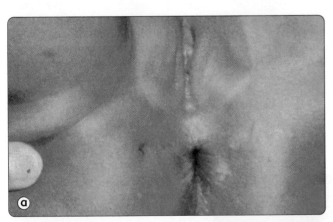

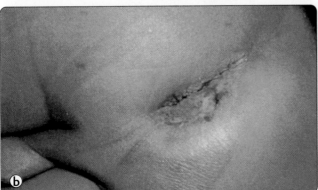

Fig 9.13 Sexual abuse. **(a)** Abrasions, contusions, and punctate tears of the perineum and perianal area can be observed in this prepubescent girl. **(b)** Severe, perianal lacerations, contusions, and abrasions are apparent in this prepubescent boy subjected to sodomy.

A bleeding diathesis, which may present with increased bruising, may be quickly excluded by a platelet count and coagulation studies. Insect bites may resemble cigarette burns and, in rare instances, osteogenesis imperfecta may simulate child abuse.

GRAFT-VERSUS-HOST DISEASE

Graft-versus-host disease (GVHD) is an immunologic disorder caused by injury induced by immunocompetent, histoincompatible donor cells in a compromised recipient. Susceptible immunodeficiency states include the normal developing fetus, congenital immunodeficiency, and acquired immunodeficiency.

When GVHD develops *in utero* in normal fetuses, viable maternal lymphocytes enter the fetal circulation by spontaneous maternal–fetal transfusion. Affected infants usually show signs of chronic disease at delivery. In infants with congenital immunodeficiencies, particularly T-cell deficiencies and severe combined immunodeficiency, the development of GVHD may be the first symptom of the immunodeficiency, which develops about 7–10 days after therapeutic blood transfusion (Fig 9.14a). In many nurseries, sick infants receive irradiated blood that eliminates the risk of accidental infusion of viable lymphocytes. The most common group of children at risk for GVHD includes patients with acquired immunodeficiencies that result from chemotherapy, lymphoreticular malignancy, and bone marrow transplantation (Figs 9.14b–d and 9.15). Virtually every allogenic transplant patient experiences mild GVHD at least.

Acute disease usually begins with a widespread, symmetric, pruritic, morbilliform rash within 2–6 weeks and up to 100 days after the introduction of donor cells (Fig 9.14c,d). The face, neck, and the sides of the palms, soles, and digits are commonly involved. Hepatic involvement is evident by the presence of elevated liver enzymes, and gastrointestinal symptoms include nausea and vomiting, and often progress to bloody diarrhea.

Chronic disease appears 100–400 days after the introduction of donor cells and may occur without antecedent acute symptoms. Chronic GVHD is a multisystem disease with autoimmune-like findings. Early in its course, the skin is involved with diffuse hypo- and hyperpigmentation, a lichenoid rash that resembles lichen planus, and scaly patches. Occasionally, patients develop a diffuse erythroderma. Untreated patients may eventually develop poikiloderma with atrophy, ulcerations, and progressive, widespread sclerodermatous changes (see Fig 9.15). Other findings include mucositis, cicatricial alopecia, vitiligo, dystrophic nails, Sjögren syndrome, and chronic pulmonary, cardiac, and gastrointestinal disease.

Fortunately, in transplant patients aggressive, immunosuppressive therapy with cyclosporine, tacrolimus, prednisone, cyclophosphamide, and other agents usually prevents the development of serious GVHD. Routine irradiation of blood products before transfusion also reduces the risk of GVHD in transplant patients and other immunodeficient individuals. In infants with congenital immunodeficiency, mortality is high despite intensive supportive care.

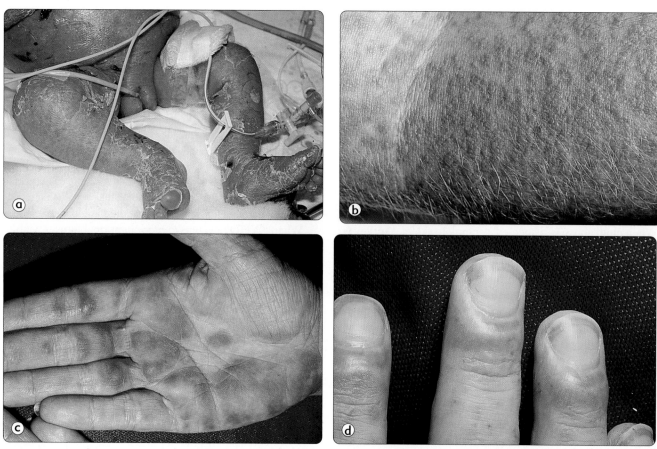

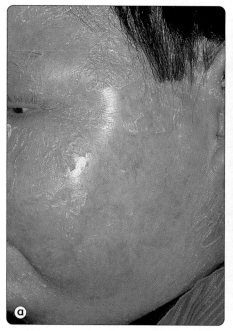

Fig 9.14 Acute graft-versus-host disease. **(a)** A newborn with severe combined immunodeficiency developed graft-versus-host disease after a transfusion with nonirradiated, packed red blood cells. Note the diffuse erythema and scaling. **(b, c, d)** Severe skin disease developed 3 weeks after allogenic bone marrow transplantation in an adolescent with acute myelogenous leukemia. **(b)** A widespread morbilliform rash became confluent in the skin creases and over the thighs. Necrotic vesicles developed in the center of many red papules, reminiscent of erythema multiforme. Painful, violaceous nodules and plaques appeared on **(c)** the palms and soles, over the knuckles, and **(d)** around the nails.

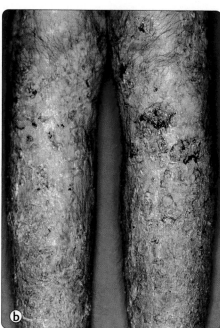

Fig 9.15 Chronic graft-versus-host disease. **(a)** Widespread atrophy, scaling, and fibrosis developed over a year after bone-marrow transplantation. This 14-year-old boy had experienced only minimal acute disease following his transplant. **(b)** Recurrent erosions, ulcers, and crusts formed on the arms, trunk, and legs in this 16-year-old boy with chronic disease.

ACQUIRED IMMUNODEFICIENCY SYNDROME

Although the prevalence of AIDS is relatively low in children, the recent epidemic, which has spread to heterosexual women of childbearing age, has resulted in a rise in pediatric cases. In some areas human immunodeficiency virus (HIV) seroprevalence among pregnant women exceeds 3%. The rate of transmission from untreated, asymptomatic mothers ranges from 15 to 35%. Other sources of infection in children include exposure to contaminated blood products, sexual transmission, and intravenous drug use.

Infected infants rarely develop overt disease during the first 3 months of life. However, before 1 year of age nonspecific symptoms commonly include poor growth, generalized lymphadenopathy, hepatosplenomegaly, chronic oral thrush, and recurrent upper respiratory, middle ear, and gastrointestinal infections. At least 50% of infected infants show central nervous system involvement, with neurodevelopmental delay or loss of milestones, acquired microcephaly, spastic diplegia, and quadriplegia. Pulmonary disease is the most common manifestation of pediatric AIDS, and affects over 75% of children during the first several years of life. Interstitial pneumonitis caused by *Pneumocystis carinii* is reported in

60% of patients. Lymphoid interstitial pneumonitis associated with Epstein–Barr virus infection occurs in about half of patients who survive the first year. Other important opportunistic pathogens include cytomegalovirus, *Candida*, *Mycobacterium avium-intracellulare*, and *Cryptococcus neoformans*. Patients are also susceptible to bacteremia, severe soft-tissue infection, pneumonitis, and meningitis from encapsulated bacterial organisms, such as *Streptococcus pneumoniae* or *Hemophilus influenzae*.

Skin lesions

Cutaneous findings may provide an early clue to diagnosis. Persistent diaper candidiasis and oral thrush, recalcitrant to topical therapy, occur commonly and prompt a search for HIV infection, especially in a child with growth failure or maternal risk factors. Many children are unable to localize common, usually self-limiting, viral infections. Widepsread, recurrent herpetic gingivostomatitis and disseminated cutaneous herpes simplex, as well as chronic herpes infections, are a frequent problem. Recurrent, localized herpes zoster and disseminated zoster have also been reported. Widespread, recalcitrant warts or molluscum contagiosum may be the first sign of AIDS in an otherwise asymptomatic child (Fig 9.16). Persistent and widespread dermatophyte

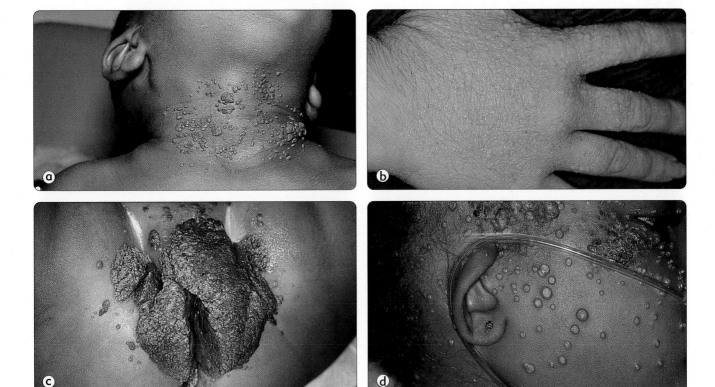

Fig 9.16 Acquired immunodeficiency syndrome (AIDS). **(a)** Multiple, recalcitrant warts developed on the neck of a 2-year-old infant with AIDS. **(b)** This adolescent was plagued with disseminated, flat warts, demonstrated here by virtually confluent papules on the top of the hand. **(c)** Large, recalcitrant, genital warts were associated with bleeding and recurrent bacterial infections in this toddler. **(d)** Severe molluscum contagiosum became chronically irritated and secondarily infected in this 6-year-old girl with AIDS. When her lymphocyte count rebounded on antiviral therapy, the molluscum regressed.

infections that involve the skin, nails, and hair may occur. Disseminated, deep, fungal infections with cutaneous involvement, including cryptococcosis and histoplasmosis, have been described. Skin lesions produced by these fungi may simulate an indolent, bacterial folliculitis or molluscum.

Crusted scabies infestations, with thick, widespread, scaly papules and patches, require rapid identification to prevent spread to parents, teachers, and healthcare workers (Fig 9.17). As in adults, the prevalence of seborrheic dermatitis, particularly widespread, erosive lesions, appears to be high in children with AIDS. Cutaneous manifestations of nutritional deficiencies, which include zinc deficiency dermatitis, pellagra, and scurvy, have been noted, particularly in children with chronic gastrointestinal disease.

An increased frequency of drug eruptions has been reported in adults and children with AIDS. This is a serious problem in patients who require chronic prophylaxis against *Pneumocystis* with trimethoprim–sulfamethoxazole. The incidence of morbilliform drug rashes in adults on this regimen approaches 75%.

Other cutaneous findings in children with AIDS include ecchymoses from idiopathic thrombocytopenic purpura and chronic leukocytoclastic vasculitis. Although cutaneous Kaposi sarcoma is reported frequently in adults, in whom it is an AIDS-defining illness, it occurs only rarely in children.

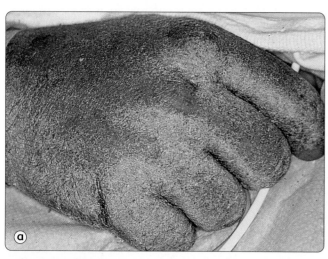

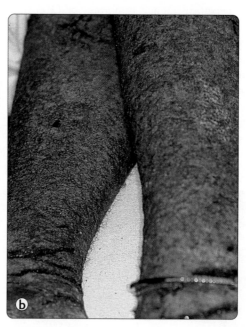

Fig 9.17 Crusted scabies. A widespread, thick, scaly, crusted eruption shown on (**a**) the right hand and (**b**) the legs developed in an adolescent with severe neurologic involvement from AIDS. Scrapings demonstrated multiple scabies mites.

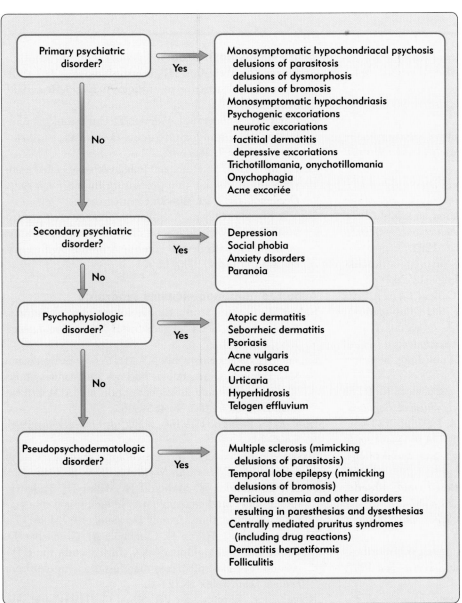

Psychodermatologic disorders. (Modified from Koo and Smith, 1991.)

BIBLIOGRAPHY

Psychodermatology

Koblenzer CS. *Psychocutaneous disease*. Harcourt Brace Javonavich, Orlando, 1987.

Koo JJM. Psychodermatology. In: *Current concepts*, Upjohn, Kalamazoo, 1989, pp. 3–45.

Koo JJM, Smith LL. Obsessive–compulsive disorders in the pediatric dermatology practice. *Pediatr Dermatol*. 1991, **8**:107–13.

Child abuse and neglect

American Academy of Pediatrics Section on Child Abuse and Neglect. *A guide to references and resources in child abuse and neglect*. Elk Grove Village, 1994.

Botash AS. Examination for sexual abuse in prepubertal children: an update. *Pediatr Ann*. 1997, **26**:312–20.

Briere J, Berliner L, Bulkley JA, Jenny C, Reid T. *The APSAC handbook on child maltreatment*. Sage Publications, Thousand Oaks, 1996.

Brodeur AE, Monteleone JA. *Child maltreatment, a clinical guide and reference*. GW Medical Publishing, St Louis, 1994.

Carrasco MM, Davis HW. Child abuse and neglect. In: Davis HW, Zitelli BJ (eds), *Atlas of pediatric physical diagnosis*, 3rd edn. Mosby–Yearbook, St Louis, 1997, pp. 133–78.

Giardino AP, Christian CW, Giardino ER. *A practical guide to the evaluation of abuse and neglect*. Sage Publications, Thousand Oaks, 1997.

Helfer RE, Kempe RS (eds). *The battered child*, 4th edn. University of Chicago Press, Chicago, 1987.

Hobbs CJ, Wynne JM. *Physical signs of child abuse, a colour atlas*. WB Saunders, London, 1996.

Look KM, Look RM. Skin scraping, cupping and moxibustion that may mimic physical abuse. *J Forens Sci*. 1997, **42**:103–5.

Monteleone JA. *Child maltreatment, a comprehensive photographic reference identifying potential child abuse*. GW Medical Publishing, St Louis, 1994.

Graft-versus-host disease

Anderson KC, Weinstein HJ. Transfusion-associated graft-versus-host disease (review article). *N Engl J Med*. 1990, **323**:315–21.

Andrews ML, Robertson I, Weedon D. Cutaneous manifestations of chronic graft-versus-host disease. *Aust J Dermatol*. 1997, **38**:53–62.

Berger RS, Dixon SL. Fulminant transfusion-associated graft-versus-host disease in a premature infant. *J Am Acad Dermatol*. 1989, **20**:945–50.

Farre A, Scerri L, Stevens A, Millard LG. Acute graft-versus-host disease with cutaneous intracellular vacuolization in an infant with severe combined immunodeficiency. *Pediatr Dermatol*. 1995, **12**:311–3.

Acquired immunodeficiency syndrome

Italian Multicenter Study. Epidemiology, clinical features, and prognostic factors of pediatric HIV infection. *Lancet*. 1988, **ii**:1043–6.

Kaplan MH, Sadick N, McNutt NS, McItzer M, Sarngadharan MG, Pahwa S. Dermatologic findings and manifestations of acquired immunodeficiency syndrome (AIDS). *J Am Acad Dermatol*. 1987, **16**:485–506.

Lambert JS. Pediatric HIV infection. *Curr Opin Pediatr*. 1996, **8**:606–14.

Myskowski PL, Ahkami R. Dermatologic complications of HIV infection. *Med Clin North Am*. 1996, **80**:1415–35.

Prose NS, Mendez H, Menikoff H, Miller HJ. Pediatric human immunodeficiency virus infection and its cutaneous manifestations. *Pediatr Dermatol*. 1987, **4**:267–74.

Ramos-Gomez FJ, Hilton JF, Camchola AJ, Greenspan D, Greenspan JS, Maldonado YA. Risk factors for HIV-related orofacial soft-tissue manifestations in children. *Pediatr Dent*. 1996, **18**:121–6.

Tschachler E, Bergstresser PR, Stingl G. HIV-related skin diseases. *Lancet*. 1996, **348**:659–63.

Zuckerman G, Metrou M, Bernstein LJ, Crain EF. Neurologic disorders and dermatologic manifestations in HIV-infected children. *Pediatr Emerg Care*. 1991, **7**: 99–105.

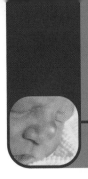

Index

Note: Numbers in **boldface** type refer to figure numbers.